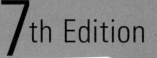

7th Edition

ECGs MADE EASY

BARBARA AEHLERT, MSEd, BSPA, RN

ELSEVIER

Elsevier

3251 Riverport Lane
St. Louis, MO 63043

Notice

Practitioners and researchers must always rely on their own experience and knowledge in evaluating and using any information, methods, compounds, or experiments described herein. Because of rapid advances in the medical sciences, in particular, independent verification of diagnoses and drug dosages should be made. To the fullest extent of the law, no responsibility is assumed by Elsevier, authors, editors, or contributors for any injury and/or damage to persons or property as a matter of products liability, negligence, or otherwise or from any use or operation of any methods, products, instructions, or ideas contained in the material herein.

Senior Content Strategist: Sandra Clark/Kelly Skelton
Director, Content Development: Laurie Gower
Senior Content Development Specialist: Elizabeth McCormac
Publishing Services Manager: Deepthi Unni
Senior Book Designer: Brian Salisbury

Printed in Canada.

Last digit is the print number: 9 8 7 6 5 4 3 2 1

to
Deepak C. Patel, MD
whose knowledge, humor, and genuine compassion for his patients are unparalleled.

Reviewers for the Seventh Edition

Kanayo K.C. Egwatu, Sr. MD
Education/Clinical Laboratory
Woodruff Medical Training and Testing
Tucker, Georgia

Christopher Hanifin, EdD, PA-C
Department Chair
Department of Physician Assistant
Seton Hall University
South Orange, New Jersey

Jennifer Lunny, RN, MSN/Ed.
Associate Professor of Nursing
Nursing Department
Broward College
Coconut Creek, Florida

Andrea N. Pifher, MHSc, RRT-ACCS, RCP
Assistant Professor
Allied Health, Respiratory Care Program
Columbus State Community College
Columbus, Ohio

Preface to the Seventh Edition

Many years ago, as a green but enthusiastic nurse preparing to shift from medical-surgical nursing to critical care, I signed up for a course in basic ECG recognition. It was a daunting experience. My instructor was extremely knowledgeable and kind, and I studied diligently throughout the course, yet I struggled to crack the code of heart rhythm interpretation. To make matters worse, I couldn't find any resources in which these complex concepts were presented in a practical, helpful way. Although I passed the course, I repeated it a few months later because I simply did not retain the content presented the first time, and I could not apply that information when viewing my patients' ECGs.

After completing the second course, I promised myself that I would someday teach this information in a simpler way. That promise became my life's work. Since then, I've been looking for better ways in which to present the skill of basic ECG recognition to those who will apply that knowledge every working day:

- Paramedics
- Nursing and medical students
- ECG monitor technicians
- Nurses and other allied health personnel working in emergency departments, critical care units, post-anesthesia care units, operating rooms, and telemetry units

This book can be used alone or as part of a formal course of instruction in basic dysrhythmia recognition. The book's content focuses on the essentials of ECG interpretation. Each ECG rhythm is described and accompanied by a sample rhythm strip. Then the discussion turns to possible signs and symptoms related to each rhythm and, where appropriate, currently recommended treatment. At the end of each chapter, additional rhythm strips and their descriptions are provided for practice. (All rhythm strips shown in this text were recorded in lead II unless otherwise noted.) The Stop and Review exercises at the end of each chapter are self-assessment activities that allow you to check your learning.

I've made every attempt to supply content consistent with current literature, including current resuscitation guidelines. However, medicine is a dynamic field. Recommendations change as medical research evolves, technology improves, and new medications, procedures, and devices are developed. As a result, be sure to learn and follow local protocols as defined by your medical advisors. Neither I nor the publisher can assume responsibility or liability for loss or damage resulting from using information contained within.

I genuinely hope this book is helpful to you, and I wish you success in your studies and clinical practice.

Best regards,
Barbara Aehlert

Acknowledgments

I would like to thank the following healthcare professionals who provided many of the rhythm strips used in this book: Andrew Baird, CEP; James Bratcher; Joanna Burgan, CEP; Holly Button, CEP; Gretchen Chalmers, CEP; Thomas Cole, CEP; Brent Haines, CEP; Paul Honeywell, CEP; Timothy Klatt, RN; Bill Loughran, RN; Andrea Lowrey, RN; Joe Martinez, CEP; Stephanos Orphanidis, CEP; Jason Payne, CEP; Steve Ruehs, CEP; Patty Seneski, RN; David Stockton, CEP; Jason Stodghill, CEP; Dionne Socie, CEP; Kristina Tellez, CEP; and Fran Wojculewicz, RN.

About the Author

Barbara Aehlert, MSEd, BSPA, RN, has been a registered nurse for over 40 years, with clinical experience in medical/surgical nursing, critical care nursing, prehospital education, and nursing education. Barbara enjoys teaching basic dysrhythmia recognition.

Contents

Anatomy and Physiology

LEARNING OBJECTIVES

After reading this chapter, you should be able to:

1. Describe the location of the heart.
2. Identify the surfaces of the heart.
3. Describe the cardiac muscle layers.
4. Identify and describe the chambers of the heart and the vessels that enter or leave each.
5. Identify and describe the location of the atrioventricular and semilunar valves.
6. Explain atrial kick.
7. Name the heart's primary branches and areas supplied by the right and left coronary arteries.
8. Define and explain acute coronary syndromes.
9. Compare and contrast the effects of sympathetic and parasympathetic stimulation of the heart.
10. Identify and discuss each phase of the cardiac cycle.
11. Beginning with the right atrium, describe blood flow through the normal heart and lungs to the systemic circulation.
12. Identify and explain the components of blood pressure and cardiac output.

KEY TERMS

acute coronary syndrome (ACS): Distinct conditions caused by a similar sequence of pathologic events—a temporary or permanent blockage of a coronary artery. These conditions are characterized by an excessive demand or inadequate supply of oxygen and nutrients to the heart muscle associated with plaque disruption, thrombus formation, and vasoconstriction. ACSs consist of three major syndromes: unstable angina, non–ST-elevation myocardial infarction, and ST-elevation myocardial infarction.

afterload: The pressure or resistance against which the ventricles must pump to eject blood.

angina pectoris: Chest discomfort or other related symptoms of sudden onset that may occur because the heart's increased oxygen demand temporarily exceeds the blood supply.

atria: Two upper chambers of the heart (singular, atrium).

atrial kick: Blood pushed into the ventricles because of atrial contraction.

atrioventricular (AV) valve: The valve located between each atrium and ventricle; the tricuspid separates the right atrium from the right ventricle, and the mitral (bicuspid) separates the left atrium from the left ventricle.

blood pressure: Force exerted by the blood against the arteries' walls as the ventricles of the heart contract and relax.

cardiac output (CO): The amount of blood pumped into the aorta each minute by the left ventricle; defined as the stroke volume multiplied by the heart rate.

chordae tendineae (tendinous cords): Thin strands of fibrous connective tissue that extend from the AV valves to the papillary muscles that prevent the AV valves from bulging back into the atria during ventricular systole (contraction).

chronotropy: A change in (heart) rate.

diastole: Phase of the cardiac cycle in which the atria and ventricles relax between contractions and blood enters these chambers. When the term is used without reference to a specific chamber of the heart, ventricular diastole is implied.

dromotropy: Refers to the speed of impulse transmission through the conduction system.

dysrhythmia: Any disturbance or abnormality in a regular rhythmic pattern; any cardiac rhythm other than sinus rhythm.

ejection fraction: The percentage of blood pumped out of a ventricle with each contraction.

endocardium: Innermost layer of the heart that lines the inside of the myocardium and covers the heart valves.

epicardium: Also known as the visceral pericardium; the external layer of the heart wall that covers the heart muscle.

heart failure: A condition in which the heart cannot pump enough blood to meet the body's metabolic needs; it may result from any condition that impairs preload, afterload, cardiac contractility, or heart rate.

inotropy: Refers to a change in myocardial contractility.

ischemia: Decreased supply of oxygenated blood to a body part or organ.

Continued

KEY TERMS—cont'd

mediastinum: Middle area of the thoracic cavity; contains the heart, great vessels, trachea, and esophagus, among other structures; extends from the sternum to the vertebral column.

myocardial infarction (MI): Death of some mass of the heart muscle caused by prolonged ischemia.

myocardium: Middle and thickest layer of the heart; contains the cardiac muscle fibers that cause contraction of the heart and contains the conduction system and blood supply.

papillary muscles: Muscles attached to the chordae tendineae of the AV valves and the heart's ventricular muscle that help prevent the AV valves from bulging too far into the atria.

pericardium: A double-walled sac that encloses the heart and helps protect it from trauma and infection.

peripheral resistance: Resistance to the flow of blood determined by blood vessel diameter and the tone of the vascular musculature.

preload: Force exerted by the blood on the walls of the ventricles at the end of diastole.

semilunar (SL) valves: Valves shaped like half-moons that separate the ventricles from the aorta and pulmonary artery.

septum: An internal wall of connective tissue.

stroke volume (SV): The amount of blood ejected from the left ventricle with each heartbeat.

sulcus: Groove.

systole: Contraction of the heart (usually referring to ventricular contraction), during which blood is propelled into the pulmonary artery and aorta; when the term is used without reference to a specific chamber of the heart, ventricular systole is implied.

tone: A term that may be used when referring to the normal state of balanced tension in body tissues.

venous return: Amount of blood flowing into the right atrium each minute from the systemic circulation.

ventricles: The two lower chambers of the heart.

LOCATION, SIZE, AND SHAPE OF THE HEART

The heart is a hollow muscular organ that lies in the space between the lungs (i.e., the **mediastinum**) in the middle of the chest (Fig 1.1). It sits behind the sternum and just above the diaphragm. About two-thirds of the heart lies to the left of the sternum's midline between the second and sixth ribs. The remaining third lies to the right of the sternum.

The adult heart is about the size of its owner's fist. The heart's weight is about 0.45% of a man's body weight and about 0.40% of a woman's. A person's heart size and weight are influenced by age, body weight and build, physical exercise frequency, and heart disease.

SURFACES OF THE HEART

The front (anterior) surface of the heart lies behind the sternum and costal cartilages. Most of the anterior surface is formed by the right atrium and the right **ventricle**, with the left ventricle contributing a small portion (Fig. 1.2). Because the heart is tilted slightly toward the left in the chest, the right ventricle is the heart area that lies most directly behind the sternum. The anterior surfaces of the right and left ventricles are separated by the left anterior descending (LAD) artery (Gosling et al., 2017).

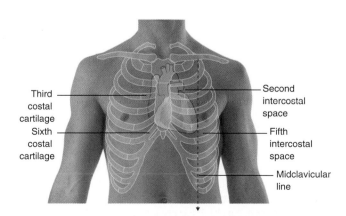

Fig. 1.1 Anterior view of the chest wall of a man showing skeletal structures and the surface projection of the heart. (From Drake, R., Vogl, A. W., & Mitchell, A. W. M. (2015). *Gray's anatomy for students* (3rd ed.). New York: Churchill Livingstone.)

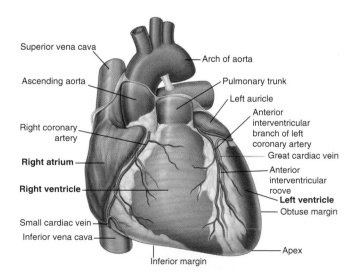

Fig. 1.2 The anterior surface of the heart. (From Drake, R., Vogl, A. W., & Mitchell, A. W. M. (2015). *Gray's anatomy for students* (3rd ed.). New York: Churchill Livingstone.)

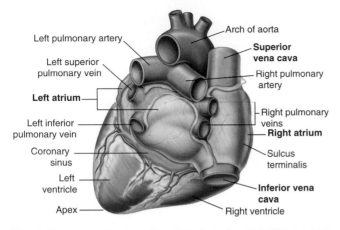

Fig. 1.3 The base of the heart. (From Drake, R., Vogl, A. W., & Mitchell, A. W. M. (2015). *Gray's anatomy for students* (3rd ed.). New York: Churchill Livingstone.)

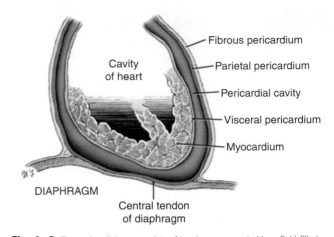

Fig. 1.4 The pericardial sac consists of two layers separated by a fluid-filled space. The visceral pericardium is attached directly to the heart's surface. The parietal pericardium forms the outer layer of the sac. (From Nagelhout, J. J., & Elisha, S. (2018). *Nurse anesthesia* (6th ed.). St. Louis Elsevier.)

The heart's inferior surface, also called the diaphragmatic surface, is formed by the left and right ventricles and a small portion of the right atrium. The left ventricle makes up most of the inferior surface (Gosling et al., 2017). The right and left ventricles are separated by a groove containing the posterior interventricular vessels.

The heart's base, or upper portion, is formed by the left atrium, a small portion of the right atrium, and portions of the superior and inferior venae cavae and the pulmonary veins (Fig. 1.3). The heart's apex, or lower portion, is formed by the left ventricle's tip and is positioned at about the level of the left fifth intercostal space at the midclavicular line.

COVERINGS OF THE HEART

The **pericardium** is a double-walled sac that encloses the heart and helps protect it from trauma and infection. The pericardial sac's tough outer layer is called the fibrous parietal pericardium (Fig. 1.4). It anchors the heart to some of the structures around it, such as the sternum and diaphragm, through ligaments. This helps prevent excessive movement of the heart in the chest with changes in body position.

The pericardium's inner layer, the serous pericardium, consists of two layers: parietal and visceral. The parietal layer lines the inside of the fibrous pericardium. The visceral layer (i.e., the epicardium) attaches to the large vessels that enter and exit the heart and forms the heart's outer surface. Between the visceral and parietal layers is a space (the pericardial space) that generally contains about 20 mL of serous (pale yellow and transparent) fluid. This fluid acts as a lubricant, preventing friction as the heart beats.

The right and left phrenic nerves, which innervate the diaphragm, pass through the fibrous pericardium as they descend to the diaphragm. Because these nerves supply sensory fibers to the fibrous pericardium, the parietal serous pericardium, and the mediastinal pleura, discomfort related to conditions affecting the pericardium may be felt in the areas above the shoulders or lateral neck.

⏱ ECG Pearl

If the pericardium becomes inflamed (pericarditis), excess pericardial fluid can be quickly generated in response to the inflammation. Pericarditis can result from a bacterial or viral infection, rheumatoid arthritis, tumors, and destruction of the heart muscle in a heart attack, among other causes.

Heart surgery or trauma to the heart, such as a stab wound, can cause a rapid buildup of blood in the pericardial space. The buildup of excess blood or fluid in the pericardial space compresses the heart, which can affect the heart's ability to relax and fill with blood between heartbeats. If the heart cannot adequately fill with blood, the amount of blood the ventricles can pump out to the body (cardiac output) will be decreased. As a result, the amount of blood returning to the heart is also decreased. These changes can result in a life-threatening condition called *cardiac tamponade*. The amount of blood or fluid in the pericardial space needed to impair the heart's ability to fill depends on the rate at which the buildup of blood or fluid occurs and the pericardium's ability to stretch and accommodate the increased volume of fluid.

STRUCTURE OF THE HEART

Layers of the Heart Wall

The heart walls consist of three tissue layers: the endocardium, myocardium, and epicardium (Table 1.1). The heart's innermost layer, the **endocardium**, lines the heart's inner chambers, valves, chordae tendineae (tendinous cords), and papillary muscles. The heart's conduction system's terminal components can be found within this layer (Anderson & Roden, 2010). The endocardium is continuous with the innermost layer of the arteries, veins, and capillaries of the body, thereby creating a continuous, closed circulatory system.

TABLE **1.1**	Layers of the Heart Wall
Heart Layer	**Description**
Epicardium	External layer of the heart
	Coronary arteries, blood capillaries, lymph capillaries, nerve fibers nerves, and fat are found in this layer
Myocardium	Middle and thickest layer of the heart
	Muscular component of the heart; responsible for the heart's pumping action
Endocardium	Innermost layer of the heart
	Lines heart's inner chambers, valves, chordae tendineae, and papillary muscles
	Continuous with the innermost layer of arteries, veins, and capillaries of the body

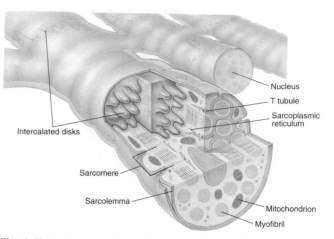

Fig. 1.5 Cardiac muscle fiber. Unlike other types of muscle fibers, the cardiac muscle fiber is typically branched and forms junctions, called intercalated disks, with adjacent cardiac muscle fibers. (From Patton, K. T., & Thibodeau, G. A. (2019). *Anthony's textbook of anatomy & physiology* (21st ed.). St. Louis Elsevier.)

The **myocardium** (middle layer) is a thick, muscular layer consisting of cardiac muscle fibers (cells) responsible for the heart's pumping action. The myocardium makes up about 30% of the total left ventricular mass (Anderson & Roden, 2010). The innermost half of the myocardium is called the subendocardial area. The outermost half is called the subepicardial area. The myocardium's muscle fibers are separated by connective tissues that have a rich supply of capillaries and nerve fibers.

The heart's outermost layer is called the **epicardium** and contains blood capillaries, lymph capillaries, nerve fibers, and fat. The main coronary arteries lie on the epicardial surface of the heart. They feed this area first before entering the myocardium and supplying the heart's inner layers with oxygenated blood. **Ischemia** is a decreased supply of oxygenated blood to a body part or organ. The heart's subendocardial area is at the greatest risk of ischemia because it has a high oxygen demand and is fed by the coronary arteries' most distal branches.

CARDIAC MUSCLE

Cardiac muscle fibers make up the walls of the heart and surround the heart's chambers. Each muscle fiber is made up of many muscle cells. Within each cell are mitochondria, the energy-producing parts of the cell, and bundles of myofibrils, which are long, tube-like structures packed closely together. Myofibrils are made up of many sarcomeres responsible for the contraction of muscle fibers and thousands of myofilaments. Each myofilament is made up of protein molecules. Myosin and actin are protein molecules that help to produce a contraction. Tropomyosin and troponin are protein molecules that inhibit myosin-actin interactions. When electrically stimulated, the contractile filaments slide together, changing the muscle fiber length and enabling contraction.

Intercalated disks join cardiac muscle cells together end to end (Fig. 1.5). Gap junctions, which are like tunnels that join cell membranes, are present in the intercalated disks and allow electrical impulses to move rapidly from one fiber to

another. The arrangement of the cardiac muscle fibers and intercalated disks allows cardiac muscle to function as a *syncytium*, which means that all fibers will become stimulated when one cardiac muscle fiber is stimulated (Koeppen & Stanton, 2018). The heart consists of two syncytia: atrial and ventricular. The atrial syncytium consists of the walls of the right and left atria. The ventricular syncytium consists of the walls of the right and left ventricles. The atrial and ventricular syncytia are separated by fibrous tissue. The presence of two syncytia allows the atria to contract a short time before ventricular contraction (Hall, 2016). Usually, impulses can be conducted from the atrial syncytium into the ventricular syncytium only through the atrioventricular (AV) junction, which is a part of the heart's electrical system.

Heart Chambers

The heart has four chambers, two atria and two ventricles. The thickness of a heart chamber is related to the amount of pressure or resistance that the chamber's muscle must overcome to eject blood.

The outside surface of the heart has grooves called sulci. The coronary arteries and their major branches lie in these grooves. The coronary **sulcus** (groove) encircles the outside of the heart and separates the atria from the ventricles. It contains the coronary blood vessels and epicardial fat.

ATRIA

The heart's two upper chambers are the right and left **atria** (singular, *atrium*) (Fig. 1.6). An earlike flap called an auricle (meaning "little ear") protrudes from each atrium.

Because the atria's purpose is to *receive* blood, think of them as holding tanks or reservoirs for blood for their respective ventricles. The right atrium receives blood low in oxygen from the superior vena cava (which carries blood from the head and upper extremities), the inferior vena cava

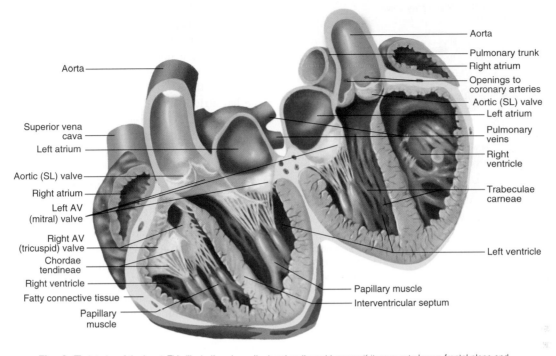

Fig. 1.6 Interior of the heart. This illustration shows the heart as it would appear if it were cut along a frontal plane and opened like a book. The heart's front portion lies to the reader's right; the back portion of the heart lies to the left. The four chambers of the heart—two atria and two ventricles—are easily seen. *AV,* Atrioventricular; *SL,* semilunar. (From Patton K. T., & Thibodeau, G. A. (2019). *Anatomy & physiology* (10th ed.). St. Louis: Elsevier.)

(which carries blood from the lower body), and the coronary sinus (which is the largest vein that drains the heart). The left atrium receives freshly oxygenated blood from the lungs via the right and left pulmonary veins.

The atria have thin walls because they encounter little resistance when pumping blood to the ventricles. Blood is pumped from the atria through an **atrioventricular (AV) valve** and into the ventricles. The valves of the heart are discussed later in this chapter.

VENTRICLES

The heart's two lower chambers are the right and left ventricles. Their purpose is to *pump* blood. The right ventricle pumps blood through the blood vessels of the lungs and then into the left atrium. The left ventricle pumps blood out to the body. Because the ventricles must pump blood either to the lungs (the right ventricle) or to the rest of the body (the left ventricle), the ventricles have a much thicker myocardial layer than the atria.

When the left ventricle contracts, it normally produces an impulse that can be felt at the heart's apex (apical impulse). This palpable impulse occurs because the left ventricle rotates forward as it contracts. In a normal heart, this causes the apex of the left ventricle to hit the chest wall. You may be able to see the apical impulse in thin individuals. The apical impulse is also called the point of maximal impulse because it is the site where the left ventricular contraction is most strongly felt.

Heart Valves

The heart has a skeleton, which is made up of four rings of thick connective tissue. This tissue surrounds the bases of the pulmonary trunk, the aorta, and the heart valves. The inside of the rings provides secure attachments for the heart valves. The outside of the rings provides for the attachment of the myocardium (Fig. 1.7). The heart's skeleton also helps form the partitions (septa) that separate the atria from the ventricles.

There are four one-way valves in the heart: two AV valves and two **semilunar (SL)** valves. The valves open and close in a specific sequence and help produce the pressure gradient needed between the chambers to ensure a smooth flow of blood through the heart and prevent the backflow of blood.

ATRIOVENTRICULAR VALVES

AV valves separate the atria from the ventricles. The tricuspid valve is the AV valve that lies between the right atrium and the right ventricle. It consists of three separate cusps or flaps (Fig. 1.8). The mitral valve, also called the bicuspid valve, has only two cusps and lies between the left atrium and left ventricle (Fig. 1.9). The mitral valve is so named because of its resemblance to a miter, which is a double-cusp bishop's hat, when open.

The AV valves open when a forward pressure gradient forces blood in a forward direction. They close when a backward pressure gradient pushes blood backward. The AV valves require almost no backflow to cause closure (Hall, 2016).

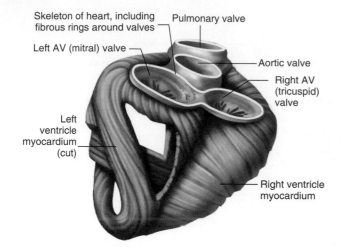

Fig. 1.7 Skeleton of the heart. This posterior view shows part of the ventricular myocardium with the heart valves still attached. Each heart valve's rim is supported by a fibrous structure, called the skeleton of the heart, which encircles all four valves. *AV,* Atrioventricular. (From Patton K. T., & Thibodeau, G. A. (2019). *Anatomy & physiology* (10th ed.). St. Louis: Elsevier.)

The flow of blood from the superior and inferior venae cavae into the atria usually is continuous. About 80% of this blood flows directly through the atria and into the ventricles before the atria contract (passive filling) (Hall, 2016). As the atria fill with blood, the pressure within the atrial chamber rises. This pressure forces the tricuspid and mitral valves open, and the ventricles begin to fill, gradually increasing the pressure within the ventricles. When the atria contract,

an additional 20% of the returning blood is added to the ventricles (Hall, 2016). This additional contribution of blood resulting from atrial contraction is called **atrial kick**.

On the right side of the heart, blood low in oxygen empties from the right atrium into the right ventricle. On the left side of the heart, freshly oxygenated blood empties from the left atrium into the left ventricle. When the ventricles then contract (i.e., systole), the pressure within the ventricles rises sharply. The tricuspid and mitral valves completely close when the pressure within the ventricles exceeds that of the atria.

Chordae tendineae (tendinous cords) are thin strands of connective tissue. On one end, they are attached to the underside of the AV valves. On the other end, they are attached to small mounds of myocardium called **papillary muscles**. Papillary muscles project inward from the lower portion of the ventricular walls. When the ventricles contract and relax, so do the papillary muscles. The papillary muscles adjust their tension on the chordae tendineae, preventing them from bulging too far into the atria. Thus, the chordae tendineae and papillary muscles serve as anchors. Because the chordae tendineae are thin and string-like, they are sometimes called "heart strings."

SEMILUNAR VALVES

The pulmonic and aortic valves are **SL valves**. The SL valves prevent the backflow of blood from the aorta and pulmonary arteries into the ventricles. The SL valves have three cusps shaped like half-moons. The SL valves' openings are smaller

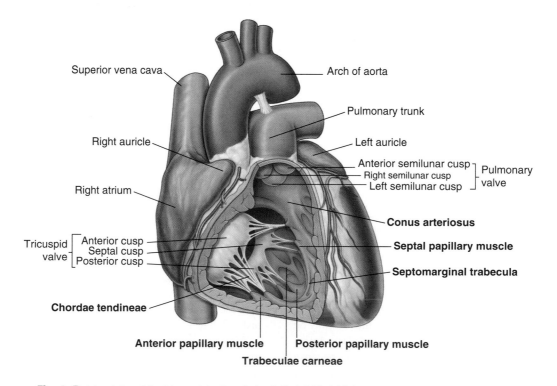

Fig. 1.8 Internal view of the right ventricle. (From Drake, R., Vogl, A. W., & Mitchell, A. W. M. (2015). *Gray's anatomy for students* (3rd ed.). New York: Churchill Livingstone.)

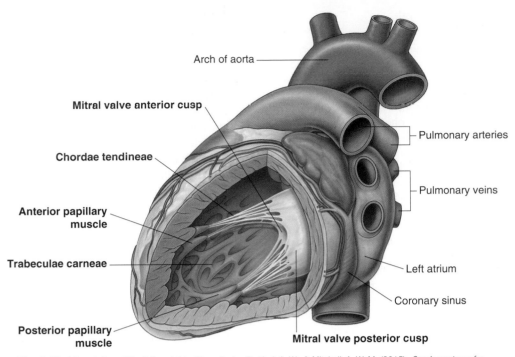

Fig. 1.9 Internal view of the left ventricle. (From Drake, R., Vogl, A. W., & Mitchell, A. W. M. (2015). *Gray's anatomy for students* (3rd ed.). New York: Churchill Livingstone.)

than the AV valves' openings, and the flaps of the SL valves are smaller and thicker than the AV valves. Unlike the AV valves, the SL valves are not attached to chordae tendineae.

When the ventricles contract, the SL valves open, allowing blood to flow out of the ventricles. When the right ventricle contracts, blood low in oxygen flows through the pulmonic valve into the pulmonary trunk, which divides into the right and left pulmonary arteries. When the left ventricle contracts, freshly oxygenated blood flows through the aortic valve into the aorta and out to the body (Fig. 1.10). The SL valves close as ventricular contraction ends, and the pressure in the pulmonary artery and aorta exceeds that of the ventricles.

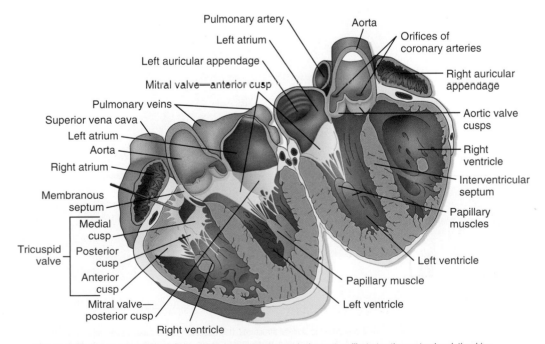

Fig. 1.10 Drawing of a heart split perpendicular to the interventricular septum illustrates the anatomic relationships of the atrioventricular and aortic valves' leaflets. (From Koeppen, B. M., & Stanton, B. A. (2018). *Berne & Levy physiology* (7th ed.). Philadelphia: Elsevier.)

⊙ ECG Pearl

Improper valve function can hamper blood flow through the heart. *Valvular heart disease* is the term used to describe a malfunctioning heart valve. Types of valvular heart disease include the following:

- *Valvular prolapse.* If a valve flap inverts, it is said to have *prolapsed*. Prolapse can occur if one valve flap is larger than the other. It can also occur if the chordae tendineae stretch markedly or rupture.
- *Valvular regurgitation.* Blood can flow backward, or regurgitate, if one or more of the heart's valves does not close properly. Valvular regurgitation is also known as *valvular incompetence* or *valvular insufficiency.*
- *Valvular stenosis.* If a valve narrows, stiffens, or thickens, it is said to be *stenosed*. The heart must work harder to pump blood through a stenosed valve.
- Papillary muscles receive their blood supply from the coronary arteries. If a papillary muscle ruptures because of an inadequate blood supply (as in myocardial infarction), the attached valve cusps will not completely close and may result in a *murmur*. If a papillary muscle in the left ventricle ruptures, the mitral valve's leaflets may invert (i.e., prolapse). This may result in blood leaking from the left ventricle into the left atrium (e.g., regurgitation) during ventricular contraction. Blood flow to the body (i.e., cardiac output) could decrease as a result.

HEART SOUNDS

Heart sounds occur because of vibrations in the heart's tissues caused by the closing of the heart's valves. Vibrations are created as blood flow is suddenly increased or slowed with the contraction and relaxation of the heart chambers and with the opening and closing of the valves.

The first heart sound, known as S_1, is the result of closure of the tricuspid and mitral (AV) valves and reflects the start of ventricular contraction. S_1 ("lub") is heard loudest at the apex of the heart. The second heart sound (i.e., S_2) is caused by closure of the pulmonic and aortic (SL) valves and reflects the start of ventricular relaxation. S_2 ("dub") is heard loudest at the base of the heart.

A third heart sound (S_3) is a low-frequency sound produced by ventricular filling. It is a normal variant in children and healthy young adults, but when heard in people older than 40 years of age, it is generally considered abnormal and is often associated with heart failure. An S_1–S_2–S_3 sequence is called a ventricular gallop or gallop rhythm. It sounds like "Kentucky"—*Ken* (S_1) *-tuck* (S_2) *-y* (S_3).

Turbulent blood flow within the cardiac chambers and vessels can produce heart murmurs. An inflamed pericardium can produce a pericardial friction rub, which sounds like rough sandpaper.

The location of the heart's AV and SL valves for auscultation is shown in Fig. 1.11. A summary of the heart's

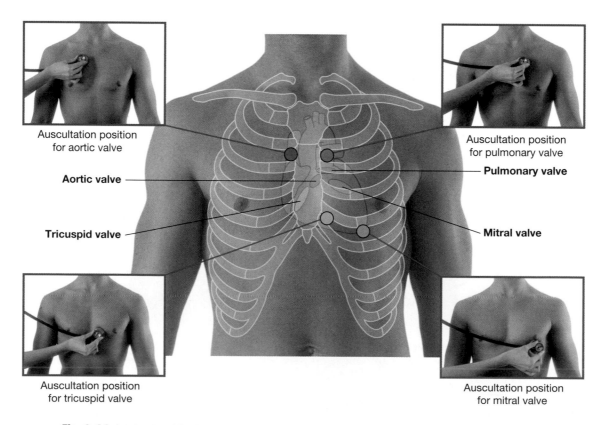

Fig. 1.11 Anterior view of the chest wall showing skeletal structures, heart, location of the heart valves, and where to listen to heart sounds. (From Drake, R., Vogl, A. W., & Mitchell, A. W. M. (2015). *Gray's anatomy for students* (3rd ed.). New York: Churchill Livingstone.)

TABLE 1.2	Heart Valves and Auscultation Points		
Valve Name	**Valve Type**	**Location**	**Auscultation Point**
Tricuspid	Atrioventricular	Separates the right atrium and right ventricle	Just to the left of the lower part of the sternum near the fifth intercostal space
Mitral (bicuspid)	Atrioventricular	Separates the left atrium and left ventricle	Heart apex in the left fifth intercostal space at the midclavicular line
Pulmonic (pulmonary)	Semilunar	Between the right ventricle and pulmonary artery	Left second intercostal space close to the sternum
Aortic	Semilunar	Between the left ventricle and aorta	Right second intercostal space close to the sternum

valves and auscultation points for heart sounds appears in Table 1.2.

The Heart's Blood Supply

The coronary circulation consists of coronary arteries and veins. The right and left coronary arteries encircle the myocardium like a crown, or corona.

CORONARY ARTERIES

The main coronary arteries lie on the outer (i.e., epicardial) surface of the heart. Coronary arteries that run on the surface of the heart are called epicardial coronary arteries. They branch into progressively smaller vessels, eventually becoming arterioles and then capillaries. Thus, the epicardium has a rich blood supply to draw from. Branches of the main coronary arteries penetrate the heart's muscle mass and supply the subendocardium with blood. The diameter of these "feeder branches" (i.e., collateral circulation) is much narrower. The tissues supplied by these branches get enough blood and oxygen to survive, but they do not have much extra blood flow.

To ensure that it has an adequate blood supply, the heart provides itself with a fresh supply of oxygenated blood before supplying the rest of the body. This freshly oxygenated blood is supplied mainly by the branches of two vessels: the right and left coronary arteries. The right and left coronary arteries are the very first branches off the base of the aorta. The openings to these vessels lie just beyond the cusps of the aortic SL valve. When the left ventricle contracts (systole), the pressure within the left ventricle pushes blood into the arteries that branch from the aorta, causing the arteries to fill. However, the coronary arteries are compressed during ventricular contraction, reducing blood flow to the heart's tissues. Thus, the coronary arteries fill when the aortic valve is closed, and the left ventricle is relaxed (i.e., diastole).

The three major epicardial coronary arteries include the LAD artery, circumflex (Cx) artery, and right coronary artery (RCA). A person is said to have coronary artery disease (CAD) if there is more than 50% diameter narrowing (i.e., stenosis) in one or more of these vessels.

Right Coronary Artery

The RCA originates from the right side of the aorta (Fig. 1.12). It travels along the groove between the right atrium and the right ventricle. A branch of the RCA supplies the following structures:

- Right atrium
- Right ventricle
- Inferior surface of the left ventricle in about 85% of individuals
- Posterior surface of the left ventricle in 85%
- Sinoatrial (SA) node in about 60%
- AV bundle in 85% to 90%

Left Coronary Artery

The left coronary artery (LCA) originates from the aorta's left side (see Fig. 1.12). The first segment of the LCA is called the left main coronary artery. It is about the diameter of a soda straw and less than 1 inch (2.5 cm) long. The left main coronary artery supplies oxygenated blood to its two primary branches: the LAD, which is also called the *anterior interventricular artery*, and the Cx. These vessels are slightly smaller than the left main coronary artery.

The LAD is on the outer (i.e., epicardial) surface on the front of the heart. It travels along the groove that lies between the right and left ventricles (i.e., the anterior interventricular sulcus) toward the heart's apex. In most patients, the LAD travels around the left ventricle's apex and ends along the left ventricle's inferior surface. In the remaining patients, the LAD does not reach the inferior surface. Instead, it stops at or before the heart's apex. Occlusion of the proximal LAD coronary artery has been referred to as the "widow maker" because of its association with sudden cardiac arrest when it is blocked.

The major branches of the LAD are the septal and diagonal arteries. The LAD supplies blood to the following:
- The anterior surface of the left ventricle
- Part of the lateral surface of the left ventricle
- The anterior two-thirds of the interventricular septum

The Cx coronary artery circles around the left side of the heart in a groove on the back of the heart that separates the left atrium from the left ventricle called the coronary sulcus (see Fig. 1.12). The Cx supplies blood to the following:
- The left atrium
- Part of the lateral surface of the left ventricle
- The inferior surface of the left ventricle in about 15% of individuals
- The posterior surface of the left ventricle in 15%

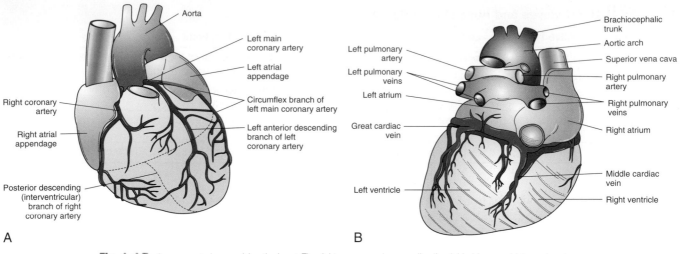

Fig. 1.12 Coronary arteries supplying the heart. The right coronary artery supplies the right atrium, ventricle, and posterior aspect of the left ventricle in most individuals. The left coronary artery divides into the left anterior descending and circumflex arteries, which perfuse the left ventricle. A, Anterior view. B, Posterior view. (From Banasik, J. L., Copstead, L. C., & Banasik, J. L. (2019). *Pathophysiology* (6th ed.). St. Louis: Elsevier.)

- The SA node in about 40%
- The AV bundle in 10% to 15%

A summary of the heart's areas supplied by the three major coronary arteries is shown in Table 1.3.

Coronary Artery Dominance

The coronary artery that forms the posterior descending artery is considered the *dominant* coronary artery. In most people, a branch of the RCA becomes the posterior descending artery, which is described as a right-dominant system. If the Cx branches and ends at the posterior descending artery, the coronary artery arrangement is described as a left-dominant system. In some people, neither coronary artery is dominant. If damage to the left ventricle's posterior wall is suspected, a cardiac catheterization usually is necessary to determine which coronary artery is involved.

ACUTE CORONARY SYNDROMES

Acute coronary syndrome (ACS) is a term that refers to distinct conditions caused by a similar sequence of pathologic events involving abruptly reduced coronary artery blood flow. This sequence of events results in conditions that range from myocardial ischemia or injury to death (i.e., necrosis) of the heart muscle.

The usual cause of an ACS is the rupture of an atherosclerotic plaque. Arteriosclerosis is a chronic disease of the arterial system characterized by abnormal thickening and hardening of the vessel walls. Atherosclerosis is a form of arteriosclerosis. The thickening and hardening of the vessel walls are caused by a buildup of fat-like deposits (e.g., plaque) in the inner lining of large and middle-sized muscular arteries. As the fatty deposits build up, the artery's opening slowly narrows, and blood flow to the muscle

TABLE **1.3**	Coronary Arteries	
Coronary Artery	**Portion of Myocardium Supplied**	**Portion of Conduction System Supplied**
Right	Right atrium	Sinoatrial (SA) node (about 60%)[a]
	Right ventricle	Atrioventricular (AV) bundle (85% to 90%)[a]
	Inferior surface of left ventricle (about 85%)[a]	
	Posterior surface of left ventricle (85%)[a]	
Left anterior descending	Anterior surface of left ventricle	Most of right bundle branch
	Part of lateral surface of left ventricle	Part of left bundle branch
	Anterior two-thirds of interventricular septum	
Circumflex	Left atrium	SA node (about 40%)[a]
	Part of lateral surface of left ventricle	AV bundle (10% to 15%)[a]
	Inferior surface of left ventricle (about 15%)[a]	
	Posterior surface of left ventricle (15%)[a]	

[a]Of the population.

decreases. The extent of arterial narrowing and the amount of blood flow reduction are critical determinants of coronary artery disease.

Angina pectoris is chest discomfort or other related symptoms that occur suddenly when the heart's increased oxygen demand temporarily exceeds the blood supply. Angina is a symptom of myocardial ischemia, and it most often occurs in patients with CAD that involves at least one coronary artery. However, it can be present in patients with normal coronary arteries. Angina also occurs in people with uncontrolled high blood pressure or valvular heart disease.

Partial or intermittent blockage of a coronary artery may result in no clinical symptoms (i.e., silent ischemia), angina, a heart attack, which is also called a **myocardial infarction (MI)**, or sudden death. The area supplied by a blocked coronary artery goes through a sequence of events that have been identified as zones of ischemia, injury, and infarction. Each zone is associated with characteristic ECG changes that will be discussed later in this book. When myocardial ischemia or infarction is suspected, an understanding of coronary artery anatomy and the heart areas that each vessel supplies helps you predict which coronary artery is blocked and anticipate problems associated with blockage of that vessel.

If the blocked coronary vessel is quickly opened to restore blood flow and oxygen to the injured area, no tissue death occurs. Methods of restoring blood flow may include giving clot-busting drugs (i.e., fibrinolytics) or performing endovascular therapies.

⊘ ECG Pearl

When myocardial cells die, such as during myocardial infarction, substances in intracardiac cells pass through broken cell membranes and leak into the bloodstream. These substances are called inflammatory markers, cardiac biomarkers, or serum cardiac markers, and include creatine kinase myocardial band (CK-MB), myoglobin, troponin I, and troponin T. Blood tests are used to measure their levels in the blood and determine if an infarction has occurred. The diagnosis of an acute coronary syndrome is made based on the patient's assessment findings and his or her symptoms and history, the presence of cardiovascular risk factors, serial electrocardiogram results, blood test results (i.e., cardiac biomarkers), and other diagnostic test results.

CORONARY VEINS

The coronary (cardiac) veins travel alongside the arteries. Blood that has passed through the myocardial capillaries is drained by branches of the cardiac veins that join the coronary sinus. The coronary sinus is the largest vein that drains the heart (see Fig. 1.12). It lies in the groove (sulcus) that separates the atria from the ventricles. The coronary sinus receives blood from the great, middle, and small cardiac veins; a vein of the left atrium; and the left ventricle's posterior vein. The coronary sinus drains into the right atrium. The anterior cardiac veins do not join the coronary sinus but empty directly into the right atrium.

The Heart's Nerve Supply

The myocardium can produce its own electrical impulses without signals from an outside source, such as a nerve. Because there are times when the body needs to increase or decrease its heart rate (HR) and/or force of contraction, it is beneficial that both divisions of the autonomic nervous system send fibers to the heart. The sympathetic division prepares the body to function under stress (i.e., the "fight-or-flight" response). The parasympathetic division conserves and restores body resources (i.e., the "rest and digest" response).

SYMPATHETIC STIMULATION

Sympathetic (accelerator) nerves innervate specific areas of the heart's electrical system, atrial muscle, and the ventricular myocardium. When sympathetic nerves are stimulated, the neurotransmitters norepinephrine and epinephrine are released. Remember: The job of the sympathetic division is to prepare the body for emergency or stressful situations. Therefore, the release of norepinephrine and epinephrine results in the following predictable actions:

- Dilation of pupils
- Dilation of smooth muscles of bronchi to improve oxygenation
- Increased HR, force of contraction, conduction velocity, blood pressure, and cardiac output (CO)
- Increased sweating
- Mobilization of stored energy to ensure an adequate supply of glucose for the brain and fatty acids for muscle activity
- Shunting of blood from skin and blood vessels of internal organs to skeletal muscle
- Sympathetic (i.e., adrenergic) receptors are located in different organs and have different physiologic actions when stimulated. There are five main types of sympathetic receptors: alpha$_1$, alpha$_2$, beta$_1$, beta$_2$, and beta$_3$.
- Alpha$_1$ receptors are found in the eyes, blood vessels, bladder, and male reproductive organs. The stimulation of alpha$_1$ receptor sites results in constriction.
- Alpha$_2$ receptor sites are found in parts of the digestive system and on presynaptic nerve terminals in the peripheral nervous system. Stimulation of alpha$_2$ receptor sites results in decreased secretions, peristalsis, and suppression of norepinephrine release.
- Beta receptor sites are divided into beta$_1$, beta$_2$, and beta$_3$. Beta$_1$ receptors are found in the heart and kidneys. Stimulation of beta$_1$ receptor sites in the heart results in increased HR, contractility, and, ultimately, irritability of cardiac cells. Beta-blockers are medications used to slow HR and AV node conduction, reduce blood pressure, decrease myocardial contractility, and decrease myocardial oxygen consumption (Fig. 1.13). Stimulation of beta$_1$ receptor sites in the kidneys results in the release of renin into the blood. Renin promotes the production of angiotensin, a potent vasoconstrictor. Beta$_2$ receptor sites are found in the arterioles of the heart, lungs, and skeletal

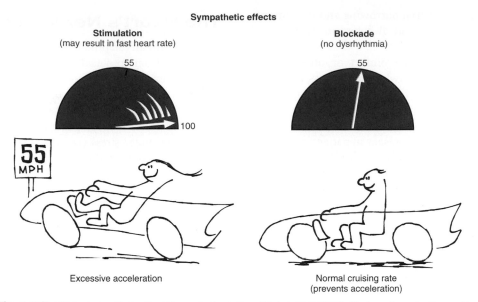

Sympathetic effects

Stimulation
(may result in fast heart rate)

Blockade
(no dysrhythmia)

Excessive acceleration

Normal cruising rate
(prevents acceleration)

Fig. 1.13 Effects of sympathetic stimulation on the heart. (From Wiederhold, R. (1999). *Electrocardiography: The monitoring and diagnostic leads* (2nd ed.). Philadelphia: Saunders.)

muscle. Stimulation of beta$_2$ receptor sites results in dilation. Beta$_3$ receptor sites are found in fat cells. When stimulated, they promote the breakdown of fats and other lipids.

⟳ ECG Pearl

Remember: Beta$_1$ receptors affect the heart (you have one heart); beta$_2$ receptors affect the lungs (you have two lungs).

PARASYMPATHETIC STIMULATION

Parasympathetic (inhibitory) nerve fibers supply the SA node, atrial muscle, and the heart's AV bundle by the vagus nerves. Acetylcholine (ACh) is a chemical messenger (neurotransmitter) released when parasympathetic nerves are stimulated. ACh binds to parasympathetic receptors. The two main types of parasympathetic (i.e., cholinergic) receptors are nicotinic and muscarinic receptors. Nicotinic receptors are located in skeletal muscle and muscarinic receptors are found in smooth muscle. Parasympathetic stimulation has the following actions:

- Slows the rate of discharge of the SA node (Fig. 1.14)
- Slows conduction through the AV node
- Decreases the strength of atrial contraction
- Can cause a small decrease in the force of ventricular contraction

Atropine sulfate is an example of a medication used to increase HR and AV conduction velocity by blocking the vagus nerve's effects on the SA and AV nodes.

BARORECEPTORS AND CHEMORECEPTORS

Baroreceptors are specialized nerve tissue (sensors). They are found in the internal carotid arteries and the aortic arch.

These sensory receptors detect changes in blood pressure. When stimulated, they cause a reflex response in either the sympathetic or the parasympathetic divisions of the autonomic nervous system. For example, if the blood pressure decreases, the body will try to compensate by:

- Constricting peripheral blood vessels
- Increasing the HR (chronotropy)
- Increasing the force of myocardial contraction (inotropy)

These compensatory responses occur because of a response by the sympathetic division. This is called a sympathetic or adrenergic response. If the blood pressure increases, the body will decrease sympathetic stimulation and increase the parasympathetic division's response. This is called a parasympathetic or cholinergic response. The baroreceptors will adjust to a new normal after a few days of exposure to a specific pressure.

Chemoreceptors in the internal carotid arteries and aortic arch detect changes in the concentration of hydrogen ions (pH), oxygen, and carbon dioxide in the blood. The response to these changes by the autonomic nervous system can be sympathetic or parasympathetic.

Chronotropy, **inotropy**, and **dromotropy** are terms used to describe effects on HR, myocardial contractility, and speed of conduction through the AV node. These terms are explained in Box 1.1.

THE HEART AS A PUMP

An internal wall of connective tissue called a **septum** separates the right and left sides of the heart. The interatrial septum separates the right and left atria. The interventricular septum separates the right and left ventricles. The septa separate the heart into two functional pumps. The right

Parasympathetic effects

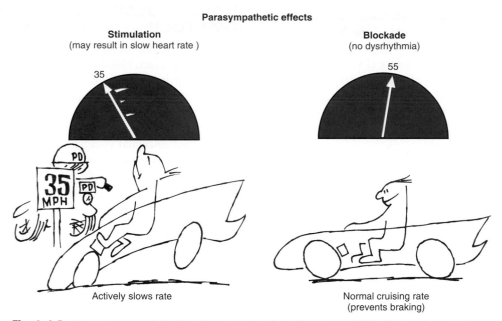

Stimulation (may result in slow heart rate)	Blockade (no dysrhythmia)
35	55
Actively slows rate	Normal cruising rate (prevents braking)

Fig. 1.14 Effects of parasympathetic stimulation on the heart. (From Wiederhold, R. (1999). *Electrocardiography: The monitoring and diagnostic leads* (2nd ed.). Philadelphia: Saunders.)

Box 1.1	**Terminology Chronotropic Effect**

- Refers to a change in heart rate.
- A positive chronotropic effect refers to an increase in heart rate.
- A negative chronotropic effect refers to a decrease in heart rate.

Inotropic Effect
- Refers to a change in myocardial contractility.
- A positive inotropic effect results in an increase in myocardial contractility.
- A negative inotropic effect results in a decrease in myocardial contractility.

Dromotropic Effect
- Refers to the speed of impulse transmission through the conduction system.
- A positive dromotropic effect results in an increase in conduction velocity.
- A negative dromotropic effect results in a decrease in conduction velocity.

---

atrium and right ventricle make up one pump. The left atrium and left ventricle make up the other (Fig. 1.15).

The heart's right side, called the pulmonary circulation, is a low-pressure system whose job is to pump unoxygenated blood from the body to and through the lungs to the left side of the heart.

The heart's left side, called the systemic circulation, receives oxygenated blood from the lungs and pumps it out to the rest of the body. Blood is carried from the heart to the

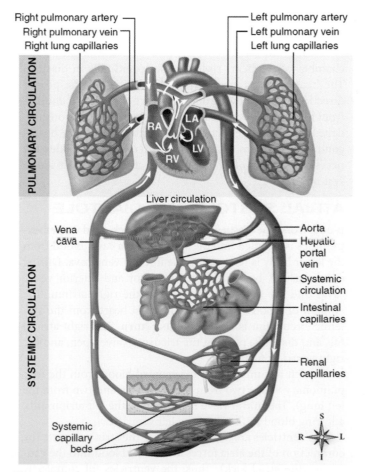

Fig. 1.15 The pulmonary circulation routes blood flow to and from the gas-exchange tissues of the lungs. The systemic circulation routes blood flow to and from the oxygen-consuming tissues of the body. (From Patton, K. T., & Thibodeau, G. A. (2019). *Anthony's textbook of anatomy and physiology* (21st ed.). St. Louis: Elsevier.)

body's organs through arteries, arterioles, and capillaries. Blood is returned to the right side of the heart through venules and veins.

The left ventricle is a high-pressure chamber. Its wall is much thicker than the right ventricle (the right ventricle is about 3–5 mm thick; the left ventricle is about 13–15 mm). This is because the left ventricle must overcome a lot of pressure and resistance from the arteries and contract forcefully to pump blood out to the body.

Cardiac Cycle

The cardiac cycle refers to a repetitive pumping process that includes all of the events associated with blood flow through the heart. The cycle has two phases for each heart chamber: systole and diastole. **Systole** is the period during which the chamber contracts and blood is ejected. **Diastole** is the period of relaxation during which the chambers fill. The myocardium receives its fresh supply of oxygenated blood from the coronary arteries during ventricular diastole.

The cardiac cycle depends on the cardiac muscle's ability to contract and on the condition of the heart's conduction system. The heart's efficiency as a pump may be affected by abnormalities of the cardiac muscle, the valves, or the conduction system.

During the cardiac cycle, the pressure within each chamber of the heart rises in systole and falls in diastole. The heart's valves ensure that blood flows in the proper direction. Blood flows from one heart chamber to another from higher to lower pressure. These pressure relationships depend on the careful timing of contractions. The heart's conduction system (discussed in Chapter 2) provides the necessary timing of events between atrial and ventricular systole.

ATRIAL SYSTOLE AND DIASTOLE

Blood from the tissues of the head, neck, and upper extremities is emptied into the superior vena cava. Blood from the lower body is returned to the inferior vena cava. During atrial diastole, blood from the superior and inferior venae cavae and the coronary sinus enters the right atrium. The amount of blood flowing into the right heart from the systemic circulation is called **venous return**. The right atrium fills and distends, pushing the tricuspid valve open, and the right ventricle fills.

The left atrium receives oxygenated blood from the four pulmonary veins (two from the right lung and two from the left lung). The mitral valve flaps open as the left atrium fills, allowing blood to flow into the left ventricle.

The ventricles are 80% filled before the atria contract. The contraction of the atria forces additional blood into the ventricles (the atrial kick). Thus, the ventricles fill completely with blood during atrial systole. The atria then enter a period of atrial diastole, which continues until the start of the next cardiac cycle.

VENTRICULAR SYSTOLE AND DIASTOLE

Ventricular systole occurs as atrial diastole begins. As the ventricles contract, blood is propelled through the systemic and pulmonary circulation and toward the atria. The term *isovolumetric contraction* (meaning "having the same volume") describes the brief period between the start of ventricular systole and the SL valves' opening. During this period, the ventricular volume remains constant as the pressure within the chamber rises sharply.

When the right ventricle contracts, the tricuspid valve closes. The right ventricle expels the blood through the pulmonic valve into the pulmonary trunk. The pulmonary trunk divides into a right and left pulmonary artery, each of which carries blood to one lung (i.e., the pulmonary circuit). Blood flows through the pulmonary arteries to the lungs. Blood low in oxygen passes through the pulmonary capillaries. There, it comes in direct contact with the alveolar-capillary membrane, where oxygen and carbon dioxide are exchanged. Blood then flows into the pulmonary veins and then to the left atrium.

When the left ventricle contracts, the mitral valve closes to prevent backflow of blood. Blood leaves the left ventricle through the aortic valve to the aorta, which is the systemic arterial circulation's primary vessel. Blood is distributed throughout the body (i.e., the systemic circuit) through the aorta and its branches. Blood continues to move in one direction because pressure pushes it from the high-pressure (i.e., arterial) side. Valves in the veins prevent backflow on the lower pressure (i.e., venous) side as blood returns to the heart.

When the SL valves close, the heart begins a period of ventricular diastole. During ventricular diastole, the ventricles are relaxed and begin to fill passively with blood. The cardiac cycle begins again with atrial systole and the completion of ventricular filling. The cardiac cycle and blood flow through the heart are shown in Fig. 1.16.

Blood Pressure

The pulse and blood pressure reflect the mechanical activity of the heart. **Blood pressure** is the force exerted by the circulating blood volume on the walls of the arteries. The volume of blood in the arteries is directly related to arterial blood pressure.

Blood pressure is equal to CO × peripheral resistance. CO is discussed later. **Peripheral resistance** is the resistance to the flow of blood determined by blood vessel diameter and the tone of the vascular musculature. **Tone** is a term that may be used when referring to the normal state of balanced tension in body tissues.

Blood pressure is affected by conditions or medications that affect peripheral resistance or CO (Fig. 1.17). For example, an increase in either CO or peripheral resistance typically increases blood pressure. Conversely, a decrease in either will result in a decrease in blood pressure.

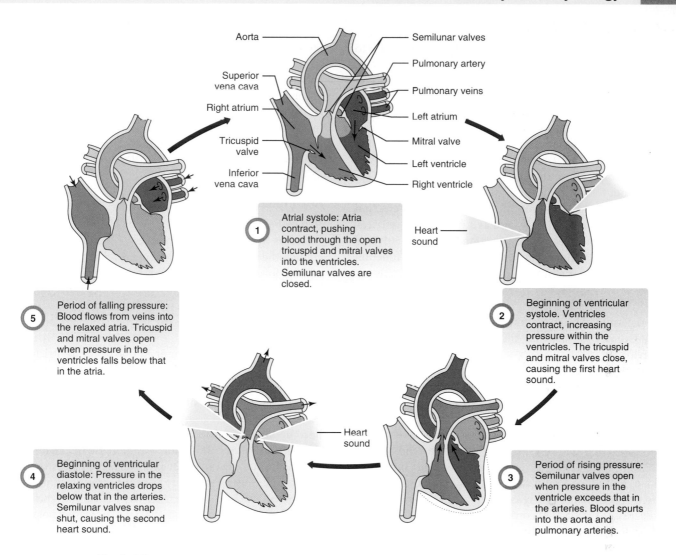

Fig. 1.16 Blood flow through the heart during the cardiac cycle. (From Solomon, E. (2016). *Introduction to human anatomy and physiology* (4th ed.). St. Louis: Saunders.)

The labels and numbered steps in the figure read:

Aorta · Semilunar valves · Pulmonary artery · Pulmonary veins · Superior vena cava · Left atrium · Right atrium · Mitral valve · Tricuspid valve · Left ventricle · Inferior vena cava · Right ventricle

1 Atrial systole: Atria contract, pushing blood through the open tricuspid and mitral valves into the ventricles. Semilunar valves are closed.

2 Beginning of ventricular systole. Ventricles contract, increasing pressure within the ventricles. The tricuspid and mitral valves close, causing the first heart sound.

3 Period of rising pressure: Semilunar valves open when pressure in the ventricle exceeds that in the arteries. Blood spurts into the aorta and pulmonary arteries.

4 Beginning of ventricular diastole: Pressure in the relaxing ventricles drops below that in the arteries. Semilunar valves snap shut, causing the second heart sound.

5 Period of falling pressure: Blood flows from veins into the relaxed atria. Tricuspid and mitral valves open when pressure in the ventricles falls below that in the atria.

Heart sound

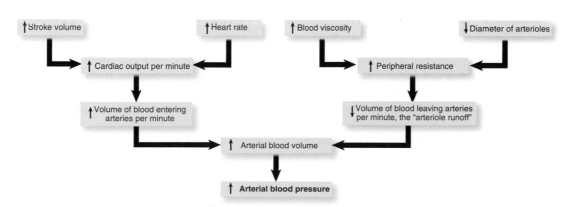

↑Stroke volume · ↑Heart rate · ↑Blood viscosity · ↓Diameter of arterioles

↑ Cardiac output per minute · ↑ Peripheral resistance

↑Volume of blood entering arteries per minute · ↓Volume of blood leaving arteries per minute, the "arteriole runoff"

↑ Arterial blood volume

↑ **Arterial blood pressure**

Fig. 1.17 Relationship between arterial blood volume and blood pressure. Arterial blood pressure is directly proportional to arterial blood volume. Cardiac output (CO) and peripheral resistance (PR) are directly proportional to arterial blood volume, but for opposite reasons: CO affects blood entering the arteries, and PR affects blood leaving the arteries. If cardiac output increases, the amount of blood entering the arteries increases and tends to increase blood volume in the arteries. If peripheral resistance increases, it decreases the amount of blood leaving the arteries, increasing the amount of blood left in them. Thus, an increase in either CO or PR results in an increase in arterial blood volume, which increases arterial blood pressure. (From Patton, K. T., & Thibodeau, G. A. (2019). *Anthony's textbook of anatomy and physiology* (21st ed.). St. Louis: Elsevier.)

CARDIAC OUTPUT

Cardiac output (CO) is the amount of blood pumped into the aorta each minute by the left ventricle (Pappano & Wier, 2019). Four factors determine CO: HR, myocardial contractility, preload, and afterload. CO is defined as the **stroke volume (SV)**, which is the amount of blood ejected from the left ventricle with each heartbeat, multiplied by the HR.

Each ventricle holds about 150 mL of blood when it is full. They usually eject about half this volume (70–80 mL) with each contraction. In a healthy average adult, the CO at rest is about 5 L/min. The percentage of blood pumped out of a ventricle with each contraction is called the **ejection fraction**. Ejection fraction is used as a measure of ventricular function. A normal ejection fraction is between 50% and 65%. A person is said to have impaired ventricular function when the ejection fraction is less than 40%.

Stroke Volume

SV is determined by the following:
- The degree of ventricular filling when the heart is relaxed (preload)
- The pressure against which the ventricle must pump (afterload)
- The myocardium's contractile state (contracting or relaxing)

Preload, which is also called the end-diastolic volume, is the force exerted on the ventricles' walls at the end of diastole. The volume of blood returning to the heart influences preload. More blood returning to the right atrium (e.g., increased venous return) increases preload. Less blood returning decreases preload. According to the Frank-Starling law of the heart, the greater the cardiac muscle stretch (within limits), the greater the resulting contraction. Heart muscle fibers stretch in response to the increased volume (preload) before contracting. Stretching of the muscle fibers allows the heart to eject the additional volume with increased force, thereby increasing SV. So in a normal heart, the greater the preload, the greater the force of ventricular contraction, and the greater the SV, resulting in increased CO.

This ability to adjust is essential so that the heart can alter its pumping capacity in response to changes in venous return. For example, during exercise, the heart muscle fibers stretch in response to increased volume (preload) before contracting. However, if the ventricle is stretched beyond its physiologic limit, CO may fall because of volume overload and overstretching of the muscle fibers. **Heart failure** is a condition in which the heart cannot pump enough blood to meet the body's metabolic needs. It may result from any condition that impairs preload, afterload, cardiac contractility, or HR.

Afterload is the pressure or resistance against which the ventricles must pump to eject blood. Afterload is influenced by the following:
- Arterial blood pressure
- The ability of the arteries to become stretched (arterial distensibility)
- Arterial resistance

The lower the resistance (lower afterload), the more easily blood can be ejected. Increased afterload (increased resistance) increases the heart's workload. Conditions that contribute to increased afterload include an increased thickness of the blood (viscosity) and high blood pressure.

Abnormal heart rhythms (**dysrhythmias**), such as atrial flutter and atrial fibrillation (discussed in Chapter 4), impede normal atrial contraction. Ineffectual atrial contraction can result in a loss of atrial kick, decreased stroke volume, and a subsequent decrease in CO.

Heart Rate

Remember that an increase in SV *or* HR may increase CO. Increases in HR shorten all phases of the cardiac cycle, including the time the ventricles spend relaxing. If the length of time for ventricular relaxation is shortened, there is less time for them to fill adequately with blood. If the ventricles do not have time to fill, the following occur:
- The amount of blood sent to the coronary arteries is reduced.
- The amount of blood pumped out of the ventricles will decrease (i.e., CO).
- Signs of myocardial ischemia may be seen.

The concentrations of extracellular ions also affect HR. Excess potassium (i.e., hyperkalemia) causes the heart to become dilated and flaccid (limp), slows the HR, and can dramatically alter conduction. An increase in calcium (i.e., hypercalcemia) has an effect almost exactly opposite that of potassium, causing the heart to go into spastic contraction. Decreased calcium levels (i.e., hypocalcemia) make the heart flaccid, similar to the effect of increased potassium levels.

Other factors that influence HR include hormone levels (e.g., epinephrine, norepinephrine), medications, stress, anxiety, fear, and body temperature. HR increases when body temperature increases and decreases when body temperature decreases.

An increase in the force of the heart's contractions (and, subsequently, SV) may occur because of many conditions, including norepinephrine and epinephrine release from the adrenal medulla, insulin and glucagon release from the pancreas, and medications (e.g., calcium, digitalis, dopamine, dobutamine). A decrease in contraction force may result from many conditions, including severe hypoxia, decreased pH, elevated carbon dioxide levels (hypercapnia), and medications (e.g., calcium blockers, beta-blockers).

Factors that increase CO include increased body metabolism, exercise, and the body's age and size. Factors that may decrease CO include shock, hypovolemia, and heart failure. Signs and symptoms of decreased CO appear in Box 1.2. Heart failure may result from any condition that impairs preload, afterload, cardiac contractility, or HR. As the heart begins to fail, the body's compensatory mechanisms attempt to improve CO by manipulating one or more of these factors.

Box **1.2**	Signs and Symptoms of Decreased Cardiac Output

- Acute drop in blood pressure
- Acute changes in mental status
- Cold, clammy skin
- Color changes in the skin and mucous membranes
- Crackles (rales)
- Dyspnea
- Dysrhythmias
- Fatigue
- Orthopnea
- Restlessness

Now that we have discussed CO, SV, and HR, let us review a vital point. Remember that an increase in HR *or* SV may increase CO. Consider the following examples:

1. A patient has an SV of 80 mL/beat. His HR is 70 beats per minute (beats/min). Is his CO normal, decreased, or increased? Substitute numbers into the formula you already learned: CO = SV × HR. 5600 mL/min = 80 mL/beat × 70 beats/min. CO is normally between 4 and 8 L/min. This patient's CO is within normal limits.

2. Now, let us see what an increase in HR does. If the patient's HR increases to 180 beats/min and his SV remains at 80 mL/beat, what happens to his CO? Using our formula again (CO = SV × HR) and substituting numbers, we end up with 14,400 mL/min = 80 mL/beat × 180 beats/min. This patient's CO is increased.

3. What happens to CO if the patient's HR is 70 beats/min but his SV drops to 50 mL/beat? Using our formula one more time (CO = SV × HR) and substituting numbers, we end up with 3500 mL/min = 50 mL/beat × 70 beats/min. This patient's CO is decreased. If the patient's HR increased to 90 beats/min to compensate for his failing pump, what would happen to his CO? (4500 mL/min = 50 mL/beat × 90 beats/min). According to our example, the patient's CO would increase—at least temporarily.

REFERENCES

Anderson, M. E., & Roden, D. M. (2010). Basic cardiac electrophysiology and anatomy. In M. H. Crawford, J. P. DiMarco, & W. J. Paulus (Eds.), *Cardiology* (3rd ed.) (pp. 653–665). Philadelphia, PA: Elsevier.

Gosling, J. A., Harris, P. F., Humpherson, J. R., Whitmore, I., & Willan, P. L. (2017). Thorax. In J. A. Gosling, P. F. Harris, J. R. Humpherson, I. Whitmore, & P. L. Willan (Eds.), *Human anatomy, color atlas and textbook* (6th ed.) (pp. 25–70). London: Elsevier.

Hall, J. E. (2016). The heart. In *Guyton and Hall textbook of medical physiology* (13th ed.) (pp. 107–166). Philadelphia, PA: Saunders.

Koeppen, B. M., & Stanton, B. A. (2018). Elements of cardiac function. In B. M. Koeppen, & B. A. Stanton (Eds.), *Berne & Levy physiology* (7th ed.) (pp. 304–344). Philadelphia, PA: Elsevier.

Pappano, A. J., & Wier, W. G. (2019). Control of cardiac output. In *Cardiovascular physiology* (11th ed.) (pp. 176–200). Philadelphia, PA: Elsevier.

STOP & REVIEW

Identify one or more choices that best complete the statement or answer the question.

1. Which of the following influence a person's heart size and weight?
   a. Age
   b. Body weight
   c. Heart disease
   d. Physical exercise frequency

2. Select the areas of the heart that make up its anterior surface.
   a. Left atrium
   b. Right atrium
   c. Left ventricle
   d. Right ventricle

3. The inferior surface of the heart is formed mainly by the
   a. right and left atria.
   b. right and left ventricles.
   c. left atrium and left ventricle.
   d. right atrium and right ventricle.

4. The pericardium
   a. is a thick, single-layer of tissue.
   b. protects the heart from trauma and infection.
   c. uses ligaments to anchor the heart to the sternum and diaphragm.
   d. contains about 20 mL of serous fluid that prevents friction as the heart beats.

5. The right atrium
   a. pumps blood to the lungs.
   b. pumps blood to the systemic circulation.
   c. receives blood from the right and left pulmonary veins.
   d. receives blood from the superior and inferior vena cavae and the coronary sinus.

6. When a ventricle relaxes in the normal heart, blood is prevented from flowing back into it by
   a. the mitral valve.
   b. a semilunar valve.
   c. the tricuspid valve.
   d. an atrioventricular valve.

7. Which of the following separate the atria from the ventricles?
   a. Aortic valve
   b. Mitral valve
   c. Pulmonic valve
   d. Tricuspid valve

8. Select the correct statements about the heart's coronary arteries.
   a. The circumflex (Cx) artery is a branch of the left coronary artery.
   b. The main coronary arteries lie on the epicardial surface of the heart.
   c. The septal and diagonal arteries are major branches of the right coronary artery (RCA).
   d. The right coronary artery supplies the sinoatrial (SA) node and atrioventricular (AV) bundle in most of the population.
   e. Occlusion of the Cx artery has been referred to as the "widow maker" because of its association with sudden cardiac arrest when it is blocked.

9. Which of the following factors determine cardiac output?
   a. Age
   b. Gender
   c. Preload
   d. Afterload
   e. Heart rate
   f. Myocardial contractility

Questions 10 Through 12 Pertain to the Following Scenario

A 65-year-old man presents with a sudden onset of substernal chest pain that radiates to his left arm and jaw and nausea. He states that his symptoms began while at rest. The patient has a history of coronary artery disease and had a three-vessel coronary artery bypass graft last year. His medications include diltiazem (Cardizem) and nitroglycerin. He has no known allergies.

10. Based on the information presented, this patient is most likely experiencing a(n)
    a. stroke.
    b. cardiac arrest.
    c. valvular prolapse.
    d. acute coronary syndrome.

11. Your assessment reveals that the patient is anxious, his skin is pale and sweaty, and his heart rate is faster than normal for his age. The patient's assessment findings are most likely
    a. the result of a blocked cerebral blood vessel.
    b. the result of the improper closure of one or more heart valves.
    c. caused by sympathetic stimulation and the release of norepinephrine.
    d. caused by parasympathetic stimulation and the release of acetylcholine.

12. Why might the patient's rapid heart rate be a cause for concern?

    a. Rapid heart rates predispose the patient to valvular heart disease.

    b. Rapid heart rates shorten diastole and can result in decreased cardiac output.

    c. Rapid heart rates lengthen systole but decrease myocardial contractility, which can lead to shock.

    d. Rapid heart rates are usually accompanied by pulmonary congestion, which leads to heart failure.

Matching

Match the terms below with their descriptions by placing the letter of each correct answer in the space provided.

a. Baroreceptors

b. Diastole

c. Left coronary artery

d. Right ventricle

e. Inotropy

f. Cardiac output

g. Blood pressure

h. Atrioventricular valves

i. Pericardium

j. Chronotropy

k. Right coronary artery

l. Chemoreceptors

m. Semilunar valves

n. Left ventricle

o. Ejection fraction

_____ **13.** Term that refers to a change in myocardial contractility

_____ **14.** Their closure at the end of systole prevents the backward flow of blood into the ventricles

_____ **15.** Double-walled sac containing a small amount of serous fluid that reduces friction as the heart beats

_____ **16.** The percentage of blood pumped out of a ventricle with each contraction

_____ **17.** This vessel supplies the SA node and AV node in most of the population

_____ **18.** Sensory receptors that detect changes in blood pressure

_____ **19.** Stroke volume multiplied by the heart rate

_____ **20.** Pumps oxygenated blood to the systemic circulation

_____ **21.** The anterior descending and circumflex are branches of this vessel

_____ **22.** Detect changes in the concentration of hydrogen ions, oxygen, and carbon dioxide in the blood

_____ **23.** Their closure causes the first heart sound (S1)

_____ **24.** Pumps blood low in oxygen to the pulmonary circulation

_____ **25.** The force exerted by the circulating blood volume on the walls of the arteries

_____ **26.** Phase of the cardiac cycle during which the greatest flow of blood enters the heart's chambers

_____ **27.** Term that refers to a change in rate

STOP & REVIEW ANSWERS

1. **A, B, C, D.** A person's heart size and weight are influenced by age, body weight and build, physical exercise frequency, and heart disease.

2. **B, C, D.** The front (anterior) surface of the heart lies behind the sternum and costal cartilages. Most of the anterior surface is formed by the right atrium and the right ventricle, with the left ventricle contributing a small portion.

3. **B.** The heart's inferior surface, also called the *diaphragmatic surface*, is formed by the left and right ventricles and a small portion of the right atrium. The left ventricle makes up most of the inferior surface.

4. **B, C, D.** The pericardium is a double-walled sac that encloses the heart and helps protect it from trauma and infection. The *fibrous parietal pericardium* is the sac's outer layer that anchors the heart to some of the structures around it, such as the sternum and diaphragm, through ligaments. The pericardium's inner layer, the *serous pericardium*, consists of two layers: parietal and visceral. The parietal layer lines the inside of the fibrous pericardium. The visceral layer (i.e., the epicardium) attaches to the large vessels that enter and exit the heart and forms the heart's outer surface. Between the visceral and parietal layers is a space (the pericardial space) that generally contains about 20 mL of serous fluid that acts as a lubricant, preventing friction as the heart beats.

5. **D.** The right atrium receives blood low in oxygen from the superior vena cava (which carries blood from the head and upper extremities), the inferior vena cava (which carries blood from the lower body), and the coronary sinus, which is the largest vein that drains the heart. The left atrium receives freshly oxygenated blood from the lungs via the right and left pulmonary veins. The right ventricle pumps blood to the lungs. The left ventricle pumps blood to the systemic circulation.

6. **B.** The semilunar valves prevent backflow of blood from the aorta and pulmonary arteries into the ventricles. When the right ventricle relaxes, blood is prevented from flowing back into it by the pulmonic valve. When the left ventricle relaxes, blood is prevented from flowing back into it by the aortic valve.

7. **B, D.** Atrioventricular valves separate the atria from the ventricles. The tricuspid valve is the AV valve that lies between the right atrium and the right ventricle. The mitral valve, also called the *bicuspid valve*, lies between the left atrium and left ventricle.

8. **A, B, D.** The main coronary arteries lie on the outer (i.e., epicardial) surface of the heart. The three major epicardial coronary arteries include the left anterior descending (LAD) artery, Cx artery, and RCA. The RCA supplies the SA node and AV bundle in most of the population. The left main coronary artery supplies oxygenated blood to its two primary branches: the LAD artery and the Cx artery. The septal and diagonal arteries are branches of the LAD. Occlusion of the proximal LAD coronary artery has been referred to as the "widow maker" because of its association with sudden cardiac arrest when it is blocked.

9. **C, D, E, F.** Four factors determine CO: HR, myocardial contractility, preload, and afterload.

10. **D.** Based on the information presented, this patient is most likely experiencing an acute coronary syndrome (ACS). ACS refers to distinct conditions caused by a similar sequence of pathologic events—a temporary or permanent blockage of a coronary artery.

11. **C.** This patient's assessment findings are typical of those experiencing an ACS and are most likely caused by sympathetic stimulation and norepinephrine and epinephrine release. Recall that the autonomic nervous system's sympathetic division prepares the body to function under stress ("fight-or-flight" response). The effects of norepinephrine and epinephrine include increases in heart rate, force of contraction, blood pressure, cardiac output, and sweating. Additional effects include the shunting of blood from the skin and blood vessels of internal organs to skeletal muscle.

12. **B.** The coronary arteries fill when the aortic valve is closed and the left ventricle is relaxed (i.e., diastole). If the length of time for ventricular relaxation is shortened (as with rapid heart rates), there is less time for them to fill adequately with blood. If the ventricles do not have time to fill, the amount of blood sent to the coronary arteries is reduced, the amount of blood pumped out of the ventricles will decrease (i.e., cardiac output), and signs of myocardial ischemia may be seen.

Matching

13. ANS: e
14. ANS: m
15. ANS: i
16. ANS: o
17. ANS: k
18. ANS: a
19. ANS: f
20. ANS: n
21. ANS: c
22. ANS: l
23. ANS: h
24. ANS: d
25. ANS: g
26. ANS: b
27. ANS: j

Basic Electrophysiology

2

LEARNING OBJECTIVES

After reading this chapter, you should be able to:

1. Describe the basic types of cardiac cells in the heart, where they are found, their function, and their primary characteristics.
2. Define the events comprising the cardiac action potential and correlate them with the waveforms produced on the electrocardiogram (ECG).
3. Define the terms *action potential*, *polarization*, *depolarization*, *repolarization*, *effective refractory period*, and *relative refractory period*.
4. Describe the normal sequence of electrical conduction through the heart.
5. Describe the location, function, and, when appropriate, the following structures' intrinsic rates: the sinoatrial node, the atrioventricular bundle, and the Purkinje fibers.
6. Differentiate the primary mechanisms responsible for producing cardiac dysrhythmias.
7. Explain the purpose of ECG monitoring.
8. Identify the limitations of the ECG.
9. Differentiate between the frontal plane and the horizontal plane leads.
10. Describe the correct anatomic placement of the standard limb leads, the augmented leads, and the chest leads.
11. Relate the cardiac surfaces or areas represented by the ECG leads.
12. Identify the numeric values assigned to the small and the large boxes on ECG paper.
13. Identify how heart rates, durations, and amplitudes can be determined from ECG recordings.
14. Define and describe the significance of each of the following as they relate to cardiac electrical activity: P wave, QRS complex, T wave, U wave, PR segment, TP segment, ST segment, PR interval, QRS duration, and QT interval.
15. Recognize the ECG changes that may reflect evidence of myocardial ischemia, injury, and infarction.
16. Define the term *artifact* and explain the methods used to minimize its occurrence.
17. Describe a systematic approach to the analysis and interpretation of cardiac dysrhythmias.

KEY TERMS

accessory pathway: An extra bundle of working myocardial tissue that forms a connection between the atria and ventricles outside the normal conduction system.

action potential: A cycle consisting of several phases that reflects the difference in the concentration of charged particles across the cell membrane at any given time.

altered automaticity: A condition in which cardiac cells not normally associated with the property of automaticity begin to depolarize spontaneously or when escape pacemaker sites increase their firing rate beyond that considered normal.

amplitude: Height (voltage) of a waveform on the electrocardiogram.

artifact: Distortion of an electrocardiographic tracing by electrical activity that is noncardiac in origin (e.g., electrical interference, poor electrical conduction, patient movement).

atrioventricular (AV) bundle: The bundle of His.

atrioventricular (AV) node: A group of cells that conduct an electrical impulse through the heart; located in the floor of the right atrium immediately behind the tricuspid valve and near the opening of the coronary sinus; delays the electrical impulse to allow the atria to contract and complete filling of the ventricles.

augmented limb lead: Leads aVR, aVL, and aVF; these leads record the difference in electrical potential at one location relative to zero potential rather than relative to the electrical potential of another extremity.

automaticity: Ability of cardiac pacemaker cells to spontaneously initiate an electrical impulse without being stimulated from another source (such as a nerve).

axis: Imaginary line joining the positive and negative electrodes of a lead.

baseline: Straight line recorded on electrocardiographic graph paper when no electrical activity is detected.

Continued

KEY TERMS—cont'd

biphasic: Waveform that is partly positive and partly negative.

bipolar limb lead: Electrocardiographic lead consisting of a positive and negative electrode.

bradycardia: Heart rate slower than 60 beats per minute (beats/min) (from *brady*, meaning "slow").

bundle of His: Fibers located in the upper portion of the interventricular septum that receive an electrical impulse from the AV node and conduct the impulse to the right and left bundle branches.

complex: Several waveforms.

conduction system: A system of pathways in the heart composed of specialized electrical (pacemaker) cells.

conductivity: Ability of a cardiac cell to receive an electrical stimulus and conduct that impulse to an adjacent cardiac cell.

contractility: Ability of cardiac cells to shorten, causing cardiac muscle contraction in response to an electrical stimulus.

current: The flow of electrical charge from one point to another.

depolarization: Movement of ions across a cell membrane, causing the inside of the cell to become more positive; an electrical event expected to result in contraction.

ectopic: Impulse(s) originating from a source other than the sinoatrial node.

effective refractory period (ERP): The interval from the beginning of the action potential until the myocardial fiber can conduct another action potential; during this period, cardiac cells cannot be stimulated to conduct an electrical impulse, no matter how strong the stimulus; also called the absolute refractory period.

electrode: An adhesive pad that contains a conductive gel and is applied at specific locations on the patient's chest wall and extremities and connected by cables to an electrocardiogram machine.

electrocardiogram (ECG): A graphic display of the heart's electrical activity.

excitability: The ability of cardiac cells to respond to a stimulus.

ground electrode: Third ECG electrode (the first and second are the positive and negative electrodes), which minimizes electrical activity from other sources.

His-Purkinje system: Portion of the conduction system consisting of the bundle of His, bundle branches, and Purkinje fibers.

indicative changes: Electrocardiographic changes observed in leads that look directly at the affected area of the heart; indicative changes are significant when they are seen in two anatomically contiguous leads.

inherent: Natural, intrinsic.

interval: Waveform and a segment; in pacing, the period, measured in milliseconds, between any two designated cardiac events.

intrinsic rate: Rate at which a pacemaker of the heart normally generates impulses.

isoelectric line: Absence of electrical activity; observed on the ECG as a straight line.

J point: Point where the QRS complex and ST segment meet.

lead: Electrical connection attached to the body to record electrical activity.

millivolt (mV): Difference in electrical charge between two points in a circuit.

myocardial cells: Working cells of the myocardium that contain contractile filaments and form the muscular layer of the atrial walls and the thicker muscular layer of the ventricular walls.

pacemaker cells: Specialized cells of the heart's electrical conduction system, capable of spontaneously generating and conducting electrical impulses.

permeable: Ability of a membrane channel to allow passage of electrolytes when it is open.

polarized: Period after repolarization of a cell (also called the *resting state*) when the outside of the cell is positive and the interior of the cell is negative.

PR interval: P wave plus the PR segment; reflects depolarization of the right and left atria (P wave) and the spread of the impulse through the AV node, AV bundle, right and left bundle branches, and the Purkinje fibers (PR segment).

P wave: First wave in the cardiac cycle; represents atrial depolarization and the spread of the electrical impulse throughout the right and left atria.

QRS complex: Several waveforms (i.e., the Q wave, the R wave, and the S wave) that represent the spread of an electrical impulse through the ventricles (i.e., ventricular depolarization).

QT interval: The period from the beginning of the QRS complex to the end of the T wave.

R wave: On an ECG, the first positive deflection in the QRS complex, representing ventricular depolarization; in pacing, R wave refers to the entire QRS complex, denoting an intrinsic ventricular event.

reciprocal changes: Electrocardiographic changes observed in leads opposite the affected area of the heart; also called mirror image changes.

reentry: A disorder of impulse conduction that results from the spread of an impulse through tissue already stimulated by that same impulse.

refractoriness: Period of recovery that cells need after being discharged before they can respond to a stimulus.

relative refractory period (RRP): Corresponds with the downslope of the T wave; during this period, cardiac cells can be stimulated to depolarize if the stimulus is strong enough.

repolarization: Movement of ions across a cell membrane in which the inside of the cell is restored to its negative charge.

segment: Line between waveforms; named by the waveform that precedes and follows it.

sinoatrial (SA) node: Normal pacemaker of the heart that normally discharges at a rhythmic rate of 60 to 100 beats/min.

ST segment: Portion of the ECG representing the end of ventricular depolarization (end of the R wave) and the beginning of ventricular repolarization (T wave).

T wave: Waveform that follows the QRS complex and represents ventricular repolarization.

tachycardia: Heart rate greater than 100 beats/min (tachy, fast).

TP segment: Interval between two successive PQRST complexes during which electrical activity of the heart is absent; begins with the end of the T wave through the onset of the following P wave and represents the period from the end of ventricular repolarization to the onset of atrial depolarization.

triggered activity: A disorder of impulse formation that occurs when escape pacemaker and myocardial working cells fire more than once after stimulation by a single impulse resulting in atrial or ventricular beats that occur alone, in pairs, in runs, or as a sustained ectopic rhythm.

unipolar lead: Lead that consists of a single positive electrode and a reference point.

voltage: Difference in electrical charge between two points.

waveform: Movement away from the baseline in either a positive or negative direction.

CARDIAC CELLS

Types of Cardiac Cells

In general, cardiac cells have either a mechanical (i.e., contractile) or an electrical (i.e., pacemaker) function. **Myocardial cells** are also called working cells or mechanical cells, and they contain contractile filaments. When these cells are electrically stimulated, these filaments slide together and cause the myocardial cell to contract. These myocardial cells form the thin muscular layer of the atrial walls and the thicker muscular layer of the ventricular walls (i.e., the myocardium).

Pacemaker cells are also referred to as conducting cells or automatic cells. They are specialized cells of the electrical conduction system that can form electrical impulses spontaneously and alter the speed of electrical conduction (Wagner, 2012).

Properties of Cardiac Cells

When a nerve is stimulated, a chemical (i.e., a neurotransmitter) is released. The chemical crosses the space between the end of the nerve and the muscle membrane (i.e., the neuromuscular junction). The neurotransmitter binds to receptor sites on the muscle membrane and stimulates the receptors. An electrical impulse develops and travels along the muscle membrane, resulting in contraction; thus, a skeletal muscle normally contracts only after a nerve stimulates it.

Most atrial and ventricular working cells cannot conduct an impulse without an outside stimulus (Peterson, 2018). In contrast, the heart's pacemaker cells can generate an electrical impulse without being stimulated from another source. This property is called **automaticity**. Cardiac muscle is electrically irritable because of an ionic imbalance across the membranes of cells. **Excitability** (i.e., irritability) is a cardiac cell's ability to respond to a stimulus, such as a chemical, mechanical, or electrical source. **Conductivity** is a cardiac cell's ability to receive an electrical impulse and conduct it to an adjacent cardiac cell. All cardiac cells possess this characteristic. The intercalated disks present in the membranes of cardiac cells are responsible for the property of conductivity. They allow an impulse in any part of the myocardium to spread throughout the heart. The speed with which the impulse is conducted can be altered by sympathetic and parasympathetic stimulation and medications. **Contractility** (i.e., inotropy) is myocardial cells' ability to shorten, thereby causing cardiac muscle contraction in response to an electrical stimulus. The strength of the heart's contraction can be increased or decreased with certain medications.

CARDIAC ACTION POTENTIAL

Before we discuss the cardiac action potential, think about how a battery releases energy. A battery has two terminals; one terminal is positive and the other is negative. Charged particles exert forces on each other, and opposite charges attract. Electrons, which are negatively charged particles, are produced by a chemical reaction inside the battery. If a wire is connected between the two terminals, the circuit is completed, and the stored energy is released, allowing electrons to flow quickly from the negative terminal along the wire to the positive terminal. If no wire is connected between the terminals, the chemical reaction does not occur, and no current flow occurs. **Current** is the flow of electrical charge from one point to another.

Separated electrical charges of opposite polarity (i.e., positive vs. negative) have potential energy. The measurement of this potential energy is called **voltage**. Voltage is measured between two points. In the battery example, the current flow is caused by the voltage, or potential difference, between the two terminals. Voltage is measured in units of volts or millivolts.

Human body fluids contain electrolytes, which are elements or compounds that break into charged particles (i.e., ions) when melted or dissolved in water or another solvent. Differences in the composition of ions between the intracellular and extracellular fluid compartments are essential for normal body function, including the heart's activity. Body fluids that contain electrolytes conduct an electric current in much the same way as the wire in the battery example. Electrolytes move about in body fluids and carry a charge, just as electrons moving along a wire conduct a current.

In the body, ions spend much time moving back and forth across cell membranes (Fig. 2.1). As a result, a slight difference in the concentrations of charged particles across the membranes of cells is normal; thus, potential energy (i.e., voltage) exists because of the imbalance of charged particles. This imbalance makes the cells excitable. The voltage (i.e., the difference in electrical charges) across the cell membrane is the membrane potential. The threshold potential is the voltage level at which the cell discharges and conducts an electrical impulse.

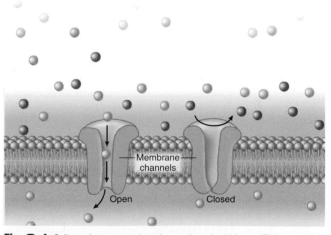

Fig. 2.1 Cell membranes contain pathways through which specific ions or other small, water-soluble molecules can cross. (From Patton, K. T. (2019). *Anatomy & physiology* (10th ed.). St. Louis: Elsevier.)

Electrolytes are quickly moved from one side of the cell membrane to the other using pumps. These pumps require energy in the form of adenosine triphosphate (ATP) when movement occurs against a concentration gradient. The energy expended by the cells to move electrolytes across the cell membrane creates a flow of current. This flow of current is expressed in volts or millivolts (mV). Voltage appears on an **electrocardiogram** (ECG) as waveforms. A cardiac cell's **action potential** reflects the rapid sequence of voltage changes across the cell membrane during the electrical cardiac cycle.

Depolarization and Repolarization

When a cardiac cell is at rest, the cell membrane's inner surface is covered by negatively charged ions while positively charged ions envelop the external surface. Under these conditions, the cell is said to be polarized.

Depolarization is the movement of ions across a cell membrane, causing the inside of the cell to become more positive (Fig. 2.2). Depolarization, an electrical event, must occur before the heart can contract and pump blood, which is a mechanical event. The stimulus that alters the electrical charges across the cell membrane may be electrical, mechanical, or chemical. An impulse normally begins in the pacemaker cells found in the SA node of the heart. A chain reaction (a wave of depolarization) occurs from cell to cell in the heart's electrical conduction system until all the cells have been stimulated and depolarized. The chain reaction is made possible because of the gap junctions that exist between the cells. These junctions permit ions to flow from one cell into the next. Eventually, the impulse is spread from the pacemaker cells to the working myocardial cells, which contract when stimulated. Depolarization proceeds from the heart's innermost layer (i.e., the endocardium) to the outermost layer (i.e., the epicardium). When the atria are stimulated, a P wave is recorded on the ECG; thus, the P wave represents atrial depolarization. When the ventricles are stimulated, a QRS complex is recorded on the ECG; therefore, the QRS complex represents ventricular depolarization (Fig. 2.3).

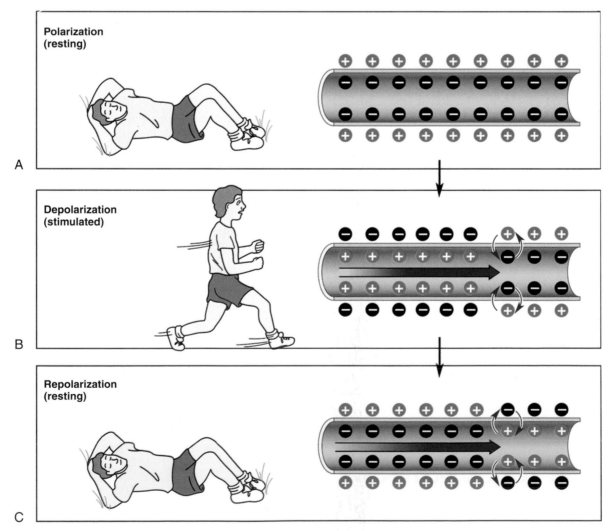

Fig. 2.2 A, Polarization. B, Depolarization. C, Repolarization. (From Herlihy, B. (2018). *The human body in health and illness* (6th ed.). St Louis: Elsevier.)

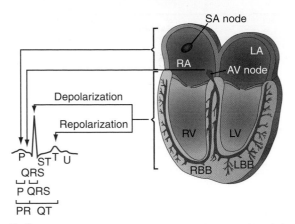

Fig. 2.3 Schematic representation of the electrocardiogram and its relationship to cardiac electrical activity. (From McCance, K. L., & Huether, S. E. (2019). *Pathophysiology* (8th ed.). St. Louis: Elsevier.)

ECG Pearl

Depolarization is not the same as contraction. Depolarization is an electrical event that is expected to result in contraction, which is a mechanical event. It is possible to see organized electrical activity on the cardiac monitor even when the assessment of the patient reveals no palpable pulse. This clinical situation is called *pulseless electrical activity*.

After the cell depolarizes, it quickly begins to recover and restore its electrical charges to normal. The movement of charged particles across a cell membrane in which the inside of the cell is restored to its negative charge is called **repolarization**. As the cell returns to its polarized (i.e., resting) state, contractile proteins in the working myocardial cells separate (i.e., relax). The cell can be stimulated again if another electrical impulse arrives at the cell membrane. Repolarization proceeds from the epicardium to the endocardium. On the ECG, the ST segment and T wave represents ventricular repolarization (see Fig. 2.3).

Action Potentials

There are two main types of action potentials in the heart: fast potentials and slow potentials. The action potential configuration varies depending on the cardiac cell's location and function (Fig. 2.4).

FAST POTENTIALS

The fast response action potential occurs in atrial and ventricular working myocardial cells and His-Purkinje fibers (Issa et al., 2019c), which are specialized conducting fibers that will be discussed later. The cardiac action potential is divided into several phases, which reflect the permeability of the cell membrane to different electrolytes (Fig. 2.5).

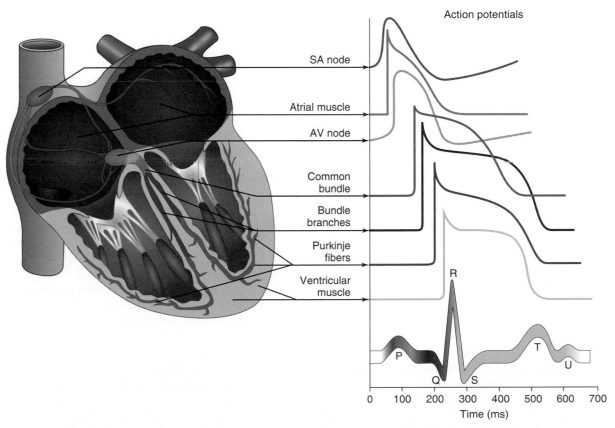

Fig. 2.4 Cardiac action potentials from the sinoatrial node to the ventricular myocardium. (From Dowd, F. J., Johnson, B. S., & Mariotti, A. J. (2017). *Pharmacology and therapeutics for dentistry* (7th ed.). St. Louis: Elsevier.)

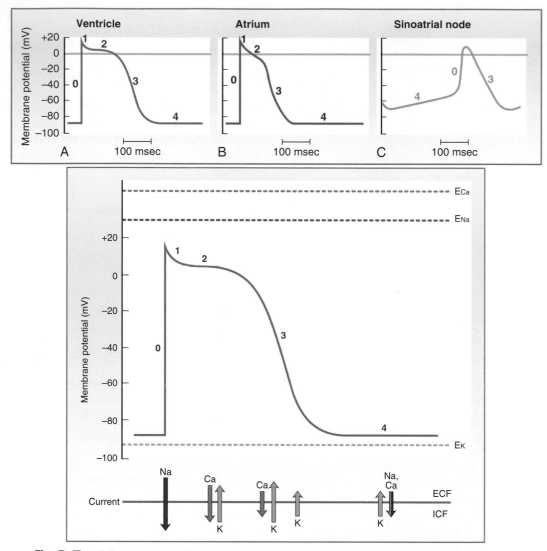

Fig. 2.5 A–C, Cardiac action potentials in the ventricle, atrium, and sinoatrial node. The numbers correspond to the phases of the action potentials. D, Currents responsible for the ventricular action potential. The length of the arrows shows the relative size of each ionic current. *E*, Equilibrium potential; *ECF*, extracellular fluid; *ICF*, intracellular fluid. (From Costanzo, L. S. (2018). *Physiology* (6th ed.). Philadelphia: Elsevier.)

Phase 0 of the fast response action potential, called the upstroke, spike, or overshoot, begins when the cell receives an impulse. The cell rapidly depolarizes in response to an influx of sodium (Na^+). The speed of phase 0 depolarization determines the velocity of impulse conduction. Medications that block the influx of Na^+ (e.g., lidocaine, procainamide) decrease the rate of phase 0 depolarization, slowing impulse conduction through the His-Purkinje system and myocardium (Burchum, 2016).

The upstroke is followed by a period of repolarization, which is divided into three phases. During phase 1 (i.e., initial repolarization), the Na^+ channels partially close, slowing the flow of Na^+ into the cell. At the same time, chloride (Cl^-) enters the cell, and potassium (K^+) leaves it through K^+ channels. The result is a decrease in the number of positive electrical charges within the cell, which produces a small negative deflection in the action potential. During phase 2

(i.e., the plateau phase), calcium (Ca^{++}) enters the cell. The cells of the atria, ventricles, and Purkinje fibers have many Ca^{++} channels. Medications that block the influx of Ca^{++} into the cell (e.g., beta-blockers, calcium blockers) decrease contractility. Rapid repolarization occurs during phase 3. This phase begins with the downslope of the action potential. The rapid movement of K^+ out of the cell causes the inside to become progressively more electrically negative. The cell gradually becomes more sensitive to external stimuli until its original sensitivity is restored. Repolarization is complete by the end of phase 3. Medications that block the movement of K^+ out of the cell (e.g., amiodarone) delay repolarization, prolonging the effective refractory period (discussed later).

Phase 4 is the resting membrane potential (i.e., return to resting state). During phase 4, the Na^+/K^+ pump is activated to move Na^+ out of the cell and K^+ back into the cell. Relaxation of the cardiac muscle occurs mainly during phase 4. The cell remains polarized until another stimulus reactivates the cell membrane.

SLOW POTENTIALS

The second type of cardiac action potential, the slow response action potential, occurs in the heart's normal pacemaker (i.e., the SA node) and in the atrioventricular (AV) node, which is the specialized conducting tissue that carries an electrical impulse from the atria to the ventricles (Fig. 2.6).

Pacemaker cells reach threshold potential sooner than other cardiac cells, reflected as a steeper slope of phase 4. Under normal conditions, the phase 4 depolarization rate in the SA node cells is faster than in all other heart cells. As a result, the SA node is considered the heart's primary pacemaker because it discharges first, thereby determining heart rate. Cells in the His-Purkinje system can also exhibit phase 4 depolarization under special circumstances, such as when pathologic processes inactivate Na^+ channels (Issa et al., 2019c).

In fast response action potentials, phase 0 is caused by an influx of Na^+. In slow response action potentials, phase 0 is mostly the result of the entry of Ca^{++} into the cell. (Calcium also triggers contraction in all myocardial working cells.) Compared with the fast response action potential, the upstroke of the slow response action potential is less steep, and it has a smaller amplitude. These findings indicate that conduction velocity is much slower in slow-response fibers than in fast-response fibers (Pappano & Wier, 2019). Medications that suppress calcium influx during phase 0 (e.g., beta-blockers, calcium blockers [verapamil, diltiazem], adenosine) can slow AV conduction, resulting in heart rate changes.

Phase 1 is absent in the slow-response action potential, and the transition from the plateau phase (phase 2) to repolarization (i.e., phase 3) is less distinct. As in the other cardiac tissues, repolarization is mainly dependent on K^+.

ECG Pearl

The heart typically beats at a regular rate and rhythm. If this pattern is interrupted, an abnormal heart rhythm can result. Health care professionals use the terms *arrhythmia* and *dysrhythmia* interchangeably to refer to an abnormal heart rhythm. Medications used to correct irregular heartbeats and slow down hearts that beat too fast are called *antiarrhythmics*. Although there is no universally accepted classification scheme for antiarrhythmic agents, a commonly used system is to classify the medications by their effects on the cardiac action potential. For example, class I antiarrhythmic medications such as procainamide and lidocaine block sodium channels, interfering with phase 0 depolarization. Class IV antiarrhythmics (Ca^{++} blockers) such as verapamil and diltiazem slow the rate at which calcium passes through the cells, interfering with phase 2 in the cells of the atria, ventricles, and His-Purkinje system.

Refractory Periods

Recall that excitability is the ability of myocardial cells to respond to a stimulus. The excitability of a myocardial cell varies throughout the action potential, and these changes in excitability are reflected in refractory periods (Costanzo, 2018).

Refractoriness is a term used to describe the period of recovery that cells need after being discharged before they are once again able to respond to a stimulus. The **effective refractory period (ERP)**, also called the *absolute refractory period*, is the interval from the beginning of the action potential until the myocardial fiber can conduct another action potential (Pappano & Wier, 2019). The ERP extends over phases 0, 1, 2, and part of phase 3 of the action potential and corresponds to the time needed to reopen channels that allow the entry of Na^+ and Ca^{++} into the cell (Cunningham et al., 2017). During the ERP, the cell is unable to respond to further stimulation,

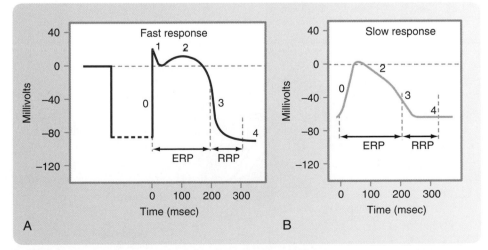

Fig. 2.6 Action potentials of fast-response (A) and slow-response (B) cardiac fibers. The phases of the action potentials are labeled. The effective refractory period (*ERP*) and the relative refractory period (*RRP*) are labeled. Note that when compared with fast-response fibers, the resting potential of slow fibers is less negative, the upstroke (phase 0) of the action potential is less steep, the amplitude of the action potential is smaller, phase 1 is absent, and the RRP extends well into phase 4 after the fibers have fully repolarized. (From Koeppen, B. M., & Stanton, B. A. (2018). *Berne & Levy physiology* (7th ed.). Philadelphia: Elsevier.)

which means that the myocardial working cells cannot contract and that the electrical conduction system's cells cannot conduct an electrical impulse or initiate a new action potential, no matter how strong the stimulus. The **relative refractory period (RRP)** begins at the end of the ERP and ends when the cell membrane is almost entirely repolarized (see Fig. 2.6). During the RRP, some cardiac cells have repolarized to their threshold potential and thus can be stimulated to respond (i.e., depolarize) to a stronger-than-normal stimulus.

CONDUCTION SYSTEM

The specialized electrical (i.e., pacemaker) cells in the heart are arranged in a system of pathways called the **conduction system** (Fig. 2.7). In the normal heart, the cells of the conduction system are interconnected. The conduction system ensures that the chambers of the heart contract in a coordinated fashion. Structures in the human heart that possess the property of automaticity and can function as pacemakers include the SA node, cells in parts of the atria, the AV bundle, and the His-Purkinje system (Issa et al., 2019b).

Sinoatrial Node

The normal heartbeat results from an electrical impulse (i.e., an action potential) that begins in the SA node. The SA node is specialized conducting tissue located in the upper posterior part of the right atrium where the superior vena cava and the right atrium meet. Pacemaker cells in the core of the SA node are responsible for spontaneously generating electrical impulses. The impulse then travels to an outer

layer of transitional cells responsible for transmitting the electrical impulse to the SA node's borders, into the right atrium, and then through the rest of the heart's electrical conduction system.

The SA node receives its blood supply from the SA node artery that runs lengthwise through the node's center. The SA node artery originates from the right coronary artery (RCA) in about 55% to 60% of people and from the circumflex (Cx) artery in the remaining 40% to 45% (Tomaselli et al., 2019). Sympathetic and parasympathetic nerve fibers richly supply the SA node.

Although the SA node is the smallest electrical area of the heart (Lederer, 2017), it is the heart's primary pacemaker because it has the fastest firing rate (specifically, the fastest rate of phase 4 depolarization) of the heart's pacemaker sites. The built-in (i.e., intrinsic) rate of the SA node is 60 to 100 beats per minute (beats/min). This rate can increase significantly, primarily through sympathetic stimulation. Heart rates faster than 150 beats/min can be problematic because: (1) the duration of diastole shortens as heart rate increases, reducing ventricular filling time and, potentially, stroke volume and (2) the heart's workload and oxygen requirements are increased, but the time for coronary artery filling, which occurs during diastole, is decreased (DeBeasi, 2003).

As the impulse leaves the SA node, it spreads from cell to cell in wavelike form across the atrial muscle. As the impulse spreads, it stimulates the right atrium and the interatrial septum. It travels along a special pathway called Bachmann's bundle to stimulate the left atrium, resulting in contraction of the right and left atria at almost the same time. Because a fibrous skeleton separates the atrial myocardium from the ventricular myocardium, the electrical stimulus affects only the atria.

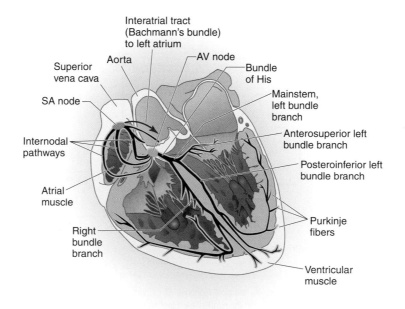

Fig. 2.7 Conduction pathways through the heart. A section through the long axis of the heart is shown. (From Boron, W. F., & Boulpaep, E. L. (2017). *Medical physiology* (3rd ed.). Philadelphia: Elsevier.)

SECONDARY PACEMAKER SITES

Areas of the heart other than the SA node can initiate beats and assume pacemaker responsibility under special circumstances. The terms *secondary*, *subsidiary*, *latent*, or *ectopic* refer to sites other than the SA node that can assume pacemaking responsibility. However, their intrinsic rates are slower than that of the SA node. Typical secondary pacemaker sites include the AV junction and Purkinje fibers' cells. Although a secondary pacemaker is typically prevented from discharging because of the dominance of the SA node's rapidly firing pacemaker cells, a secondary site may assume pacemaker responsibility in the following circumstances:

- The SA node fires too slowly because of vagal stimulation or suppression by medications.
- The SA node fails to generate an impulse because of disease, surgical removal, or suppression by medications.
- The SA node action potential is blocked because of disease in conducting pathways, failing to activate the surrounding atrial myocardium.
- The firing rate of the ectopic site becomes faster than that of the SA node.

Pacemaker cells have also been identified in several areas of the atria (Mangoni & Nargeot, 2008). An atrial pacemaker site may initiate an impulse if the SA node discharge rate is too slow. Automaticity of secondary atrial pacemakers can also be enhanced by myocardial ischemia, chronic pulmonary disease, or drugs such as digitalis and alcohol, possibly overriding normal sinus activity (Issa et al., 2019b).

Although secondary pacemakers supply a backup or safety mechanism in SA node failure, such sites can be problematic if they fire while the SA node is still functioning. For example, secondary sites may cause early (i.e., premature) beats or sustained rhythm disturbances.

Atrioventricular Node and Bundle

The **AV node** is a group of specialized conducting cells located on the right atrium floor immediately behind the tricuspid valve. The AV node has been divided into three functional regions according to their action potentials and responses to electrical and chemical stimulation (Fig. 2.8):

- The atrionodal (AN) region (also called the *transitional zone*) located between the atrium and the rest of the node
- The nodal (N) region, the middle area of the AV node where transitional cells merge with midnodal cells
- The nodal-His (NH) or lower region where the fibers of the AV node gradually join with the bundle of His

Some research suggests that the AV node itself possesses pacemaker cells, but this theory is controversial (Issa et al., 2019b). It is known that the lower portion of the AV node possesses pacemaker cells that have an intrinsic rate of 40 to 60 beats/min. Because this rate is slower than that of the SA node, the AV junction is considered a secondary pacemaker.

The **bundle of His**, also called the *common bundle* or the **AV bundle**, is a continuation of the AV node and connects the AV node with the bundle branches. The AV node and the bundle of His are called the *AV junction*. **His-Purkinje system**, or *His-Purkinje network*, refers to the bundle of His, bundle branches, and **Purkinje fibers**. In the heart's conduction system, impulse conduction is fastest in the His-Purkinje system and slowest in the SA and AV nodes.

As the impulse enters the AV junction through the internodal pathways (Fig. 2.9), conduction is markedly slowed in the AV node's nodal area before the impulse reaches the

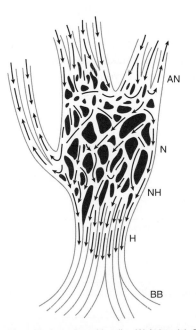

Fig. 2.8 The atrioventricular node and bundle. *AN,* Atrionodal; *BB,* bundle branches; *H,* bundle of His; *N,* nodal; *NH,* nodal-His. (From Clochesy, J. (1996). *Critical care nursing* (2nd ed.). Philadelphia: Saunders.)

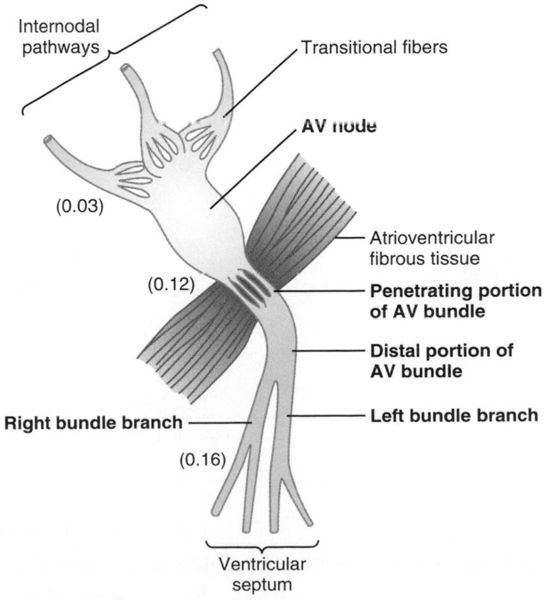

Fig. 2.9 Organization of the atrioventricular (*AV*) node and AV bundle. The numbers represent the interval of time in fractions of a second from the origin of the impulse in the sinoatrial node. (From Hall, J. E. (2016). *Guyton and Hall textbook of medical physiology* (13th ed.). Philadelphia: Elsevier.)

ventricles. If this delay did not occur, the atria and the ventricles would contract at about the same time. The conduction delay allows both atrial chambers to contract and empty blood into the ventricles before the next ventricular contraction begins, increasing the amount of blood in the ventricles and increasing stroke volume. Another vital function of the AV node is that during episodes of rapid atrial dysrhythmias, the AV node limits (i.e., blocks) the number of impulses reaching the ventricles.

Both sympathetic and parasympathetic nerve fibers supply the AV node. The AV node receives its blood supply from the RCA's posterior descending branch in 85% to 90% of the population (Tomaselli et al., 2019). In the remainder, a branch of the Cx artery provides the blood supply. There is a dual blood supply to the AV node in some patients (Tomaselli et al., 2019). Both the AV nodal artery and the first septal branch of the left anterior descending artery provide the blood supply to the bundle of His. This dual blood supply makes this portion of the conduction system less vulnerable to ischemic damage unless the ischemia is extensive (Issa et al., 2019a).

Normally, the atria and ventricles are separated by a continuous barrier of fibrous tissue, which acts as an insulator to prevent the passage of an electrical impulse through any route other than the AV node and bundle. When an atypical pathway bypasses the AV node and bundle, the abnormal route is called an **accessory pathway**.

⟳ ECG Pearl

Abnormal cardiac rhythms that develop near or within the AV node are called junctional dysrhythmias. Those that develop above the bundle of His or activate the ventricles through an accessory pathway are called supraventricular dysrhythmias. Dysrhythmias that develop below the bundle of His are called ventricular dysrhythmias.

Right and Left Bundle Branches

The bundle of His passes down the right side of the interventricular septum and then divides into the right and left bundle branches. The upper portion of the interventricular septum is supplied with blood by branches of the anterior and posterior descending coronary arteries.

The right bundle branch is thin and travels to the apex of the right ventricle. The left bundle branch spreads the electrical impulse to the interventricular septum and left ventricle. The left bundle branch is thicker than the right and splits into divisions called fascicles on the subendocardial surface of the left side of the interventricular septum.

Purkinje Fibers

The right and left bundle branches divide into smaller and smaller branches and then into a fibrous network called the Purkinje fibers, which spread out over the subendocardial surfaces of both ventricles. These fibers have pacemaker cells that have an intrinsic rate of 20 to 40 beats/min.

Purkinje fibers have a large diameter and a large concentration of gap junctions, enabling the rapid transmission of electrical impulses. The spread of an electrical impulse through the Purkinje fibers proceeds from the endocardium, where the endocardial surfaces of both ventricles are rapidly activated, to the myocardium and ventricular muscle fibers, and then finally to the epicardial surface. A summary of the conduction system is shown in Table 2.1.

CAUSES OF DYSRHYTHMIAS

Dysrhythmias result from disorders of impulse formation, disorders of impulse conduction, or both.

Disorders of Impulse Formation
ALTERED AUTOMATICITY

Altered automaticity is a condition in which one of the following occurs: (1) Cardiac cells that are generally not associated with a pacemaker function begin to depolarize spontaneously *or* (2) a pacemaker site other than the SA node increases its firing rate beyond that which is considered normal. If the rapid firing rate occurs for more than 50% of the

TABLE **2.1** Summary of the Conduction System		
Structure	Function	Intrinsic Pacemaker (beats/min)
Sinoatrial (SA) node	Primary pacemaker; initiates impulse that is normally conducted throughout the left and right atria	60 to 100
Atrioventricular (AV) node	Receives impulse from the SA node and delays the relay of the impulse to the bundle of His	
Bundle of His (AV bundle)	Receives impulse from the AV node and relays it to the right and left bundle branches	40 to 60
Right and left bundle branches	Receives impulse from the bundle of His and relays it to the Purkinje fibers	
Purkinje fibers	Receives impulse from the bundle branches and relays it to the ventricular myocardium	20 to 40

day, it is *incessant*. The rapid firing rate may also occur periodically. In these cases, it is said to be *episodic*.

Possible causes for altered automaticity include ischemia, hypoxia, electrolyte disorders, and exposure to chemicals or toxic substances. Examples of rhythms associated with altered automaticity include premature beats, accelerated idioventricular rhythm, accelerated junctional rhythm, and some forms of ventricular tachycardia.

TRIGGERED ACTIVITY

Triggered activity occurs when escape pacemaker and working cells fire more than once after stimulation by a single impulse. It results from abnormal electrical impulses that sometimes occur during repolarization (i.e., afterdepolarizations) when cells are normally quiet. Triggered activity can result in atrial or ventricular beats that occur alone, in pairs, in runs of three or more beats, or as a sustained ectopic rhythm. Causes of triggered activity include the following:

- Catecholamine increase
- Digitalis toxicity
- Hypomagnesemia
- Hypoxia
- Medications that prolong repolarization (e.g., quinidine)
- Myocardial ischemia and injury

Disorders of Impulse Conduction
CONDUCTION BLOCKS

Blockage of impulse conduction may be partial or complete. A block may occur because of trauma, drug toxicity, electrolyte disturbances, myocardial ischemia, or infarction. A partial conduction block may cause the impulse to become slowed or intermittent. In slowed conduction, all impulses are conducted, but it takes longer than normal to do so. When an intermittent block occurs, some (but not all) impulses are conducted. When a complete block exists, no impulses are conducted through the affected area. Examples of rhythms associated with disturbances in conduction include AV blocks.

REENTRY

Usually, an impulse spreads through the heart only once after it is initiated by pacemaker cells. When **reentry** occurs, also called *reactivation*, an electrical impulse is delayed, blocked, or both in one or more areas of the conduction system while being conducted normally through the rest of the system (Fig. 2.10). This results in the delayed electrical impulse entering cardiac cells that the normally conducted impulse has just depolarized. Reentry requires the following three conditions: (1) an area of unidirectional conduction block, (2) an area of delayed conduction, and (3) an area of unexcitable tissue (Peterson, 2018).

Macroreentry circuits and microreentry circuits are two main types of reentry circuits. If the reentry circuit involves conduction through a large area of the heart, such as the entire right or left atrium, it is called a *macroreentry circuit*.

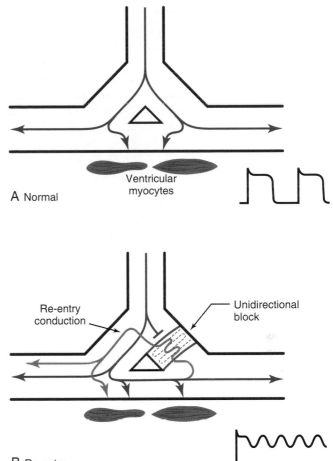

Fig. 2.10 Reentry in the presence of unidirectional block. In B, "unidirectional block" indicates an area of damage that blocks normal electrical flow but allows the impulse to find its way back against the flow where it can trigger another unintended cycle. (From Dowd, F. J., Johnson, B. S., & Mariotti, A. J. (2017). *Pharmacology and therapeutics for dentistry* (7th ed.). St. Louis: Elsevier.)

A reentry circuit involving conduction within a small area is called a *microreentry circuit*.

Common causes of reentry include hyperkalemia, myocardial ischemia, some antiarrhythmic medications, and the presence of an accessory pathway. Examples of rhythms associated with reentry include AV nodal reentrant tachycardia, AV reentrant tachycardia, and atrial flutter.

THE ELECTROCARDIOGRAM

The ECG is a graphic display of the heart's electrical activity. The first ECG was introduced by Willem Einthoven, a Dutch physiologist, in the early 1900s. When electrodes are attached to the patient's limbs or chest and connected by cables to an ECG machine, the ECG machine functions as a voltmeter, detecting and recording the voltage changes (i.e., action potentials) generated by depolarization and repolarization of the heart's cells. The voltage changes are displayed as specific waveforms and complexes (Fig. 2.11).

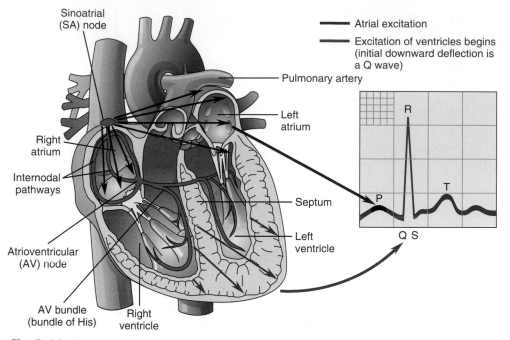

Fig. 2.11 Schematic drawing of the heart's conduction system. An impulse normally is generated in the sinoatrial node. It travels through the atria to the atrioventricular node, down the bundle of His and Purkinje fibers, and to the ventricular myocardium. Recording of the depolarizing and repolarizing currents in the heart with electrodes on the body's surface produces characteristic waveforms. (From Copstead-Kirkhorn, L. E., & Banasik, J. L. (2013). *Pathophysiology* (5th ed). St. Louis: Saunders.)

Electrocardiographic monitoring may be used for the following purposes:
- To immediately recognize sudden cardiac arrest and improve time to defibrillation (Sandau et al., 2017)
- To recognize deteriorating conditions (e.g., nonsustained dysrhythmias) that may lead to life-threatening, sustained dysrhythmias (Sandau et al., 2017)
- To assist in the diagnosis of dysrhythmias or causes of symptoms and guide appropriate management (Sandau et al., 2017)
- To monitor a patient's heart rate
- To evaluate the effects of disease or injury on heart function
- To evaluate for signs of myocardial ischemia, injury, and infarction
- To evaluate pacemaker function
- To evaluate a patient's response to medications (e.g., antiarrhythmics)
- To obtain recordings before, during, and after a medical procedure
  The ECG *can* provide information about the following:
- The orientation of the heart in the chest
- Conduction disturbances
- Electrical effects of medications and electrolytes
- The mass of cardiac muscle
- The presence of ischemic damage
  The ECG does *not* provide information about the mechanical (contractile) condition of the myocardium. Assess the patient's pulse and blood pressure to evaluate the effectiveness of the heart's mechanical activity.

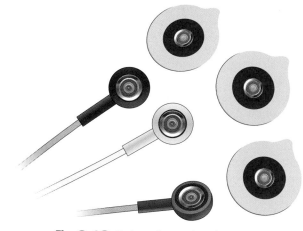

Fig. 2.12 Electrocardiogram electrodes.

Electrodes

Electrode refers to an adhesive pad containing a conductive substance in the center applied to the patient's skin (Fig. 2.12). The electrode's conductive media conducts skin surface voltage changes through wires to a cardiac monitor (i.e., electrocardiograph). Electrodes are applied at specific locations on the patient's chest wall and extremities to view the heart's electrical activity from different angles and planes.

Remove oil and dead cells from the patient's skin before applying electrodes. There are various techniques for doing so, such as a quick dry rub of the skin. Many electrode manufacturers include an abrasive area on the electrode's disposable backing for this purpose, but a gauze pad or terrycloth washcloth works well. To minimize distortion (artifact), be sure the conductive jelly in the center of the electrode is not dry, and avoid placing the electrodes directly over bony areas.

One end of a monitoring cable, also called a lead wire, is attached to the electrode and the other to an ECG machine. The cable conducts current back to the cardiac monitor. ECG cables may be coded by color, symbol, or letter. However, colors are not standard and often vary.

Leads

A **lead** is a record (i.e., tracing) of electrical activity, specifically the fluctuation in voltage differences, between positive and negative electrodes (Lederer, 2017). Each lead records the *average* current flow at a specific time in a portion of the heart. Leads allow for viewing the heart's electrical activity in the frontal and horizontal (transverse) planes (Fig. 2.13).

A 12-lead ECG views the heart in both the frontal and horizontal planes and views the left ventricle's surfaces from multiple angles. The 12-lead ECG is a useful diagnostic study you can obtain when there are changes in a patient's cardiac rhythm or condition. Indications for obtaining a 12-lead ECG are discussed in more detail in Chapter 9.

Think of each positive electrode as an eye looking in at the heart. Because the positive electrode position on the body determines the heart area seen by each lead, accurate placement of the positive electrode is essential. Each lead's view can be committed to memory or can be reasoned easily by remembering where the positive electrode is located.

⬤ ECG Pearl_____

Continuous patient monitoring is usually performed using bedside monitoring or telemetry, which is the electronic transmission of data to a distant location, such as a nurses' station. Continuous ECG monitoring may be performed using a single lead or, depending on equipment capability, three or even five leads may be used.

FRONTAL PLANE LEADS

Six leads view the heart in the frontal plane. Leads I, II, and III are called *standard limb leads*. Leads aVR, aVL, and aVF are called *augmented limb leads*.

A **bipolar lead** is an ECG lead that has a positive and negative electrode. Each lead records the difference in electrical potential (i.e., voltage) between two selected electrodes. Although all ECG leads are technically bipolar, leads I, II, and III use two different electrodes, one of which is connected to the positive input of the ECG machine and the other to the negative input (Wagner et al., 2009).

Standard Limb Leads

Leads I, II, and III make up the standard limb leads. If an electrode is placed on the right arm, left arm, and left leg, three leads are formed. The positive electrode is located at

the left wrist in lead I, and leads II and III both have their positive electrode located at the left foot. Each lead measures the difference in electrical potential between the positive pole and its corresponding negative pole.

An imaginary line that joins the positive and negative electrodes of a lead is called the lead **axis**. The axes of these three limb leads form an equilateral triangle with the heart at the center, which is called *Einthoven's triangle*. Einthoven's triangle is a way of showing that the two arms and the left leg form apices of a triangle surrounding the heart (see Fig. 2.13). The two apices at the upper part of the triangle represent the points at which the two arms connect electrically with the fluids around the heart. The lower apex is the point at which the left leg connects with the fluids (Hall, 2016).

Lead I records the difference in electrical potential between the left arm (+) and right arm (−) electrodes and views the lateral surface of the left ventricle. With normal depolarization, waveforms observed in this lead are usually positive. If negative P waves and primarily negative QRS complexes and T waves are observed in lead I, take a moment to recheck the lead wires connected to the right and left arm electrodes; the lead wires have likely been reversed (Brady et al., 2019).

Lead II records the difference in electrical potential between the left leg (+) and right arm (−) electrodes and views the inferior surface of the left ventricle. The positioning of the positive and negative electrodes in this lead most closely resembles the heart's normal current flow pathway. In the pediatric population, lead II is often used for continuous ECG monitoring because P waves are often clearly visible in this lead and because supraventricular dysrhythmias are more common than ventricular dysrhythmias (Sandau et al., 2017).

Lead III records the difference in electrical potential between the left leg (+) and left arm (−) electrodes. Waveforms observed in this lead are usually positive. Lead III views the inferior surface of the left ventricle. A summary of the standard limb leads appears in Table 2.2.

Augmented Limb Leads

Leads aVR, aVL, and aVF are limb leads that record measurements at a specific electrode with respect to a reference electrode. Frank Norman Wilson and colleagues used the term *central terminal* to describe a reference point that is the average of the limb lead electrical potentials. In the augmented leads, the Wilson central terminal (WCT) is calculated by the ECG machine's computer as an average potential of the electrical currents from the two electrodes other than the one being used as the positive electrode. For example, in lead aVL, the positive electrode is located on the patient's left arm. The ECG machine's computer calculates the central terminal by joining the electrical currents obtained from the electrodes on the patient's right arm and left leg. Lead aVL, therefore, represents the difference in electrical potential between the left arm and the central terminal. The electrical potential of the central terminal is essentially zero.

The electrical potential produced by the augmented leads usually is relatively small. The ECG machine augments (i.e.,

A FRONTAL PLANE LEADS

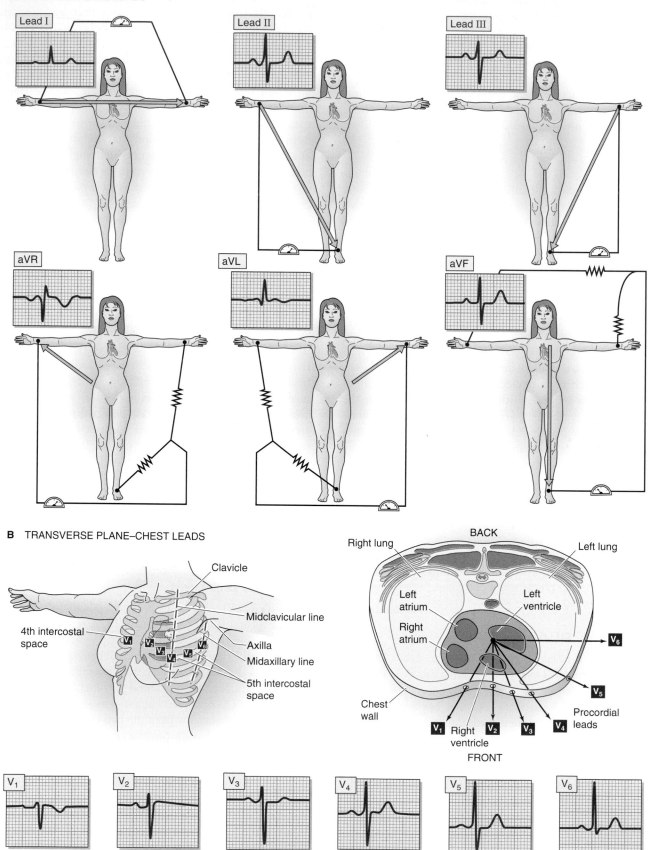

B TRANSVERSE PLANE–CHEST LEADS

Fig. 2.13 The electrocardiogram leads. (From Boron, W. F., & Boulpaep, E. L. (2017). *Medical physiology* (3rd ed.). Philadelphia: Elsevier.)

TABLE 2.2	Standard Limb Leads		
Lead	Positive Electrode	Negative Electrode	Heart Surface Viewed
I	Left arm	Right arm	Lateral
II	Left leg	Right arm	Inferior
III	Left leg	Left arm	Inferior

TABLE 2.3	Augmented Limb Leads	
Lead	Positive Electrode	Heart Surface Viewed
aVR	Right arm	None
aVL	Left arm	Lateral
aVF	Left leg	Inferior

magnifies) the amplitude of the electrical potentials detected at each extremity by about 50% over those recorded at the standard limb leads. The "a" in aVR, aVL, and aVF refers to augmented. The "V" refers to voltage, and the last letter refers to the positive electrode position. The "R" refers to the right arm, the "L" to left arm, and the "F" to left foot (i.e., leg). Therefore, the positive electrode in aVR is located on the right arm, aVL has a positive electrode at the left arm, and aVF has a positive electrode positioned on the left leg (see Fig. 2.13).

Lead aVR views the heart from the right shoulder, which is the positive electrode. Because the depolarization wave is moving away from lead aVR, waveforms in this lead are typically negative. Lead aVR was once thought to have little diagnostic value because it views current flow away from the normal direction of left ventricular depolarization (Ching & Ting, 2015). However, many clinicians believe that lead aVR reflects reciprocal (i.e., mirror image) changes from leads aVL, II, V_5, and V_6 (Gorgels et al., 2001). Research has shown value in using lead aVR in differentiating atrial tachydysrhythmias (Vorobiof & Ellestad, 2011). In patients experiencing an acute coronary syndrome (ACS), lead aVR may provide essential clues to the location of artery occlusion. Studies suggest that ST-segment elevation in this lead may be a significant indicator of left main coronary artery disease, proximal left anterior descending disease, or at least multivessel coronary artery disease (Vorobiof & Ellestad, 2011).

Lead aVL combines views from the right arm and the left leg, with the view being from the left arm and oriented to the left ventricle's lateral wall. Waveforms observed in this lead are usually positive but may be biphasic. Lead aVF combines views from the right arm and the left arm toward the left leg; it views the inferior surface of the left ventricle from the left leg. Waveforms observed in this lead are usually positive but may be biphasic. Table 2.3 summarizes the augmented limb leads.

⊙ ECG Pearl

In hospitalized patients undergoing continuous ECG monitoring, electrode placement for the limb leads has been altered and moved from the limbs to the patient's torso to allow for patient movement and minimize distortion on the ECG tracing. The right arm electrode is placed in the infraclavicular fossa close to the right shoulder, the left arm electrode is placed in the infraclavicular fossa close to the left shoulder, and the left leg electrode is placed below the rib cage on the left side of the abdomen. The ground or reference electrode can be placed anywhere, but it is usually placed on the abdomen's right side (Drew et al., 2004).

HORIZONTAL PLANE LEADS

Six chest (i.e., precordial or "V") leads view the heart in the horizontal plane (see Fig. 2.13), allowing views of the front and left side of the heart.

Chest Leads

The chest leads are V_1, V_2, V_3, V_4, V_5, and V_6 (Fig. 2.14). Each electrode placed in a "V" position is a positive electrode, measuring electrical potential with respect to the WCT.

Lead V_1 is recorded with the positive electrode in the fourth intercostal space, just to the right of the sternum. Remember, the electrode positions refer to the location of the gel. For example, the gel of the V_1 electrode, not the entire adhesive patch, is positioned in the fourth intercostal space, just to the right of the sternum. V_1 is often used for continuous ECG monitoring in adults because it is useful in diagnosing bundle branch blocks and distinguishing between ventricular tachycardia and aberrant conduction (Azland & Crijns, 2011; Sandau et al., 2017).

Lead V_2 is recorded with the positive electrode in the fourth intercostal space, just to the left of the sternum. Lead V_3 is recorded with the positive electrode on a line midway between V_2 and V_4. Lead V_4 is recorded with the positive electrode in the left midclavicular line in the fifth intercostal

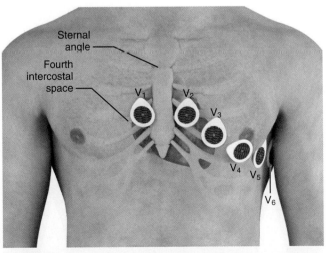

Fig. 2.14 Normal chest lead placement for a standard 12-lead electrocardiogram. If multiple or repeated electrocardiographic tracings are anticipated, mark the original lead placements on the patient's chest wall or leave stick-on leads in place after the electrocardiographic wires are removed. (From Hedges, J. R., Custalow, C. B., & Thomsen, T. W. (2019). *Roberts and Hedges' clinical procedures in emergency medicine and acute care* (7th ed.). Philadelphia: Elsevier.)

space. Lead V_5 is recorded with the positive electrode in the left anterior axillary line at the same level as V_4. Lead V_6 is recorded with the positive electrode in the left midaxillary line at the same level as V_4. Table 2.4 summarizes the chest leads.

⊙ ECG Pearl

Because their location varies, the nipples shouldn't be used as landmarks for chest electrode placement. If your patient is a woman, place the electrodes for leads V_3 through V_6 *under* the breast rather than *on* the breast.

Right Chest Leads

Other chest leads that are not part of a standard 12-lead ECG reveal specific surfaces of the heart. Right chest leads are used to evaluate the right ventricle (Fig. 2.15). Right chest

TABLE 2.4	Chest Leads	
Lead	**Positive Electrode Position**	**Heart Area Viewed**
V_1	Right side of sternum, fourth intercostal space	Interventricular septum
V_2	Left side of sternum, fourth intercostal space	Interventricular septum
V_3	Midway between V_2 and V_4	Anterior surface
V_4	Left midclavicular line, fifth intercostal space	Anterior surface
V_5	Left anterior axillary line; same level as V_4	Lateral surface
V_6	Left midaxillary line, fifth intercostal space	Lateral surface

lead placement is identical to standard chest lead placement, except that it is done on the chest's right side. Obtain a standard 12-lead ECG first; then reposition the electrodes on the right side of the chest and attach the cables for the standard chest leads to the repositioned electrodes to obtain the additional leads. If time does not permit obtaining all of the right chest leads, the lead of choice is V_4R.

Posterior Chest Leads

On a standard 12-lead ECG, no leads look directly at the posterior surface of the heart. Additional chest leads may be used for this purpose. These leads are placed farther left and toward the back. All the leads are placed on the same horizontal line as V_4 to V_6. Lead V_7 is placed at the posterior axillary line. Lead V_8 is placed at the angle of the scapula (i.e., the posterior scapular line), and lead V_9 is placed over the left border of the spine (Fig. 2.16).

Alternative Leads

Alternative lead configurations are sometimes useful in differentiating among types of dysrhythmias. For example, the Lewis lead is used to enhance the viewing of atrial activity (Fig. 2.17). The right arm (negative) electrode is applied to the right of the sternum at the second intercostal space, the left arm (positive) electrode is placed at the right fourth intercostal space, 1 inch to the right of the sternum, and the ECG machine is set to record lead I (Bakker et al., 2009).

The vertical sternal leads, also known as *Barker leads*, have been reported to record P waves larger than those seen with other leads, including the Lewis lead (Brady et al., 2019). When this lead is used, the positive electrode is placed at the xiphoid process, and the negative electrode is placed just below the suprasternal notch (see Fig. 2.17).

The modified chest leads (MCLs) are bipolar chest leads that are variations of the chest leads. Each MCL consists of a

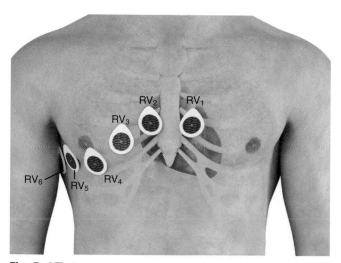

Fig. 2.15 Electrode locations for recording a right chest electrocardiogram. Right chest leads are used when a right ventricular infarction is suspected. (From Hedges, J. R., Custalow, C. B., & Thomsen, T. W. (2019). *Roberts and Hedges' clinical procedures in emergency medicine and acute care* (7th ed.). Philadelphia: Elsevier.)

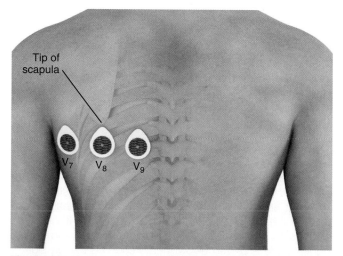

Fig. 2.16 Electrode locations for left posterior chest lead placement. (From Hedges, J. R., Custalow, C. B., & Thomsen, T. W. (2019). *Roberts and Hedges' clinical procedures in emergency medicine and acute care* (7th ed.). Philadelphia: Elsevier.)

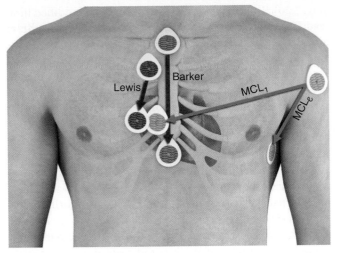

Fig. 2.17 Electrode locations for alternative electrocardiogram leads. *MCL,* Modified chest lead. (From Hedges, J. R., Custalow, C. B., & Thomsen, T. W. (2019). *Roberts and Hedges' clinical procedures in emergency medicine and acute care* (7th ed.). Philadelphia: Elsevier.)

positive and negative electrode applied to a specific location on the chest. Lead MCL$_1$ views the interventricular septum. The negative electrode is placed just below the left clavicle toward the left shoulder, and the positive electrode is placed to the right of the sternum in the fourth intercostal space (see Fig. 2.17). Leads MCL$_1$ and V$_1$ are similar but not identical. In V$_1$, the negative electrode is calculated by the ECG machine at the center of the heart. In MCL$_1$, the negative electrode is located just below the left clavicle.

Lead MCL$_6$ is a variation of the chest lead V$_6$ and views the left ventricle's low lateral wall. The negative electrode is placed below the left clavicle toward the left shoulder, and the positive electrode is placed at the fifth intercostal space, left midaxillary line.

🔄 ECG Pearl

Lead MCL$_1$ was once used to differentiate between right and left bundle blocks and distinguish ventricular tachycardia from supraventricular tachycardia with abnormal (i.e., aberrant) ventricular conduction. Because the shape (morphology) of the QRS complex in MCL$_1$ has been shown to differ in 40% of patients with ventricular tachycardia, chest lead V$_1$ should be used instead (Drew et al., 2004).

Ambulatory Cardiac Monitoring

Ambulatory cardiac monitoring, also known as ambulatory electrocardiographic (AECG) monitoring, is a noninvasive diagnostic tool used to monitor the patient's cardiac rhythm as they perform daily activities. Examples of indications for AECG monitoring include the following (Crawford et al., 1999; Mittal et al., 2011):

- To determine the association between a patient's symptoms (e.g., dizziness, palpitations, near syncope, shortness of breath, chest pain, fatigue) and cardiac rhythm disturbances

- To detect myocardial ischemia and to evaluate the efficacy of anti-ischemic medications in patients with coronary artery disease
- To assess the patient's risk of dysrhythmias after myocardial infarction; for patients with heart failure, hypertrophic cardiomyopathy, diabetic neuropathy, systemic hypertension, or valvular heart disease; for patients receiving hemodialysis; and for the preoperative evaluation of patients and after cardiac operations
- To assess the efficacy of medications on the cardiac conduction system, the patient's cardiac rhythm, or both
- To aid in correlating patient symptoms with dysrhythmias and evaluating symptomatic patients for pacemaker implantation
- To assess the function of implanted devices, such as a pacemaker or an implantable cardioverter-defibrillator
- To assess the efficacy of ablation procedures

TYPES OF AMBULATORY MONITORS

Several types of devices are used for AECG monitoring. The choice of equipment used is based on the frequency of the patient's symptoms.

Holter Monitors

A Holter monitor is a battery-powered continuous AECG recorder used when patient symptoms occur often enough to be detected during a short period (24 to 72 hours) of monitoring. Holter monitors continuously record at least two leads, and newer models can record and store up to 2 weeks of data. Electrodes and lead wires are connected to a portable, lightweight recorder attached to the patient and carried with a belt or shoulder strap (Fig. 2.18). Patients are asked to keep a log or diary while the device is in use. A typical diary consists of entries reflecting the time of day, the activity being performed, and patient symptoms. When the monitoring period is complete, the patient returns the monitor and events that have been stored on a digital flash memory device that is then scanned by a technician and interpreted by a physician. This information is then compared with the ECG

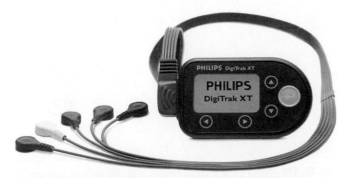

Fig. 2.18 A Holter monitor is used when patient symptoms occur often enough to be detected during a short interval of cardiac monitoring. (From Pagana, K. D., & Pagana, T. J. (2014). *Mosby's manual of diagnostic and laboratory tests* (5th ed.). St. Louis: Mosby.)

events captured by the device to determine if a relationship exists among the patient's symptoms, activities, and ECG.

Event Monitors

An event monitor is a portable recording device that intermittently records and stores ECG data for 14 to 30 days or longer. It is used when the patient's symptoms are unlikely to be captured during a 24- to 72-hour period.

A transtelephonic monitor is a small intermittent event recorder (Fig. 2.19). It has four metal electrodes on the back of the device that can record a single lead. When the patient experiences symptoms, they place the device on the center of the chest, ensure that the electrodes are firmly in contact with the skin, and then push the activation button to record and store the rhythm. The patient then transmits the ECG data via phone to a remote monitoring station, such as the provider's office. The signal is converted to a readable tracing displayed on a monitor or printed out as a single-lead rhythm strip. Disadvantages of such devices include the need for patient activation. For example, brief symptoms may resolve before the patient can push the activation button. A family member may need to activate the device if the patient experiences a syncopal episode (because the patient is physically unable to do so).

External Loop Recorders

An external loop recorder, also called a *looping memory monitor*, continuously records and stores ECG data over weeks to months. It is used when the patient's symptoms are likely to recur within a 2- to 6-week period. The recorder is connected to the patient using electrodes and lead wires

(Fig. 2.20). The device stores a single external modified limb lead ECG with a 4- to 60-minute memory buffer (Krahn et al., 2018). When a patient experiences symptoms, they activate the device, which stores the previous 3 to 14 minutes of recorded data before the event. Also, 1 to 4 minutes of data are recorded and stored after the triggered event. The captured data can subsequently be uploaded and analyzed, often providing critical information regarding the onset and termination of the dysrhythmia (Krahn et al., 2018). Newer models are equipped with a cellular phone that transmits triggered data automatically over a wireless network to a remote monitoring center.

External patch recorders permit ECG monitoring, typically for 7 to 14 days (Fig. 2.21). The device has no leads or wires; an adhesive is used to attach it to the patient's chest wall. With one type of patch-based recording system, data are recorded continuously and then later analyzed. Another patch-based recording system uses Bluetooth technology to transmit data in real-time using a smartphone-like device carried by the patient. The data are then transmitted to a central monitoring center, where it is analyzed and interpreted by trained clinicians (Krahn et al., 2018).

Mobile Cardiac Outpatient Telemetry

Mobile cardiac outpatient telemetry is used when a patient's symptoms are infrequent. It is a real-time monitoring system that automatically gathers data from a patch applied to the patient's skin and an attached sensor using Bluetooth

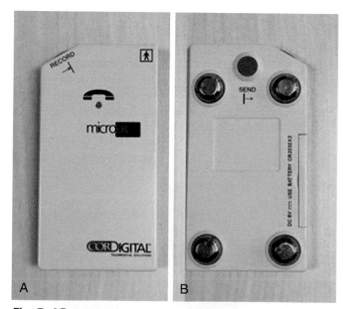

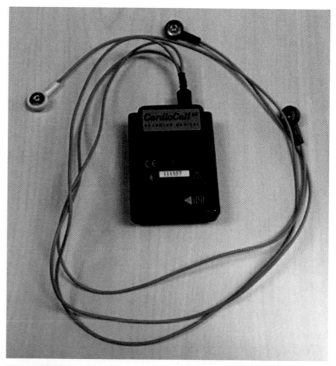

Fig. 2.19 Photograph of a cardiac event recorder, with the front panel with activation button (A) and the recording electrodes on the back (B). (From Krahn, A. D., Yee, R., Skanes, A. C., & Klein, G. J. (2018). Cardiac monitoring: Short and long-term recording. In D. P. Zipes, J. Jalife, & W. G. Stevenson (Eds.): *Cardiac electrophysiology: from cell to bedside* (7th ed.). Philadelphia: Elsevier.)

Fig. 2.20 An external loop recorder with recording electrodes. (From Krahn, A. D., Yee, R., Skanes, A. C., & Klein, G. J. (2018). Cardiac monitoring: Short and long-term recording. In D. P. Zipes, J. Jalife, & W. G. Stevenson (Eds.): *Cardiac electrophysiology: from cell to bedside* (7th ed.). Philadelphia: Elsevier.)

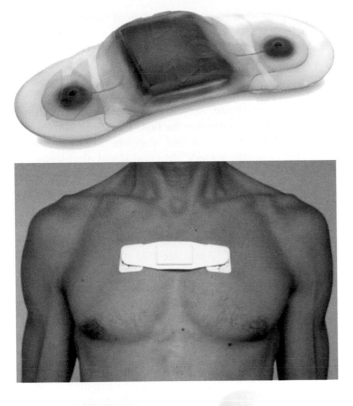

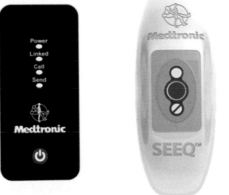

Fig. 2.21 Sample patch-based recording systems that allow both acquisition and storage of a single-lead electrocardiogram for 7 to 14 days. (From Krahn, A. D., Yee, R., Skanes, A. C., & Klein, G. J. (2018). Cardiac monitoring: Short and long-term recording. In D. P. Zipes, J. Jalife, & W. G. Stevenson (Eds.): *Cardiac electrophysiology: from cell to bedside* (7th ed.). Philadelphia: Elsevier.)

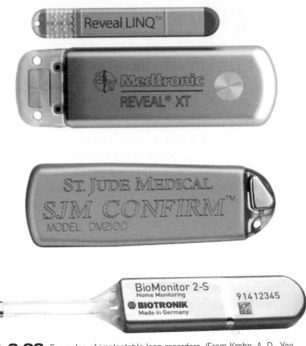

Fig. 2.22 Examples of implantable loop recorders. (From Krahn, A. D., Yee, R., Skanes, A. C., & Klein, G. J. (2018). Cardiac monitoring: Short and long-term recording. In D. P. Zipes, J. Jalife, & W. G. Stevenson (Eds.): *Cardiac electrophysiology: from cell to bedside* (7th ed.). Philadelphia: Elsevier.)

technology. When a dysrhythmia is detected, the device transmits the ECG data to a receiving center staffed with trained technicians. The patient's physician is notified of any dysrhythmias based on predetermined notification criteria. Although no patient intervention is needed to either capture or transmit when a dysrhythmia occurs, the patient is encouraged to record symptoms when they happen.

Implantable Loop Recorders

An implantable loop recorder, also called an insertable cardiac monitor, is a small ECG recording device that resembles a flash drive (Fig. 2.22). It is used when a patient's symptoms

(e.g., fainting, seizures, palpitations) are recurrent but infrequent. An insertable monitor is usually implanted under the skin on the left chest under local anesthesia. The device records a single ECG lead and has a battery life of 2 to 3 years (Shen et al., 2017). The patient or a family member can manually activate the device with a small, handheld activator placed on the chest wall over the monitor when the patient experiences symptoms. The device can also be programmed to detect and record heart rates outside a predetermined range. If no data meet the preset criteria, the information is subsequently erased; however, the data are saved to the recorder's memory for later retrieval if an event does occur. Depending on the model, stored ECG data can be sent via phone to a remote monitoring center or downloaded and analyzed in the provider's office.

Portable Handheld Electrocardiogram Monitors

Several portable handheld ECG monitors are available for home use, and the number is rising (Bansal & Joshi, 2018). Most handheld ECG monitors record in a single limb lead, and some display the ECG rhythm while recording. Some devices use electrodes and lead wires, whereas others have metal electrodes for thumb, finger, or chest contact. Saved ECG data can be transferred to other devices using software, Bluetooth, smartphones, or USB ports and then shared with the individual's provider. The US Food and Drug Administration has approved several handheld monitors, and some have shown reliability in the detection of specific dysrhythmias, such as atrial fibrillation.

ELECTROCARDIOGRAPHY PAPER

Remember that an ECG is a graphical representation of the heart's electrical activity. When you place electrodes on the patient's body and connect them to an electrocardiograph, the machine records the voltage (i.e., the potential difference) between the electrodes. The needle, or pen, of the ECG moves a specific distance depending on the voltage measured. This recording is made on ECG paper.

ECG paper is graph paper made up of small and large boxes measured in millimeters. The smallest boxes are 1 mm wide and 1 mm high (Fig. 2.23). The horizontal axis of the paper corresponds with time. Time is used to measure the duration of specific cardiac events, which is stated in seconds. Measuring how quickly or slowly an electrical impulse spreads through the heart provides essential information about the condition of the heart's conduction system and the muscle itself.

ECG paper normally records at a constant speed of 25 mm/sec. Thus, each horizontal unit (i.e., each 1-mm box) represents 0.04 second (25 mm/second × 0.04 second = 1 mm). The rate at which ECG paper goes through the printer is adjustable. A slower paper speed makes the rhythm appear faster. Increasing the paper speed to 50 mm/sec has the effect of making the rhythm appear slower. When evaluating rapid atrial or ventricular rhythms, clinicians sometimes use this technique, making it easier to see the waveforms and analyze the tachycardia. Increasing the paper speed also exaggerates any existing irregularity and makes it possible to measure intervals more accurately on the ECG (Brady et al., 2019).

Look closely at the boxes in Fig. 2.23. You can see that the lines after every five small boxes on the paper are heavier. The heavier lines indicate one large box. Because each large box is the width of five small boxes, a large box represents 0.20 second. Five large boxes, each consisting of five small boxes, represent 1 second; 15 large boxes equal 3 seconds; and 30 large boxes represent 6 seconds.

The vertical axis of the graph paper represents the voltage or amplitude of the ECG waveforms or deflections. Voltage is measured in millivolts (mV). Voltage may appear as a positive or negative value because voltage is a force with direction and amplitude. Amplitude is measured in millimeters (mm). The default value for ECG machine calibration is 10 mm/mV, which means that when the ECG machine is calibrated correctly, a 1-mV electrical signal produces a deflection that measures precisely 10 mm tall (i.e., the height of 10 small boxes) (Fig. 2.24). When a calibration marker is present, it appears at the extreme left side of the ECG tracing, before the first waveform. Some electrocardiographs print the paper speed and standardization at the bottom of the ECG paper ("25 mm/second, 10 mm/mV") instead of displaying the calibration marker (Goldberger et al., 2018).

Clinically, the height of a waveform is usually stated in mm rather than in mV. Calibration, also called standardization, can be adjusted manually, by the clinician, or automatically by the ECG machine's computer. Decreasing the calibration to 5 mm/mV can help when the QRS amplitude is so large that it encroaches on those of neighboring leads (Brady et al., 2019). Increasing the amplitude to 20 mm/mV can be valuable when analyzing waveforms.

Waveforms

A **waveform** (i.e., a deflection) is movement away from the baseline in a positive (i.e., upward) or negative (i.e., downward) direction (Box 2.1). Each waveform that you see on an ECG is related to a specific electrical event in the heart. Waveforms are named alphabetically, beginning with P, QRS, T, and occasionally U. When electrical activity is not detected, a straight line is recorded. This line is called the **baseline** or **isoelectric line**. If the wave of depolarization

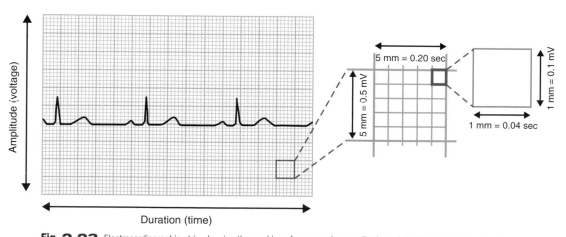

Fig. 2.23 Electrocardiographic strip showing the markings for measuring amplitude and duration of waveforms, using a standard recording speed of 25 mm/sec. (From Copstead-Kirkhorn, L. E., & Banasik, J. L. (2013). *Pathophysiology* (5th ed). St. Louis: Saunders.)

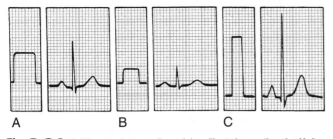

Fig. 2.24 A, When an electrocardiograph is calibrated correctly, a 1-mV electrical signal produces a deflection measuring exactly 10 mm tall (i.e., normal standardization). B, One-half standardization. C, Two times normal standardization. (From Goldberger, A. L., Goldberger, Z. D., & Shvilkin, A. (2018). *Clinical electrocardiography: a simplified approach* (9th ed.). Philadelphia: Elsevier.)

Box **2.1**	Terminology

Baseline (isoelectric line): A straight line recorded when electrical activity is not detected

Waveform: Movement away from the baseline in either a positive or negative direction

Segment: A line between waveforms; named by the waveform that precedes or follows it

Complex: Several waveforms

Interval: A waveform and a segment

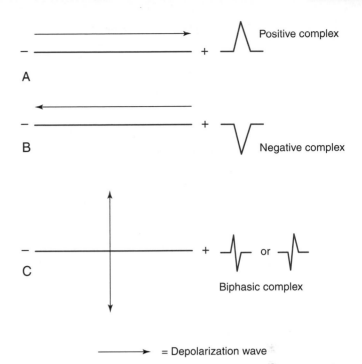

Fig. 2.25 Electrocardiographic waveforms may be positive or negative. A, A positive waveform is seen if the wave of depolarization spreads toward the lead's positive pole. B, A negative waveform is seen if the depolarization wave spreads toward the lead's negative pole (away from the positive pole). C, A biphasic (partly positive, partly negative) waveform or a straight line is seen if the mean direction of the wave of depolarization moves perpendicularly (at a right angle) to the positive electrode. (From Goldberger, A. L., Goldberger, Z. D., & Shvilkin, A. (2018). *Clinical electrocardiography: a simplified approach* (9th ed.). Philadelphia: Elsevier.)

(i.e., the electrical impulse) moves toward the positive electrode, the waveform recorded on ECG graph paper will be upright (i.e., a positive deflection) (Fig. 2.25). If the wave of depolarization moves away from the positive electrode, the waveform recorded will be inverted (i.e., a downward or negative deflection). A **biphasic** (i.e., partly positive, partly negative) waveform or a straight line is recorded when the wave of depolarization moves perpendicularly to the positive electrode. The term *equiphasic* may be used instead of *biphasic* to describe a waveform with no net positive or negative deflection.

P WAVE

The first waveform in the cardiac cycle is the *P wave* (Fig. 2.26). It is usually easiest to see P waves in the inferior leads: leads II, III, and aVF. The P wave represents the spread of the electrical impulse throughout the right and left atria (i.e., atrial depolarization). A P wave normally precedes each QRS complex. Activation of the SA node occurs before the onset of the P wave. This event is not recorded on the ECG. However, the spread of that impulse throughout the right and left atrial muscle (atrial depolarization) is observed. The beginning of the P wave is recognized as the first abrupt or gradual movement away from the baseline; its end is the point at which the waveform returns to the baseline. P wave characteristics are shown in Box 2.2.

The atria contract a fraction of a second after the P wave begins. The atria begin to repolarize at the same time as the ventricles depolarize. A waveform representing atrial

repolarization is usually not seen on the ECG because it is small and buried in the QRS complex.

Tall and pointed (i.e., peaked) or wide and notched P waves may be seen in conditions such as chronic obstructive pulmonary disease, heart failure, or valvular disease and may indicate atrial enlargement (Fig. 2.27). Enlargement of the right atrium produces an abnormally tall initial part of the P wave. The latter part of the P wave is prominent in left atrial enlargement (see Chapter 9).

P waves that begin at a site other than the SA node (i.e., ectopic P waves) may be positive or negative in lead II. If the ectopic pacemaker is in the atria, the P wave will be upright. If the ectopic pacemaker is in the AV bundle, the P wave will be negative (i.e., inverted) in lead II.

QRS COMPLEX

A **complex** consists of several waveforms. The QRS complex consists of the Q wave, R wave, and S wave (see Fig. 2.26) and represents the spread of the electrical impulse through the ventricles (i.e., ventricular depolarization) and the sum of all ventricular muscle cell depolarizations. Ventricular depolarization normally triggers the contraction of ventricular tissue. Thus, shortly after the QRS complex begins, the ventricles contract. The QRS complex is significantly larger than the P wave because ventricular depolarization involves a considerably greater muscle mass than atrial depolarization. Remember

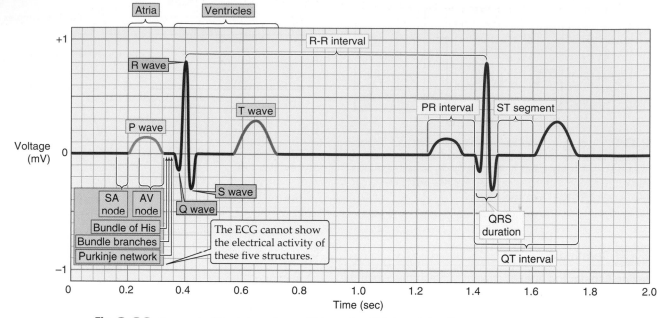

Fig. 2.26 Components of the electrocardiogram (*ECG*) recording. *AV*, Atrioventricular; *SA*, sinoatrial. (From Boron, W. F., & Boulpaep, E. L. (2017). *Medical physiology* (3rd ed.). Philadelphia: Elsevier.)

Box 2.2	Normal P-Wave Characteristics

- Smooth and rounded
- No more than 2.5 mm in height
- No more than 0.12 second in duration
- Positive in leads I, II, III, aVL, aVF, and V_2 through V_6
- May be biphasic in V_1

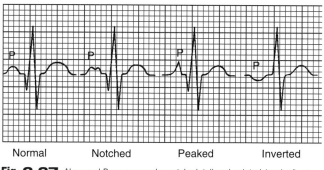

Normal   Notched   Peaked   Inverted

Fig. 2.27 Abnormal P waves may be notched, tall and pointed (peaked), or inverted (negative).

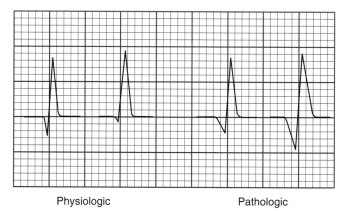

Physiologic   Pathologic

Fig. 2.28 Physiologic and pathologic Q waves. (From Phalen, T., & Aehlert, B. J. (2012). *The 12-lead ECG in acute coronary syndromes* (3rd ed.). St. Louis: Mosby.)

that atrial repolarization occurs during ventricular depolarization, but the QRS complex overshadows it on the ECG.

A QRS complex normally follows each P wave. One or even two of the three waveforms that make up the QRS complex may be absent. When it is present, the Q wave is the first downward deflection following the P wave. The Q wave represents depolarization of the interventricular septum, which normally occurs from left to right and posteriorly to anteriorly. A Q wave is *always* a negative waveform. The Q wave

begins when it leaves the isoelectric line in a downward direction and continues until it returns to the isoelectric line.

It is essential to differentiate normal (i.e., physiologic) Q waves from pathologic Q waves (Fig. 2.28). Except for leads III and aVR, a normal Q wave in the limb leads is less than 0.03 second in duration (Surawicz & Knilans, 2008). An abnormal (i.e., pathologic) Q wave is more than 0.03 second in duration or more than 30% of the following R wave height in that lead, or both (Anderson & Fang, 2020). Myocardial infarction is one possible cause of abnormal Q waves.

The QRS complex continues as a large, upright, triangular waveform known as the *R wave* (see Fig. 2.26). The R wave is the first positive (i.e., upright) waveform following the P wave. The S wave is the negative waveform following the R wave. An R wave is *always* positive, and an S wave is *always* negative. The R and S waves represent depolarization of the right and left ventricles.

In a normally conducted beat, the QRS complex represents the left ventricle's electrical activity because it is much larger than the right. Factors other than the size or mass of the left ventricle affect QRS amplitude. For example, electrode placement sites, age, gender, and race influence QRS voltage (Hancock et al., 2009).

The QRS complex may appear predominantly positive, negative, or biphasic, depending on the lead. It is predominantly positive in leads that view the heart from the left (e.g., I, aVL, V_5, V_6) and in leads that look at the heart's inferior surface (e.g., II, III, aVF). In leads that view the heart from the right side, the QRS complex is predominantly negative (e.g., aVR, V_1, V_2). The QRS usually is biphasic in leads V_3, V_4, and sometimes III.

QRS MEASUREMENT

The QRS duration is a measurement of the time required for ventricular depolarization. A QRS complex's width is most accurately determined when it is viewed and measured in more than one lead. The measurement should be taken from the QRS complex with the longest duration and clearest onset and end. The beginning of the QRS complex is measured from the point where the first wave of the complex begins to deviate from the baseline. The point at which the last wave of the complex begins to level out or distinctly change direction at, above, or below the baseline marks the QRS complex's end. In adults, the normal duration of the QRS complex is 0.11 second or less (Bagliani et al., 2019; Surawicz et al., 2009). The QRS duration in women is generally shorter than that in men by about 5 to 8 milliseconds (msec) (Mirvis & Goldberger, 2019).

If an electrical impulse does not follow the normal ventricular conduction pathway, it will take longer to depolarize the myocardium. This delay in conduction through the ventricles produces a wider QRS complex. QRS complex characteristics appear in Box 2.3.

🔆 ECG Pearl

Einthoven expressed the relationship among leads I, II, and III as the sum of any complex in leads I and III equals that of lead II. Thus, lead I + III = II. Stated another way, the voltage of a waveform in lead I plus the same waveform voltage in lead III equals the same waveform voltage in lead II. For example, when you look at leads I, II, and III, if the R wave in lead II does not appear to be the sum of the R waves' voltage in leads I and III, the leads may have been incorrectly applied.

Box 2.3	Normal QRS Complex Characteristics

- Normal duration of 0.075 to 0.11 second in adults (Ganz & Link, 2020)
- QRS amplitude varies among leads

Abnormal QRS Complexes

- In adults, the duration of an abnormal QRS complex is greater than 0.11 second.
- The duration of a QRS caused by an impulse originating in an ectopic pacemaker in the Purkinje network or ventricular myocardium is usually greater than 0.12 second and often 0.16 second or greater.
- If the impulse originates in a bundle branch, a QRS duration between 0.11 and 0.12 second in adults is called an *incomplete* bundle branch block (Surawicz et al., 2009). In adults, a QRS measuring 0.12 second or more is called a *complete* bundle branch block (Surawicz et al., 2009). Bundle branch blocks are discussed in more detail in Chapter 9.
- Low-amplitude QRS complexes measure less than 5 mm or 0.5 mV (Ganz & Link, 2020).
- Enlargement of the right ventricle produces an abnormally tall R wave; left ventricular enlargement produces an abnormally deep S wave.

QRS Variations

Although the term *QRS complex* is used, not every QRS complex contains a Q wave, R wave, and S wave. If the QRS complex consists entirely of a positive waveform, it is called an *R wave*. If the complex consists entirely of a negative waveform, it is called a *QS wave*. QS waves may be pathologic. If there are two positive deflections in the same complex, the second is called *R prime* and is written *R′*. If there are two negative deflections following an R wave, the second is called *S prime* and is written *S′*. Capital (i.e., upper case) letters are used to designate waveforms of relatively large amplitude, and small (i.e., lower case) letters are used to label relatively small waveforms (Fig. 2.29).

T WAVE

The T wave represents the repolarization of both ventricles (Fig. 2.30). The ERP is still present during the beginning of the T wave. At the peak of the T wave, the RRP has begun. It

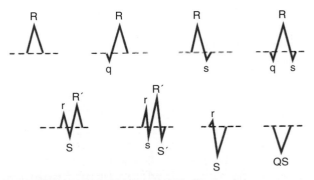

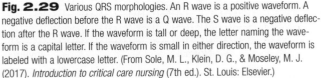

Fig. 2.29 Various QRS morphologies. An R wave is a positive waveform. A negative deflection before the R wave is a Q wave. The S wave is a negative deflection after the R wave. If the waveform is tall or deep, the letter naming the waveform is a capital letter. If the waveform is small in either direction, the waveform is labeled with a lowercase letter. (From Sole, M. L., Klein, D. G., & Moseley, M. J. (2017). *Introduction to critical care nursing* (7th ed.). St. Louis: Elsevier.)

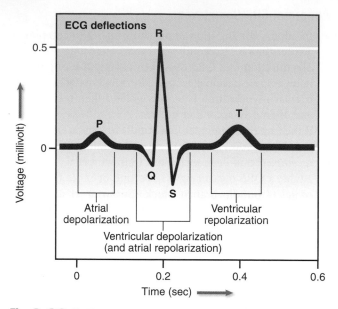

Fig. 2.30 The T wave reflects ventricular repolarization. (From McCance, K. L., & Huether, S. E. (2019). *Pathophysiology* (8th ed.). St. Louis: Elsevier.)

Box 2.4	Normal T-Wave Characteristics

- Slightly asymmetric
- Negative in aVR; may be positive or negative in leads III, aVL, and V_1
- Normally upright in leads I, II, and V_3 through V_6 (Rautaharju et al., 2009)
- Usually 0.5 mm or more in height in leads I and II
- Usually 5 mm or less in height in any limb lead or 10 mm or less in any chest lead

is during the RRP that a stronger than normal stimulus may produce ventricular dysrhythmias.

In the limb leads, lead II most commonly reveals the tallest T wave. The normal T wave is slightly asymmetric: The waveform's peak is closer to its end than the beginning, and the first half has a more gradual slope than the second half (Box 2.4). The beginning of the T wave is identified as the point where the ST segment's slope appears to become abruptly or gradually steeper. The T wave ends when it returns to the baseline. The T wave direction is usually the same as the QRS complex that precedes it. It is sometimes

challenging to determine the onset and end of the T wave. Examples of T waves are shown in Fig. 2.31.

Abnormal T Waves

- A T wave following an abnormal QRS complex usually moves in a direction opposite that of the QRS. In other words, when the QRS complex points down, the T wave points up and vice versa. This pattern may be seen with ventricular beats or rhythms and in bundle branch block.
- In a patient experiencing an ACS, T-wave inversion suggests the presence of myocardial ischemia.
- Tall, pointed (i.e., peaked) T waves are commonly seen in hyperkalemia.
- Low-amplitude T waves may be seen in hypokalemia or hypomagnesemia.
- Tall, broad T waves may be seen with internal pacemakers.
- Deeply inverted T waves may be seen with acute central nervous system events (e.g., intracranial hemorrhage, massive stroke) and therapy with tricyclic antidepressants or phenothiazines (Amsterdam et al., 2014).
- The T wave in leads I, II, aVL, and V_2 to V_6 should be described as *inverted* when the T-wave amplitude is from -1 mm to -5 mm, as *deep negative* when the amplitude is from -5 mm to -10 mm, and as *giant negative* when the amplitude is more than -10 mm. The T wave is described as *low* when its amplitude is less than 10% of the R wave amplitude in the same lead and as *flat* when the peak T-wave amplitude is between 1 mm and -1 mm in leads I, II, aVL (with an R wave taller than 3 mm), and V_4 to V_6 (Rautaharju et al., 2009).

U WAVE

A U wave is a small waveform that, when seen, follows the T wave. The U wave is thought to represent the late repolarization of the Purkinje fibers (Lederer, 2017). However, some cardiologists believe that U waves are simply two-part T waves resulting from a longer action potential duration in some ventricular myocardial cells (Patton & Thibodeau, 2019).

U waves are most easily seen when the heart rate is slow and are difficult to identify when the rate exceeds 95 beats/min (Rautaharju et al., 2009). When seen, they are generally tallest in leads V_2 and V_3 (Rautaharju et al., 2009). The normal U wave amplitude is usually less than 0.1 mV (Mirvis & Goldberger, 2019). Possible causes of

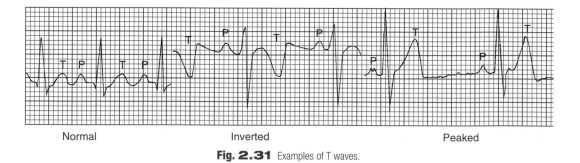

Normal   Inverted   Peaked

Fig. 2.31 Examples of T waves.

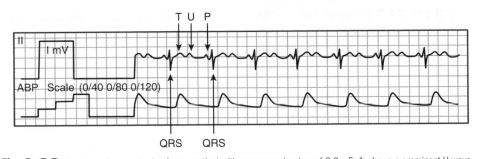

Fig. 2.32 Electrocardiogram tracing from a patient with a serum potassium of 2.6 mEq/L shows a prominent U wave. (From Urden, L. D., Stacy, K. M., & Lough, M. E. (2018). *Critical care nursing: diagnosis and management* (8th ed.). Maryland Heights, MO: Elsevier.)

prominent U waves include central nervous system disease, electrolyte imbalance (e.g., hypokalemia) (Fig. 2.32), hyperthyroidism, long QT syndrome, and medications (e.g., amiodarone, digitalis, disopyramide, phenothiazines, procainamide, quinidine).

U waves usually appear in the same direction as the T waves that precede them. Inverted U waves seen in leads V_2 through V_5 are abnormal and may appear during episodes of acute ischemia or in the presence of hypertension (Rautaharju et al., 2009).

Segments

A **segment** is a line between waveforms. It is named by the waveform that precedes or follows it.

PR SEGMENT

The PR segment is part of the PR interval (PRI), specifically, the horizontal line between the end of the P wave and the beginning of the QRS complex (Fig. 2.33). The PR segment usually is isoelectric and represents the spread of the electrical impulse from the AV node, through the AV bundle, the right and left bundle branches, and the Purkinje fibers to activate ventricular muscle. The PR segment ends when enough ventricular myocardium has been activated to begin recording the QRS complex (Mirvis & Goldberger, 2019). Most of the conduction delay during the PR segment results from slow conduction within the AV node (Wagner, 2012).

TP SEGMENT

The TP segment is the portion of the ECG tracing between the end of the T wave and the beginning of the next P wave, during which there is no electrical activity (Fig. 2.34). When the heart rate is within normal limits, the TP segment is usually isoelectric. With rapid heart rates, the TP segment is often unrecognizable because the P wave encroaches on the preceding T wave.

ST SEGMENT

The portion of the ECG tracing between the QRS complex and the T wave is the ST segment. The term *ST segment* is used regardless of whether the final wave of the QRS

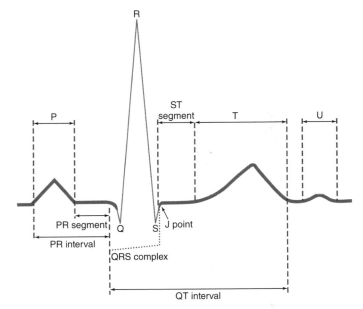

Fig. 2.33 Waveforms, segments, and intervals. (From Ignatavicius, D. D., & Workman, M. L. (2016). *Medical-surgical nursing: patient-centered collaborative care* (8th ed.). St. Louis: Elsevier.)

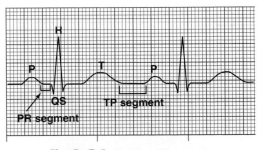

Fig. 2.34 The PR and TP segments.

complex is an R or an S wave. The ST segment represents the early part of the repolarization of the right and left ventricles. The normal ST segment begins at the isoelectric line, extends from the end of the S wave, and curves gradually upward to the beginning of the T wave.

The junction where the QRS complex and the ST segment meet is called the J point (see Fig. 2.33). To determine if ST segments are elevated or depressed, begin by identifying the onset of the QRS, which serves as the reference point. Next, locate the J point. Then compare the level of the ST segment with the reference point. Deviation is measured as the number of mm of vertical ST segment displacement (at the J point) from the reference point (Thygesen et al., 2018). It can be challenging to determine the J point in some situations (e.g., rapid heart rates, hyperkalemia, ventricular paced rhythms, bundle branch blocks). Some displacement of the ST segment from the isoelectric line is normal and dependent on age, sex, race, and ECG lead.

◐ ECG Pearl

Proper machine calibration is critical when analyzing ST segments. The ST segment criteria described here apply *only* when the monitor is adjusted to standard calibration.

Various conditions may displace the ST segment from the isoelectric line either positively or negatively. Myocardial ischemia, injury, and infarction are among the causes of ST-segment deviation (Fig. 2.35). When ECG changes of myocardial ischemia, injury, or infarction occur, they are not found in every ECG lead. Findings are considered significant if viewed in two or more leads looking at the same or adjacent heart area. If these findings are seen in leads that look directly at the affected area, they are called **indicative changes**. If findings are seen in leads opposite the affected area, they are called **reciprocal changes** (also called "mirror image" changes). Indicative changes are significant when they are seen in two anatomically contiguous leads. Two leads are contiguous if they look at the same or adjacent areas of the heart or if they are numerically consecutive chest leads (see Chapter 9).

Abnormal ST Segments

- ST-segment depression of 0.5 mm or more in a patient experiencing an ACS is suggestive of myocardial ischemia

when seen in two or more anatomically contiguous leads (Thygesen et al., 2018).

- New or presumed new ST-segment elevation of 1 mm or more at the J point in all leads other than V_2 and V_3 in a patient experiencing an ACS is suggestive of myocardial injury when observed in two or more anatomically contiguous leads (O'Gara et al., 2013). For leads V_2 and V_3, ST elevation is considered significant if it is elevated 2 mm or more in men 40 years and older, 2.5 mm or more in men younger than 40 years, or elevated 1.5 mm or more in women (Thygesen et al., 2018).
- Other causes of ST-segment changes include a normal variant, hyperkalemia, acute pericarditis, myocarditis, left ventricular aneurysm, and bundle branch block, among other causes. Pericarditis causes ST-segment elevation in all or virtually all leads.
- A horizontal ST segment (i.e., forming a sharp angle with the T wave) suggests ischemia.
- Digitalis causes a depression or scoop of the ST segment that is sometimes referred to as a "dig dip" (Fig. 2.36).

Intervals

An **interval** is made up of a waveform and a segment.

PR INTERVAL

The P wave plus the PR segment equals the PRI; thus, the PRI reflects total supraventricular activity (see Fig. 2.33).

The PRI is measured from the point where the P wave leaves the baseline to the beginning of the QRS complex. The term *PQ interval* is preferred by some because it is the period that is measured unless a Q wave is absent. The PRI changes with heart rate but normally measures 0.12 to 0.20 second in adults (Box 2.5). As the heart rate increases, the duration of the PRI shortens. A PRI is considered short if it is less than 0.12 second and long if it is more than 0.20 second.

Abnormal PR Intervals

Delays in impulse conduction through the atria, AV node, or AV bundle can result in prolongation (greater than 0.20 second) of the PRI. Conditions causing such disturbances may be inflammatory, circulatory, nervous, endocrine, or pharmacologic in origin. The P wave associated with a prolonged PRI may be normal or abnormal.

A PRI of less than 0.12 second may be seen when the impulse originates in an ectopic pacemaker in the atria close to the AV node or the AV bundle. A shortened PRI may also occur if the electrical impulse progresses from the atria to the ventricles through an abnormal conduction pathway that bypasses the AV node and depolarizes the ventricles earlier than usual.

QT INTERVAL

The **QT interval** is the period from the beginning of the QRS complex to the end of the T wave. It represents total ventricular activity; this is the time from ventricular depolarization (i.e., activation) to repolarization (i.e., recovery)

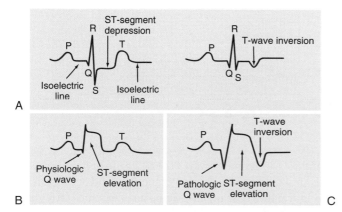

Fig. 2.35 ST segment, T wave, and Q wave changes associated with myocardial ischemia (A), injury (B), and infarction (C). (From Lewis, S. L., Bucher, L., Heitkemper, M. M., & Harding, M. M. (2017). *Medical-surgical nursing: assessment and management of clinical problems* (10th ed.). St. Louis: Elsevier.)

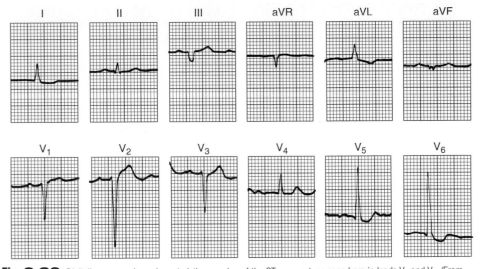

Fig. 2.36 Digitalis may produce characteristic scooping of the ST segment, as seen here in leads V_5 and V_6. (From Goldberger, A. L., Goldberger, Z. D., & Shvilkin, A. (2018). *Clinical electrocardiography: a simplified approach* (9th ed.). Philadelphia: Elsevier.)

Box 2.5	Normal PR Interval Characteristics

- Normally measures 0.12 to 0.20 second in adults; may be shorter in children and longer in older adults
- Typically shortens as heart rate increases

(see Fig. 2.33). In the absence of a Q wave, the QT interval is measured from the beginning of the R wave to the end of the T wave. The term *QT interval* is used regardless of whether the QRS complex begins with a Q wave or an R wave.

The duration of the QT interval varies with age, sex, and heart rate. As the heart rate increases, the QT interval shortens (i.e., decreases). As the heart rate decreases, the QT interval lengthens (i.e., increases). Generally, a normal QT interval is between 0.40 and 0.44 second.

A prolonged QT interval indicates a lengthened RRP. A QTc of more than 0.50 second is considered dangerous because it has been correlated with a higher risk for potentially fatal ventricular dysrhythmias (e.g., torsades de pointes [TdP]). A prolonged QT interval may be congenital or acquired. Myocardial ischemia or infarction, electrolyte disorders (e.g., hypokalemia, hypocalcemia), sudden decreases in heart rate, acute neurologic events, and medications (e.g., ibutilide, quinidine, sotalol) can prolong the QT interval.

Because of the variability of the QT interval with the heart rate, it can be measured more accurately if corrected (i.e., adjusted) for the patient's heart rate. A corrected QT interval is noted as *QTc*. In adults, the QTc is considered prolonged if it measures 0.47 second or more in men and 0.48 second or more in women (Drew et al., 2010).

Methods used to measure the QT and QTc duration include manual measurement using handheld calipers, electronic calipers built into an electrocardiographic monitoring system, and automated continuous QTc monitoring. To date, no studies have determined the best method for in-hospital monitoring of QT/QTc (Sandau et al., 2017). When measuring the QT interval, select a lead with the most well-defined T-wave end. For example, if a T wave is not clearly visible in lead II, try using lead I, V_5, or V_6 (Postema & Wilde, 2014). Avoid using a lead with U waves. Use the same lead for subsequent measurements to ensure meaningful comparisons of later tracings.

Several formulas have been used to calculate the corrected QT interval and compare this measurement at differing heart rates. Bazett's formula, in which the corrected QT interval is calculated as the QT interval divided by the R-R interval's square root (in seconds), has been widely used for many years. This formula works well with heart rates within the normal range, but studies show that it overcorrects at rapid heart rates and undercorrects at slow rates.

Document the QTc interval before starting and when increasing the dosage of medications that prolong the QR interval, and at least every 8 to 12 hours after that (Drew et al., 2010). Obtain and document QTc measurements more often if prolongation is observed.

R-R AND P-P INTERVALS

The R-R (R wave-to-R wave) and P-P (P wave-to-P wave) intervals are used to determine a cardiac rhythm's rate and regularity. The interval between two consecutive R waves is measured to evaluate the ventricular rhythm's regularity on a rhythm strip (see Fig. 2.26). The distance between succeeding R-R intervals is measured and compared. If the ventricular rhythm is regular, the R-R intervals will measure the same. Atrial regularity is similarly evaluated, except the interval between two consecutive P waves is measured and compared with succeeding P-P intervals.

Artifact

Accurate ECG rhythm recognition requires a tracing in which the waveforms and intervals are free of distortion. Distortion of an ECG tracing by electrical activity that is

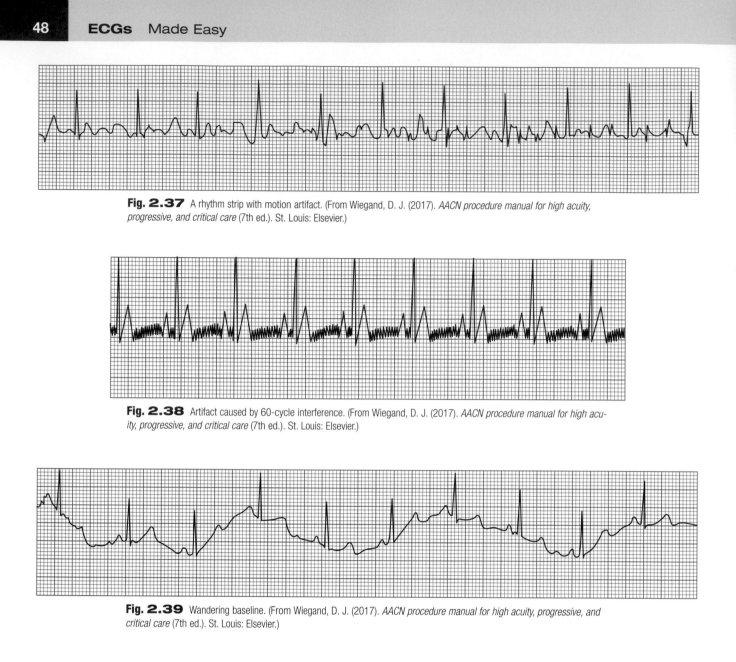

Fig. 2.37 A rhythm strip with motion artifact. (From Wiegand, D. J. (2017). *AACN procedure manual for high acuity, progressive, and critical care* (7th ed.). St. Louis: Elsevier.)

Fig. 2.38 Artifact caused by 60-cycle interference. (From Wiegand, D. J. (2017). *AACN procedure manual for high acuity, progressive, and critical care* (7th ed.). St. Louis: Elsevier.)

Fig. 2.39 Wandering baseline. (From Wiegand, D. J. (2017). *AACN procedure manual for high acuity, progressive, and critical care* (7th ed.). St. Louis: Elsevier.)

noncardiac in origin is called **artifact** (Fig. 2.37). Because artifact can mimic various cardiac dysrhythmias, including ventricular fibrillation, it is essential to evaluate the patient before beginning any medical intervention.

Proper preparation of the patient's skin and evaluation of monitoring equipment (e.g., electrodes, wires) before use can minimize the problems associated with artifact. Electrodes may adhere poorly if the patient's skin is especially hairy because the gel comes into contact with hair instead of skin. Skin contact is necessary for adequate signal penetration. If necessary, remove excessive chest hair from the areas where the electrodes are to be applied.

Artifact may result from external or internal sources. Possible external artifact causes include loose electrodes, broken ECG cables or broken lead wires, external chest compressions, and 60-cycle interference (Fig. 2.38). If 60-cycle interference is observed, check for the crossing of cable wires with other electrical wires (e.g., a bed control) or frayed and

broken wires. Verify that all electrical equipment is properly grounded and that the cable electrode connections are clean.

Internal artifact may result from patient movement, shivering, muscle tremors (e.g., seizures, Parkinson disease), or hiccups (Wung, 2017). A wandering baseline may occur because of normal respiratory movement (particularly when electrodes have been applied directly over the ribs) or because of poor electrode contact with the patient's skin (Fig. 2.39). Consider clipping the ECG cable to the patient's clothing to minimize excessive movement.

SYSTEMATIC RHYTHM INTERPRETATION

A systematic approach to rhythm analysis that is consistently applied when analyzing a rhythm strip is essential (Box 2.6). If you do not develop such an approach, you are more likely

Box 2.6	Systematic Rhythm Interpretation

1. Assess regularity (atrial and ventricular).
2. Assess rate (atrial and ventricular).
3. Identify and examine waveforms.
4. Assess intervals (e.g., PR, QRS, QT) and examine ST segments.
5. Interpret the rhythm and assess its clinical significance.

to miss something important. Begin analyzing the rhythm strip from left to right.

Assess Regularity

The waveforms on an ECG strip are evaluated for regularity by measuring the distance between the P waves and the QRS complexes.

ECG Pearl

Conflicting information about regularity exists among textbooks related to electrocardiography. Some texts indicate that a rhythm is irregular if the R-R or P-P intervals vary by more than 0.04 second, 0.06 second, 0.08 second, 0.12 second, or even 0.16 second, depending on the author. Because most texts agree that *any* deviation in regularity is, by definition, an irregular rhythm, that is the criteria used concerning regularity throughout this text.

VENTRICULAR REGULARITY

To determine if the ventricular rhythm is regular or irregular, measure the distance between two consecutive R-R intervals. Place one point of a pair of handheld calipers or make a mark on a piece of paper on an R wave (Fig. 2.40). Place the other point of the calipers or make a second mark on the paper at an identical point on the R wave of the next QRS complex. Without adjusting the calipers, evaluate each succeeding R-R interval. If paper is used, lift the paper and move it across the rhythm strip. Compare the distance measured with the other R-R intervals. If the ventricular rhythm is regular, the R-R intervals will be equal (measure the same). If the intervals are unequal, the ventricular rhythm is considered irregular.

You can also determine regularity by counting the small squares between intervals and comparing the intervals. Many ECG monitoring systems are equipped with electronic calipers used in the same way as physical calipers or paper and pencil.

ATRIAL REGULARITY

To determine if the atrial rhythm is regular or irregular, follow the same procedure previously described to evaluate ventricular regularity but measure the distance between two consecutive P-P intervals (instead of R-R intervals) and compare that distance to the other P-P intervals. If the atrial rhythm is regular, the P-P intervals will be equal. If the intervals are unequal, the atrial rhythm is considered irregular.

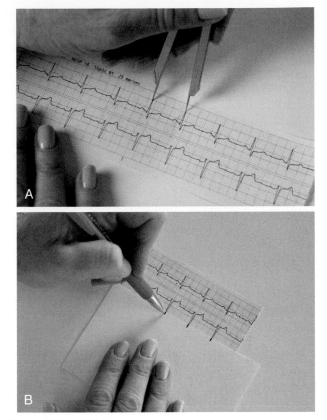

Fig. 2.40 A, Establishing ventricular regularity with handheld calipers. B, Establishing ventricular regularity with paper and pencil. (From Sole, M. L., & Klein, D., & Moseley, M. (2014). *Introduction to critical care nursing* (6th ed.). Philadelphia: Saunders.)

For accuracy, the R-R or P-P intervals should be evaluated across an entire 6-second rhythm strip.

Assess Rate

Calculating the heart rate is essential because deviations from normal can affect the patient's ability to maintain an adequate blood pressure and cardiac output. Although the atrial and ventricular rates are usually the same, they differ in some dysrhythmias; therefore, you must calculate both rates.

A tachycardia (tachy means "fast") exists in adults if the rate is more than 100 beats/min. Some dysrhythmias with very rapid ventricular rates (faster than 150 beats/min) require medication or a shock to the heart to stop the rhythm. A **bradycardia** exists if the rate is less than 60 beats/min (*brady* means "slow") in adults. Many patients tolerate a heart rate of 50 to 60 beats/min but become symptomatic when the rate drops below 50 beats/min.

Several methods are used for calculating heart rate. A discussion of each method follows.

SIX-SECOND METHOD

Most ECG paper is printed with 1-second or 3-second markers on the top or bottom of the paper. On ECG paper, 5 large boxes = 1 second, 15 large boxes = 3 seconds, and 30 large boxes = 6 seconds. To determine the ventricular rate, count the number of complete QRS complexes within 6 seconds, and multiply that number by 10 to find the number of complexes in 1 minute (Fig. 2.41). The 6-second method, also called the rule of 10, can be used for regular and irregular rhythms. This is the simplest, quickest, and most commonly used method of rate measurement, but it also is the most inaccurate.

LARGE BOX METHOD

The large box method of rate determination is also called the rule of 300. To determine the ventricular rate, count the number of large boxes between an R-R interval and divide into 300 (Fig. 2.42). Alternately, select an R wave that falls on a dark vertical line. Number the next six consecutive dark vertical lines as follows: 300, 150, 100, 75, 60, and 50

(see Fig. 2.42). Note where the next R wave falls in relation to the six dark vertical lines already marked. This is the heart rate.

To determine the atrial rate, count the number of large boxes between a P-P interval and divide into 300 (Table 2.5). This method is best used if the rhythm is regular; however, it may be used if the rhythm is irregular and a rate range (slowest [longest R-R interval] and fastest [shortest R-R interval] rate) is given.

SMALL BOX METHOD

The small box method of rate determination is also called the rule of 1500. Each 1-mm box on the graph paper represents 0.04 second. A total of 1500 boxes represents 1 minute (60 second/min divided by 0.04 second/box = 1500 boxes/min). To calculate the ventricular rate, count

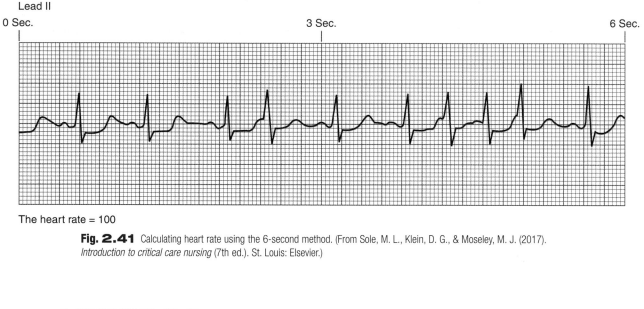

The heart rate = 100

Fig. 2.41 Calculating heart rate using the 6-second method. (From Sole, M. L., Klein, D. G., & Moseley, M. J. (2017). *Introduction to critical care nursing* (7th ed.). St. Louis: Elsevier.)

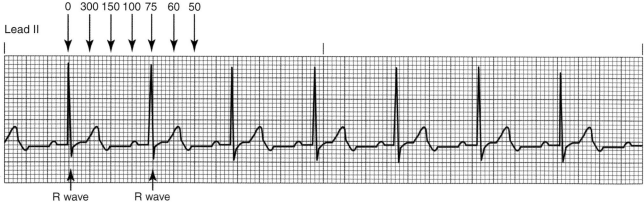

Fig. 2.42 Calculating heart rate using the large box method. To measure the ventricular rate, find an R wave that falls on a heavy dark line. Count the number of large boxes between that R wave and the one that follows it. Divide 300 by the number of large boxes between these R waves. Alternately, using the large boxes, count 300, 150, 100, 75, 60, and 50 until a second R wave occurs. This will be the heart rate. In this example, the second R wave occurs just before the arrow reading a rate of 75 beats/min; thus, the heart rate in this example is about 75 beats/min. (From Sole, M. L., Klein, D. G., & Moseley, M. J. (2017). *Introduction to critical care nursing* (7th ed.). St. Louis: Elsevier.)

TABLE 2.5	Heart Rate Determination Based on the Number of Large Boxes
Number of Large Boxes	**Heart Rate (beats/min)**
1	300
2	150
3	100
4	75
5	60
6	50
7	43
8	38
9	33
10	30

the number of small boxes between an R-R interval and divide into 1500 (Fig. 2.43). To determine the atrial rate, count the number of small boxes between a P-P interval and divide into 1500 (Table 2.6). This method is time-consuming but accurate.

⏱ ECG Pearl

Throughout this edition of the text, the 6-second method is used to calculate the heart rate when the rhythm is irregular. Electronic calipers are used when the rhythm is regular and when calculating intervals. During printing, distortion of ECGs can occur and can result in slight variations in the measurements provided in this book compared with the measurements you obtain.

Identify and Examine Waveforms

Look to see if the typical waveforms (P, Q, R, S, and T) are present. To locate P waves, look to the left of each QRS complex. Normally, one P wave precedes each QRS complex

(i.e., there is a 1:1 relationship); they occur regularly (P-P intervals are equal), and they look similar in size, shape, and position. Make a note if a P wave is absent or if P waves are present, but they appear inverted (i.e., pointed in a negative direction). Also, if there is more than one P wave before each QRS, record their number.

Next, evaluate the QRS complex. Are QRS complexes present? If so, does a QRS follow each P wave? Do the QRS complexes look alike? Assess the T waves. Does a T wave follow each QRS complex? Does a P wave follow the T wave? Are the T waves upright and of normal height? Look to see if a U wave is present. If so, note its height and direction (positive or negative).

Assess Intervals and Examine Segments
PR INTERVAL

Intervals are measured to evaluate conduction. Is a PRI present? If so, measure the PRIs and determine if they are equal. The PRI is measured from the point where the P wave leaves the baseline to the beginning of the QRS complex. Are the PRIs within normal limits? Remember that a normal PRI measures 0.12 to 0.20 seconds. If the PRIs are the same, they are said to be constant. If the PRIs are different, is a pattern present? In some dysrhythmias, the PRI duration gradually increases until a P wave appears with no QRS after it. This pattern is referred to as the lengthening of the PRI. PRIs that vary in duration and have no pattern are said to be variable.

QRS DURATION

Identify the QRS complexes and measure their duration. The beginning of the QRS is measured from the point where the first wave of the complex begins to deviate from the baseline. The point at which the last wave of the complex begins to level out at, above, or below the baseline marks the QRS

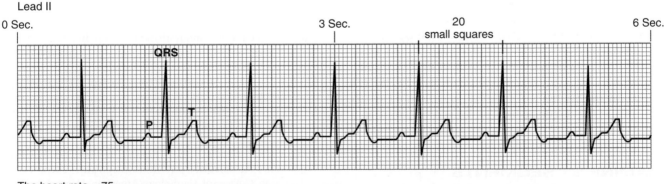

The heart rate = 75

Fig. 2.43 Calculating heart rate using the small box method. To measure the ventricular rate, find an R wave that falls on a heavy dark line. Count the number of small boxes between that R wave and the one that follows it. Divide 1500 by the number of small boxes between these R waves; this will be the heart rate (1500 ÷ 20 = 75 beats/min). (From Sole, M. L., Klein, D. G., & Moseley, M. J. (2017). *Introduction to critical care nursing* (7th ed.). St. Louis: Elsevier.)

TABLE **2.6** Heart Rate Determination Based on the Number of Small Boxes

Number of Small Boxes	Heart Rate (beats/min)	Number of Small Boxes	Heart Rate (beats/min)
5	300	28	54
6	250	29	52
7	214	30	50
8	188	31	48
9	167	32	47
10	150	33	45
11	136	34	44
12	125	35	43
13	115	36	42
14	107	37	41
15	100	38	40
16	94	39	39
17	88	40	38
18	83	41	37
19	79	42	36
20	75	43	35
21	71	44	34
22	68	45	33
23	65	46	33
24	62	47	32
25	60	48	31
26	58	49	31
27	56	50	30

complex's end. The QRS is considered narrow (i.e., normal) if it measures 0.11 second or less and wide if it measures more than 0.11 second. A narrow QRS complex is presumed to be supraventricular in origin.

QT INTERVAL

To determine the QT interval, count the number of small boxes between the beginning of the QRS complex and the end of the T wave. Then multiply that number by 0.04 second. If no Q wave is present, measure the QT interval from the beginning of the R wave to the end of the T wave. The QT interval generally measures 0.40 to 0.44 second. Recall that a corrected QT interval is calculated as the QT interval divided by the R-R interval's square root (in seconds). The QTc is considered prolonged in adults if it measures 0.47 second or more in men and 0.48 second or more in women.

EXAMINE ST SEGMENTS

Determine the presence of ST segment elevation or depression. Remember to start by identifying the onset of the QRS, which serves as the reference point. Next, locate the J

point and then compare the ST segment level with the reference point. Deviation is measured as the number of mm of vertical ST segment displacement (at the J point) from the reference point.

Interpret the Rhythm

Interpret the rhythm, specifying the site of origin (pacemaker site) of the rhythm (sinus), the mechanism (bradycardia), and the ventricular rate (for example, "Sinus bradycardia at 38 beats/min)." Assess the patient to find out how they are tolerating the rate and rhythm.

REFERENCES

Amsterdam, E. A., Wenger, N. K., Brindis, R. G., Casey Jr, D. E., Ganiats, T. G., & Zieman, S. J. (2014). 2014 AHA/ACC guideline for the management of patients with non-ST-elevation acute coronary syndromes: A report of the American College of Cardiology/American Heart Association Task Force on Practice Guidelines. *J Am Coll Cardiol, 64*(24), e139–e228.

Anderson, J. L., & Fang, J. C. (2020). ST segment elevation acute myocardial infarction and complications of myocardial infarction. In L. Goldman & A. I. Schafer (Eds.), *Goldman-Cecil medicine* (26th ed.) (pp. 388–401). Philadelphia, PA: Elsevier.

Azland, B. S., & Crijns, H. J. (2011). Diagnostic criteria of broad QRS complex tachycardia: Decades of evolution. *Europace, 13*(4), 465–472.

Bagliani, G., Brugada, J., De Ponti, R., Viola, G., Berne, P., & Leonelli, F. M. (2019). QRS variations during arrhythmias: Mechanisms and substrates. Toward a precision electrocardiology. *Card Electrophysiol Clin, 11*(2), 315–331.

Bakker, A. L., Nijkerk, G., Groenemeijer, B. E., Waalewijn, R. A., Koomen, E. M., Braam, R. L., & Wellens, H. J. (2009). The Lewis lead: Making recognition of P waves easy during wide QRS complex tachycardia. *Circulation, 119*(24), e592593.

Bansal, A., & Joshi, R. (2018). Portable out-of-hospital electrocardiography: A review of current technologies. *J Arrhythm, 34*(2), 129–138.

Brady, W. J., Harrigan, R. A., & Chan, T. C. (2019). Basic electrocardiographic techniques. In J. R. Roberts, C. B. Custalow, & T. W. Thomsen (Eds.), *Roberts and Hedges' clinical procedures in emergency medicine and acute care* (7th ed.) (pp. 275–287). Philadelphia, PA: Elsevier.

Burchum, J. R. (2016). Antidysrhythmic drugs. In J. R. Burchum & L. D. Rosenthal (Eds.), *Lehne's pharmacology for nursing care* (9th ed.) (pp. 534–555). St. Louis, MO: Saunders.

Ching, S., & Ting, S. M. (2015). The forgotten lead: aVR in left main disease. *Am J Med, 128*(12), e11–e13.

Costanzo, L. S. (2018). Cardiovascular physiology. In *Physiology* (6th ed.) (pp. 117–188). Philadelphia, PA: Elsevier.

Crawford, M. H., Bernstein, S. J., Deedwania, P. C., DiMarco, J. P., Ferrick, K. J., Garson Jr, A., … Smith Jr, S. C. (1999). ACC/AHA guidelines for ambulatory electrocardiography. A report of the American College of Cardiology/American Heart Association Task Force on Practice Guidelines (Committee to Revise the Guidelines for Ambulatory Electrocardiography). *J Am Coll Cardiol, 34*(3), 912–948.

Cunningham, S. G., Brashers, V. L., & McCance, K. L. (2017). Structure and function of the cardiovascular and lymphatic systems. In S. E. Huether, K. L. McCance, V. L. Brashers, & N. S. Rote (Eds.), *Understanding pathophysiology* (6th ed.) (pp. 569–597). St. Louis, MO: Elsevier.

DeBeasi, L. C. (2003). Anatomy of the cardiovascular system. In S. A. Price & L. M. Wilson (Eds.), *Pathophysiology: Clinical concepts of disease processes* (6th ed.) (pp. 405–415). St. Louis, MO: Mosby.

Drew, B. J., Ackerman, M. J., Funk, M., Gibler, W. B., Kligfield, P., Menon, V., … Zareba, W. (2010). Prevention of torsade de pointes in hospital settings: A scientific statement from the American Heart Association and the American College of Cardiology Foundation. *J Am Coll Cardiol, 55*(9), 934–947.

Drew, B. J., Califf, R. M., Funk, M., Kaufman, E. S., Krucoff, M. W., Laks, M. M., … Van Hare, G. F. (2004). Practice standards for electrocardiographic monitoring in hospital settings: An American Heart Association scientific statement from the Councils on Cardiovascular Nursing, Clinical Cardiology, and Cardiovascular Disease in the Young. *Circulation, 110*(17), 2721–2746.

Ganz, L., & Link, M. S. (2020). Electrocardiography. In L. Goldman & A. I. Schafer (Eds.), *Goldman-Cecil medicine* (26th ed.) (pp. 246–253). Philadelphia, PA: Elsevier.

Goldberger, A. L., Goldberger, Z. D., & Shvilkin, A. (2018). How to make basic ECG measurements. In *Goldberger's clinical electrocardiography* (9th ed.) (pp. 11–20). Philadelphia, PA: Elsevier.

Gorgels, A. P., Engelen, D. J., & Wellens, H. J. (2001). Lead aVR, a mostly ignored but very valuable lead in clinical electrocardiography. *J Am Coll Cardiol, 38*(5), 1355–1356.

Hall, J. E. (2016). The normal electrocardiogram. In *Guyton and Hall textbook of medical physiology* (13th ed.) (pp. 131–137). Philadelphia, PA: Elsevier.

Hancock, E. W., Deal, B. J., Mirvis, D. M., Okin, P., Kligfield, P., & Gettes, L. S. (2009). AHA/ACCF/HRS recommendations for the standardization and interpretation of the electrocardiogram: Part V: Electrocardiogram changes associated with cardiac chamber hypertrophy. *J Am Coll Cardiol, 53*(11), 992–1002.

Issa, Z. F., Miller, J. M., & Zipes, D. P. (2019a). Atrioventricular conduction abnormalities. In *Clinical arrhythmology and electrophysiology* (3rd ed.) (pp. 255–285). Philadelphia, PA: Elsevier.

Issa, Z. F., Miller, J. M., & Zipes, D. P. (2019b). Electrophysiological mechanisms of cardiac arrhythmias. In *Clinical arrhythmology and electrophysiology* (3rd ed.) (pp. 51–80). Philadelphia, PA: Elsevier.

Issa, Z. F., Miller, J. M., & Zipes, D. P. (2019c). Molecular mechanisms of cardiac electrical activity. In *Clinical arrhythmology and electrophysiology* (3rd ed.) (pp. 1–14). Philadelphia, PA: Elsevier.

Krahn, A. D., Yee, R., Skanes, A. C., & Klein, G. J. (2018). Cardiac monitoring: Short- and long-term recording. In D. P. Zipes, J. Jalife, & W. G. Stevenson (Eds.), *Cardiac electrophysiology: From cell to bedside* (7th ed.) (pp. 623–629). Philadelphia, PA: Elsevier.

Lederer, W. J. (2017). Cardiac electrophysiology and the electrocardiogram. In W. F. Boron & E. L. Boulpaep (Eds.), *Medical physiology* (3rd ed.) (pp. 483–506). Philadelphia, PA: Elsevier.

Mangoni, M. E., & Nargeot, J. (2008). Genesis and regulation of the heart automaticity. *Physiol Rev, 88*(3), 919–982.

Martin, D., & Wharton, J. M. (2001). Sustained monomorphic ventricular tachycardia. In P. J. Podrid & P. R. Kowey (Eds.), *Cardiac arrhythmia: Mechanisms, diagnosis, and management* (2nd ed.) (pp. 573–601). Philadelphia, PA: Lippincott Williams & Wilkins.

Mirvis, D. M., & Goldberger, A. L. (2019). Electrocardiography. In D. P. Zipes, P. Libby, R. O. Bonow, D. L. Mann, G. F. Tomaselli, & E. Braunwald (Eds.), *Braunwald's heart disease: A textbook of cardiovascular medicine* (11th ed.) (pp. 117–153). Philadelphia, PA: Elsevier.

Mittal, S., Movsowitz, C., & Steinberg, J. S. (2011). Ambulatory external electrocardiographic monitoring: Focus on atrial fibrillation. *J Am Coll Cardiol, 58*(17), 1741–1749.

O'Gara, P. T., Kushner, F. G., Ascheim, D. D., Casey Jr, D. E., Chung, M. K., de Lemos, J. A., … Zhao, D. X. (2013). 2013 ACCF/AHA guideline for the management of ST-elevation myocardial infarction. *J Am Coll Cardiol, 61*(4), e78–e140.

Pappano, A. J., & Wier, W. G. (2019). Excitation: The cardiac action potential. In *Cardiovascular physiology* (11th ed.) (pp. 10–28). Philadelphia, PA: Elsevier.

Patton, K. T., & Thibodeau, G. A. (2019). Heart. In *Anatomy & physiology* (10th ed.) (pp. 634–662). St. Louis, MO: Elsevier.

Peterson, K. (2018). Advanced dysrhythmias. In V. S. Good & P. L. Kirkwood (Eds.), *Advanced critical care nursing* (2nd ed.) (pp. 12–33). St. Louis, MO: Elsevier.

Postema, P. G., & Wilde, A. A. (2014). The measurement of the QT interval. *Curr Cardiol Rev, 10*(3), 287–294.

Rautaharju, P. M., Surawicz, B., & Gettes, L. S. (2009). AHA/ACCF/HRS recommendations for the standardization and interpretation of the electrocardiogram: Part IV: The ST segment, T and U waves, and the QT interval. *J Am Coll Cardiol, 53*(11), 982–991.

Sandau, K. E., Funk, M., Auerbach, A., Barsness, G. W., Blum, K., Cvach, M., … Wang, P. J. (2017). Update to practice standards for electrocardiographic monitoring in hospital settings: A scientific statement from the American Heart Association. *Circulation, 136*(19), e273–344.

Shen, W.-K., Sheldon, R. S., Benditt, D. G., Cohen, M. I., Forman, D. E., Goldberger, Z. D., … Yancy, C. W. (2017). 2017 ACC/AHA/HRS guideline for the evaluation and management of patients with syncope: A report of the American College of Cardiology/American Heart Association Task Force on Clinical Practice Guidelines and the Heart Rhythm Society. *J Am Coll Cardiol, 70*(5), e39–110.

Surawicz, B., & Knilans, T. K. (2008). Normal electrocardiogram: Origin and description. In *Chou's electrocardiography in clinical practice* (6th ed.) (pp. 1–28). Philadelphia, PA: Saunders.

Surawicz, B., Childers, R., Deal, B. J., & Gettes, L. S. (2009). AHA/ACCF/HRS recommendations for the standardization and interpretation of the electrocardiogram: Part III: intraventricular conduction disturbances: A scientific statement from the American Heart Association Electrocardiography and Arrhythmias Committee. *J Am Coll Cardiol, 53*(11), 976–981.

Thygesen, K., Alpert, J. S., Jaffe, A. S., Chaitman, B. R., Bax, J. J., Morrow, D. A., & White, H. D. (2018). Fourth universal definition of myocardial infarction. *J Am Coll Cardiol, 72*(18), 2231–2264.

Tomaselli, G. F., Rubart, M., & Zipes, D. P. (2019). Mechanisms of cardiac dysrhythmias. In D. P. Zipes, P. Libby, R. O. Bonow, D. L. Mann, G. F. Tomaselli, & E. Braunwald (Eds.), *Braunwald's heart disease: A textbook of cardiovascular medicine* (11th ed.) (pp. 619–647). Philadelphia, PA: Elsevier.

Vorobiof, G., & Ellestad, M. H. (2011). Lead aVR: Dead or simply forgotten? *JACC Cardiovasc Imaging, 4*(2), 187–190.

Wagner, G. (2012). Basic electrocardiography. In S. Saksena & A. J. Camm (Eds.), *Electrophysiological disorders of the heart* (2nd ed.) (pp. 125–158). Philadelphia, PA: Saunders.

Wagner, G. S., Macfarlane, P., Wellens, H., Josephson, M., Gorgels, A., Mirvis, D. M., … Gettes, L. S. (2009). AHA/ACCF/HRS recommendations for the standardization and interpretation of the electrocardiogram: Part VI: Acute ischemia/infarction; a scientific statement from the American Heart Association Electrocardiography and Arrhythmias Committee. *J Am Coll Cardiol, 53*(11), 1003–1011.

Wung, S. F. (2017). Procedure 55 Extra electrocardiographic leads. In D. J. Wiegand (Ed.), *AACN procedure manual for high acuity, progressive, and critical care* (7th ed.) (pp. 477–485). St. Louis, MO: Elsevier.

STOP & REVIEW

Identify one or more choices that best complete the statement or answer the question.

1. When an ECG machine is properly calibrated, a 1-millivolt (mV) electrical signal will produce a deflection measuring exactly _____ tall.
   a. 1 mm
   b. 5 mm
   c. 10 mm
   d. 20 mm

2. Fifteen large boxes equal an interval of _____ on ECG paper.
   a. 1 second
   b. 3 seconds
   c. 6 seconds
   d. 10 seconds

3. The QRS complex
   a. normally follows each P wave.
   b. represents ventricular depolarization.
   c. normally measures 0.20 second or less.
   d. generally represents right ventricular electrical activity.

4. The SA node
   a. is normally the heart's primary pacemaker.
   b. is supplied by sympathetic and parasympathetic nerve fibers.
   c. generates electrical impulses at a rate of 40 to 60 beats/min.
   d. is located at the junction of the superior vena cava and right atrium.

5. Which of the following surfaces of the heart are not directly viewed when using a standard 12-lead ECG?
   a. Right ventricle
   b. Lateral surface of the left ventricle
   c. Inferior surface of the left ventricle
   d. Anterior surface of the left ventricle
   e. Posterior surface of the left ventricle

6. On the ECG, total supraventricular activity is reflected by the:
   a. TP segment.
   b. PR interval (PRI).
   c. QT interval.
   d. QRS duration.

7. Which of the following are disorders of impulse formation?
   a. Reentry
   b. Triggered activity
   c. Conduction blocks
   d. Altered automaticity

8. U waves
   a. represent repolarization of the Purkinje fibers.
   b. are most easily seen when the heart rate is slow.
   c. are often associated with elevated potassium levels.
   d. usually appear in the opposite direction as the T waves that precede them.

Questions 9 Through 14 Pertain to the Following Scenario

You are caring for a 64-year-old man complaining of chest pain that he rates a 9 on a 0 to 10 scale. He says his symptoms began 20 minutes ago while moving boxes in his garage.

9. You are applying ECG leads to this patient and will be using lead V_1 for continuous monitoring. This lead is an example of a(n)
   a. chest lead.
   b. horizontal lead.
   c. standard limb lead.
   d. augmented limb lead.

10. Lead V_1 views the
   a. right ventricle.
   b. interventricular septum.
   c. lateral surface of the left ventricle.
   d. posterior surface of the left ventricle.

11. When analyzing this patient's ECG rhythm, the first areas of the rhythm strip that should be assessed are
   a. rate.
   b. P waves.
   c. intervals.
   d. regularity.
   e. segments.
   f. QRS complexes.

12. The patient's ECG shows four large squares between two consecutive R waves. Based on this information, you calculate the patient's heart rate to be _____ beats/min.
   a. 50
   b. 75
   c. 100
   d. 150

13. When analyzing the leads facing the affected area of the heart, ECG evidence of myocardial injury is displayed as
   a. inverted P waves.
   b. ST segment elevation.
   c. prolonged PRIs.
   d. ST segment depression.

14. Which of the following statements is true regarding analysis of the ST segment on this patient's ECG?
   a. ST segment displacement should be measured at a point 0.12 second after the J point.
   b. ST segment elevation viewed in lead II would be considered clinically significant if also seen in lead III or aVF.
   c. Based on this patient's age, ST segment elevation seen in lead II would be considered clinically significant if elevated more than 0.5 mm.
   d. Use the PRI as the baseline from which to evaluate the degree of ST segment displacement from the isoelectric line.

Matching

Waveforms, Segments, and Intervals

a. waveform

b. segment

c. J point

d. interval

e. 0.12 to 0.20 second

f. Q wave

g. 0.11 second or less

h. complex

i. 0.04 second

j. millimeters

k. 3 second

l. R wave

_____ **15.** A waveform and a segment

_____ **16.** In adults, the normal duration of the QRS complex

_____ **17.** The amplitude of a waveform is measured in __.

_____ **18.** This waveform is always negative

_____ **19.** Movement away from the baseline in either a positive or negative direction

_____ **20.** Normal duration of the PRI

_____ **21.** This waveform is always positive

_____ **22.** On ECG paper, each horizontal 1-mm box represents __.

_____ **23.** A line between waveforms

_____ **24.** On ECG paper, 15 large boxes represents __.

_____ **25.** The area where the QRS complex and the ST segment meet

_____ **26.** Several waveforms

The Cardiac Action Potential

a. Procainamide and lidocaine

b. Fast response

c. Depolarization

d. Verapamil and diltiazem

e. Action potential

f. Wave of depolarization

g. Slow response

h. Repolarization

_____ **27.** This type of action potential occurs in the SA and AV nodes

_____ **28.** A chain reaction that occurs from cell to cell in the heart's electrical conduction system until all the cells have been stimulated

_____ **29.** The movement of charged particles across a cell membrane in which the inside of the cell is restored to its negative charge

_____ **30.** Examples of antiarrhythmics that block sodium channels

_____ **31.** The rapid sequence of voltage changes that occur across the cell membrane during the electrical cardiac cycle

_____ **32.** This type of action potential occurs in normal atrial and ventricular myocardial cells and in the His-Purkinje fibers

_____ **33.** The movement of ions across a cell membrane causing the inside of the cell to become more positive

_____ **34.** Examples of antiarrhythmics that slow the rate at which calcium passes through the cells

Short Answer

35. List four uses for ECG monitoring.

1.

2.

3.

4.

36. List, in order, the five steps used in ECG rhythm analysis.

1.

2.

3.

4.

5.

Practice Rhythm Strips

For each of the following rhythm strips, determine regularity and rate. Next, assess the relationship between P waves and QRS complexes, labeling the P wave, QRS complex, and T wave. Finally, measure the PRI, QRS duration, and QT interval. *Not all waveforms will be present in each of the following rhythm strips.*

37.

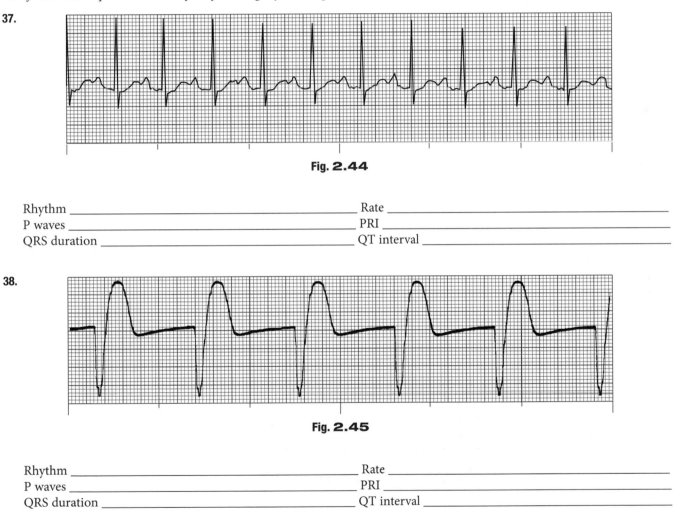

Fig. 2.44

Rhythm _____ Rate _____

P waves _____ PRI _____

QRS duration _____ QT interval _____

38.

Fig. 2.45

Rhythm _____ Rate _____

P waves _____ PRI _____

QRS duration _____ QT interval _____

39.

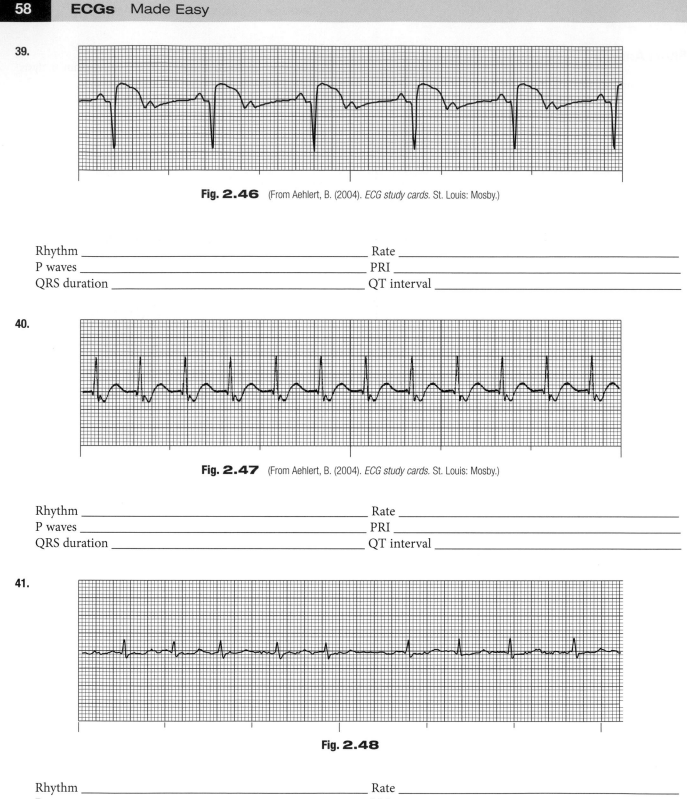

Fig. 2.46 (From Aehlert, B. (2004). *ECG study cards.* St. Louis: Mosby.)

Rhythm _____   Rate _____
P waves _____   PRI _____
QRS duration _____   QT interval _____

40.

Fig. 2.47 (From Aehlert, B. (2004). *ECG study cards.* St. Louis: Mosby.)

Rhythm _____   Rate _____
P waves _____   PRI _____
QRS duration _____   QT interval _____

41.

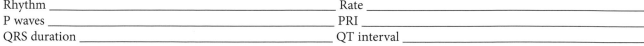

Fig. 2.48

Rhythm _____   Rate _____
P waves _____   PRI _____
QRS duration _____   QT interval _____

42.

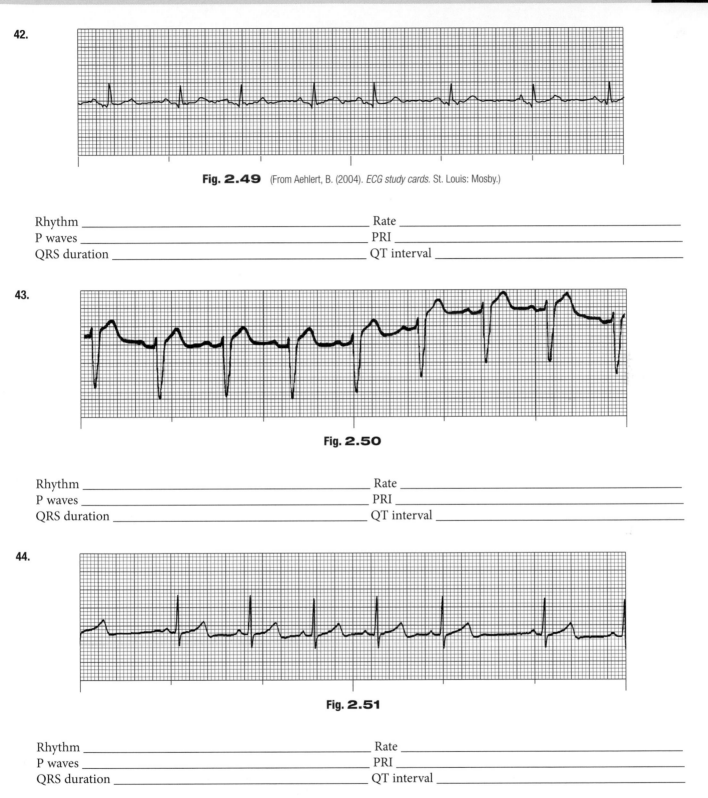

Fig. 2.49   (From Aehlert, B. (2004). *ECG study cards.* St. Louis: Mosby.)

Rhythm _____   Rate _____
P waves _____   PRI _____
QRS duration _____   QT interval _____

43.

Fig. 2.50

Rhythm _____   Rate _____
P waves _____   PRI _____
QRS duration _____   QT interval _____

44.

Fig. 2.51

Rhythm _____   Rate _____
P waves _____   PRI _____
QRS duration _____   QT interval _____

45.

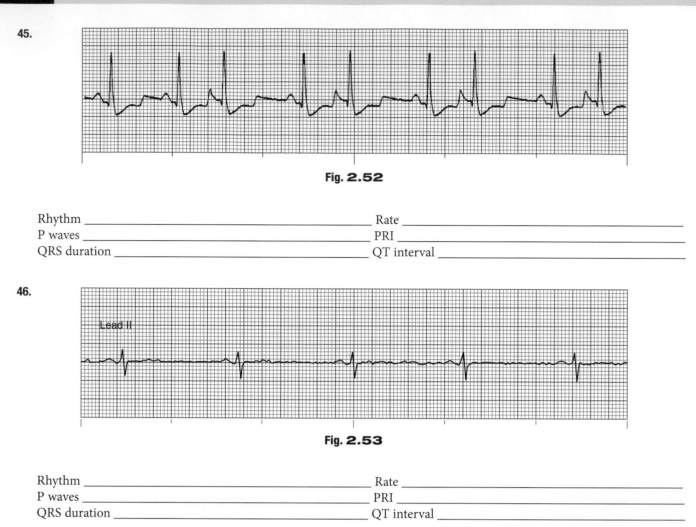

Fig. 2.52

Rhythm _____   Rate _____
P waves _____   PRI _____
QRS duration _____   QT interval _____

46.

Lead II

Fig. 2.53

Rhythm _____   Rate _____
P waves _____   PRI _____
QRS duration _____   QT interval _____

STOP & REVIEW ANSWERS

1. **C.** An ECG machine's sensitivity must be calibrated so that a 1-mV electrical signal will produce a deflection measuring exactly 10 mm tall. When properly calibrated, a small box is 1 mm high (0.1 mV), and a large box (equal to five small boxes) is 5 mm high (0.5 mV).

2. **B.** Five large boxes, each consisting of five small boxes, represent 1 second. Fifteen large boxes equal 3 seconds. Thirty large boxes represent 6 seconds.

3. **A, B.** A QRS complex normally follows each P wave. The QRS complex represents ventricular depolarization. Ventricular repolarization is recorded on the ECG as the ST segment and T wave. In adults, the normal duration of the QRS complex is 0.11 second or less. If an electrical impulse does not follow the normal ventricular conduction pathway, it will take longer to depolarize the myocardium. This delay in conduction through the ventricles produces a wider QRS complex. Because of its greater muscle mass, the QRS complex generally represents the left ventricle's electrical activity.

4. **A, B, D.** The SA node is the heart's primary pacemaker because it has the fastest firing rate of the heart's pacemaker sites. Sympathetic and parasympathetic nerve fibers richly supply the SA node. The SA node is specialized conducting tissue located in the upper posterior part of the right atrium where the superior vena cava and the right atrium meet. The SA node generates electrical impulses at a rate of 60 to 100 beats/min.

5. **A, E.** The right ventricle and posterior surface of the left ventricle are not directly viewed when using a standard 12-lead ECG. Right chest leads and posterior chest leads, respectively, are used for this purpose.

6. **B.** The P wave plus the PR segment equals the PRI; thus, the PRI reflects total supraventricular activity. The QT interval (which includes the QRS complex, ST segment, and T wave) represents total ventricular activity; this is the time from ventricular depolarization (i.e., activation) to repolarization (i.e., recovery).

7. **B, D.** Altered automaticity and triggered activity are disorders of impulse formation. Conduction blocks and reentry are disorders of impulse conduction.

8. **A, B.** A U wave is a small waveform that, when seen, follows the T wave. U waves usually appear in the same direction as the T waves that precede them. The U wave is thought to represent the late repolarization of the Purkinje fibers. However, some cardiologists believe that U

Matching

15. ANS: d
16. ANS: g
17. ANS: j
18. ANS: f

waves are simply two-part T waves resulting from a longer action potential duration in some ventricular myocardial cells. U waves are most easily seen when the heart rate is slow and are difficult to identify when the rate exceeds 95 beats/min. Possible causes of prominent U waves include central nervous system disease, electrolyte imbalance (e.g., hypokalemia), hyperthyroidism, long QT syndrome, and medications (e.g., amiodarone, digitalis, disopyramide, phenothiazines, procainamide, quinidine).

9. **A.** Lead V_1 is a chest lead and views the heart in the horizontal plane.

10. **B.** Leads V_1 and V_2 view the interventricular septum.

11. **A, D.** When analyzing a rhythm strip, begin by assessing regularity (atrial and ventricular) and rate (atrial and ventricular).

12. **B.** Using the large box (rule of 300) method to calculate heart rate, four large boxes between two consecutive R waves equals a heart rate of 75 beats/min (300 divided by 4).

13. **B.** In a patient experiencing an acute coronary syndrome, ECG evidence of myocardial injury is displayed as ST segment elevation in the leads facing the heart's affected area.

14. **B.** The onset of the QRS complex is used as the reference point from which to evaluate the degree of displacement of the ST segment from the isoelectric line. If ST segment displacement is present, note the number of millimeters of deviation (at the J point) from the reference point. When ECG changes of myocardial ischemia, injury, or infarction occur, they are not found in every ECG lead. Findings are considered significant if viewed in two or more leads looking at the same or adjacent heart area. If these findings are seen in leads that look directly at the affected area, they are called *indicative changes*. Indicative changes are significant when they are seen in two *anatomically contiguous* leads. Two leads are contiguous if they look at the same or adjacent area of the heart or they are numerically consecutive chest leads. Remember that leads II, III, and aVF view the inferior wall of the left ventricle. Therefore, in this patient situation, ST segment changes viewed in lead II would be considered clinically significant if elevated more than 1 mm and also seen in lead III or aVF.

19. ANS: a
20. ANS: e
21. ANS: l
22. ANS: i

23. ANS: b
24. ANS: k
25. ANS: c
26. ANS: h
27. ANS: g
28. ANS: f

29. ANS: h
30. ANS: a
31. ANS: e
32. ANS: b
33. ANS: c
34. ANS: d

Short Answer

35. ECG monitoring may be used for the following purposes:
- To immediately recognize sudden cardiac arrest and improve time to defibrillation
- To recognize deteriorating conditions (e.g., nonsustained dysrhythmias) that may lead to life-threatening, sustained dysrhythmias
- To assist in the diagnosis of dysrhythmias or causes of symptoms and guide appropriate management
- To monitor a patient's heart rate
- To evaluate the effects of disease or injury on heart function
- To evaluate for signs of myocardial ischemia, injury, and infarction
- To evaluate pacemaker function
- To evaluate a patient's response to medications (e.g., antiarrhythmics)
- To obtain recordings before, during, and after a medical procedure

36. 1. Assess regularity (atrial and ventricular).
2. Assess rate (atrial and ventricular).
3. Identify and examine waveforms.
4. Assess intervals (e.g., PR, QRS, QT) and examine ST segments.
5. Interpret the rhythm and assess its clinical significance.

Practice Rhythm Strip Answers

Note: The rate and interval measurements provided here were obtained using electronic calipers.

37.

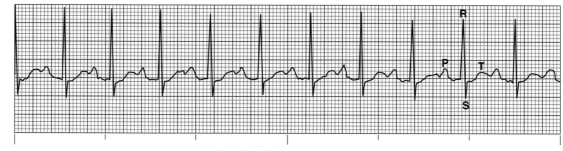

Fig. 2.54 (Answer to Fig. 2.44)

Rhythm: Regular
Rate: 110 beats/min
P waves: Uniform; upright before each QRS
PRI: 0.23 second
QRS duration: 0.07 second
QT interval: 0.30 second

38.

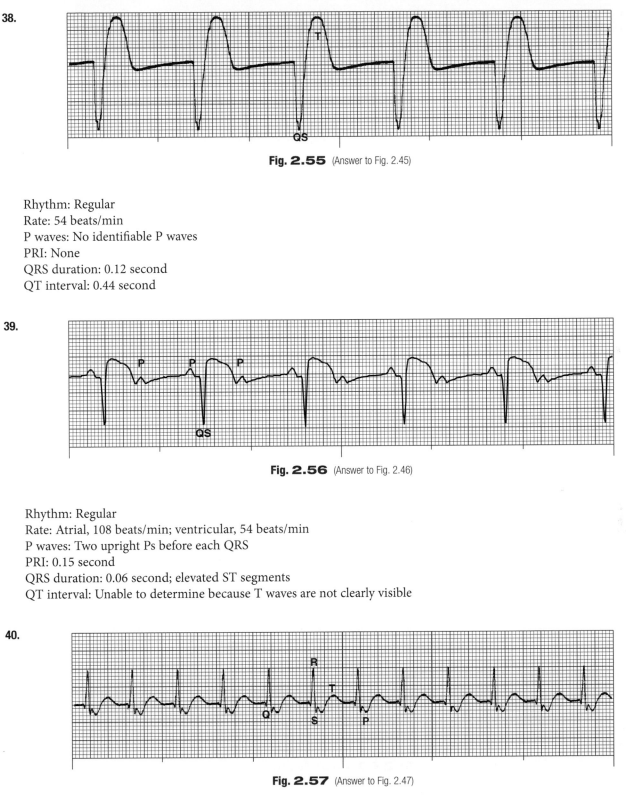

Fig. 2.55 (Answer to Fig. 2.45)

Rhythm: Regular
Rate: 54 beats/min
P waves: No identifiable P waves
PRI: None
QRS duration: 0.12 second
QT interval: 0.44 second

39.

Fig. 2.56 (Answer to Fig. 2.46)

Rhythm: Regular
Rate: Atrial, 108 beats/min; ventricular, 54 beats/min
P waves: Two upright Ps before each QRS
PRI: 0.15 second
QRS duration: 0.06 second; elevated ST segments
QT interval: Unable to determine because T waves are not clearly visible

40.

Fig. 2.57 (Answer to Fig. 2.47)

Rhythm: Regular
Rate: 119 beats/min
P waves: One inverted P appears after each QRS
PRI: None
QRS duration: 0.08 second
QT interval: 0.34 second

41.

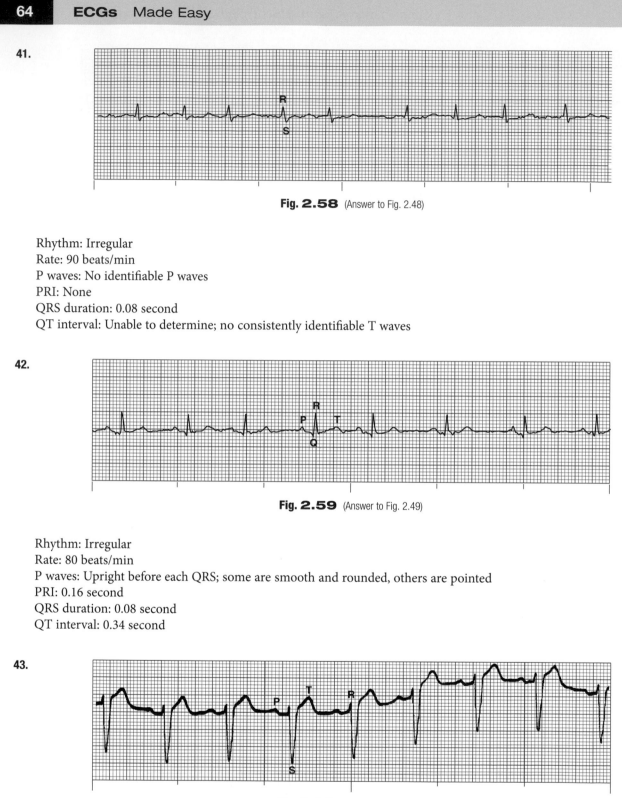

Fig. 2.58 (Answer to Fig. 2.48)

Rhythm: Irregular
Rate: 90 beats/min
P waves: No identifiable P waves
PRI: None
QRS duration: 0.08 second
QT interval: Unable to determine; no consistently identifiable T waves

42.

Fig. 2.59 (Answer to Fig. 2.49)

Rhythm: Irregular
Rate: 80 beats/min
P waves: Upright before each QRS; some are smooth and rounded, others are pointed
PRI: 0.16 second
QRS duration: 0.08 second
QT interval: 0.34 second

43.

Fig. 2.60 (Answer to Fig. 2.50)

Rhythm: Regular
Rate: 82 beats/min
P waves: Uniform; upright before each QRS
PRI: 0.20 second
QRS duration: 0.12 second; ST segment elevation
QT interval: 0.31 second

44.

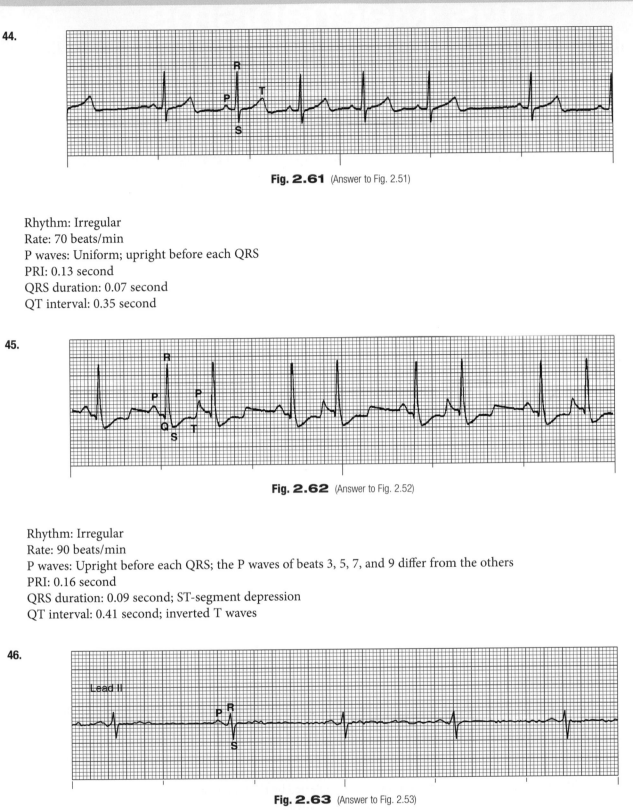

Fig. 2.61 (Answer to Fig. 2.51)

Rhythm: Irregular
Rate: 70 beats/min
P waves: Uniform; upright before each QRS
PRI: 0.13 second
QRS duration: 0.07 second
QT interval: 0.35 second

45.

Fig. 2.62 (Answer to Fig. 2.52)

Rhythm: Irregular
Rate: 90 beats/min
P waves: Upright before each QRS; the P waves of beats 3, 5, 7, and 9 differ from the others
PRI: 0.16 second
QRS duration: 0.09 second; ST-segment depression
QT interval: 0.41 second; inverted T waves

46.

Fig. 2.63 (Answer to Fig. 2.53)

Rhythm: Irregular
Rate: 50 beats/min
P waves: Upright before each QRS
PRI: 0.16 second
QRS duration: 0.08 second
QT interval: Unable to determine because T waves are not clearly visible

Sinus Mechanisms

3

LEARNING OBJECTIVES

After reading this chapter, you should be able to:

1. Describe the electrocardiogram (ECG) characteristics of a sinus rhythm.
2. Describe the ECG characteristics, possible causes, signs and symptoms, and emergency management of sinus bradycardia.
3. Describe the ECG characteristics, possible causes, signs and symptoms, and emergency management of sinus tachycardia.
4. Describe the ECG characteristics, possible causes, signs and symptoms, and emergency management of sinus arrhythmia.
5. Describe the ECG characteristics, possible causes, signs and symptoms, and emergency management of sinoatrial (SA) block.
6. Describe the ECG characteristics, possible causes, signs and symptoms, and emergency management of sinus arrest.

KEY TERMS

sinus arrhythmia: Dysrhythmia originating in the SA node that occurs when the SA node discharges irregularly; sinus arrhythmia is a normal phenomenon associated with the phases of breathing and changes in intrathoracic pressure.

sinus bradycardia: Dysrhythmia originating in the SA node with a ventricular response of less than 60 beats/min.

sinus rhythm: A normal heart rhythm; sometimes called a regular sinus rhythm (RSR) or normal sinus rhythm (NSR).

sinus tachycardia: Dysrhythmia originating in the SA node with a ventricular rate faster than 100 beats per minute (beats/min) with the maximum rate about 220 beats/min, minus the patient's age in years.

INTRODUCTION

In this chapter, you will begin learning the characteristics of specific cardiac rhythms. Study these characteristics carefully and commit them to memory. Throughout this text, all ECG characteristics pertain to adult patients unless otherwise noted.

The normal heartbeat results from an electrical impulse that starts in the SA node (Fig. 3.1). Normally, pacemaker cells within the SA node spontaneously depolarize more rapidly than other cardiac cells. As a result, the SA node usually dominates other depolarizing areas at a slightly slower rate. The impulse is sent to transitional cells at the outside edge of the SA node and then to the myocardial cells of the surrounding atrium.

A rhythm that begins in the SA node has the following characteristics:

- A positive (i.e., upright) P wave before each QRS complex
- P waves that look alike
- A constant PR interval
- A regular atrial and ventricular rhythm (usually)

An electrical impulse that begins in the SA node may be affected by the following:

- Medications
- Diseases or conditions that cause the heart rate to speed up, slow down, or beat irregularly
- Diseases or conditions that delay or block the impulse from leaving the SA node
- Diseases or conditions that prevent an impulse from being generated in the SA node

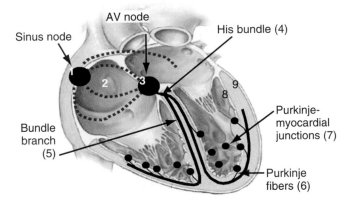

Fig. 3.1 The cardiac action potential originates in the sinoatrial (*SA*) node (1), continues in the atrial wall (2), and is delayed in the atrioventricular (*AV*) node (3). Conduction within the ventricles is initially rapid within the rapid conduction system: His bundle (4), right and left bundle branches (5), and Purkinje fibers (6). The impulse is transferred from the rapid conduction system to the working myocardium in the Purkinje-myocardial junctions (7) located in the endocardium. Within the slowly conducting working myocardium, the impulse is conducted from endocardium to epicardium. The SA node normally depolarizes faster than any other part of the heart's conduction system. As a result, the SA node usually is the heart's primary pacemaker. (From Ellenbogen, K. A., Wilkoff, B. L., Kay, G. N., Lau, C. P., & Auricchio, A. (2017). *Clinical cardiac pacing, defibrillation and resynchronization therapy* (5th ed.). Philadelphia: Elsevier.)

ECG Pearl

Most, but not all, rhythms that begin in the SA node are regular.

SINUS RHYTHM

Sinus rhythm is the name given to a normal heart rhythm. Sinus rhythm is sometimes called a regular sinus rhythm (RSR) or normal sinus rhythm (NSR). Sinus rhythm reflects normal electrical activity—that is, the rhythm starts in the SA node and then heads down the normal conduction pathway through the atria, atrioventricular (AV) node and bundle, right and left bundle branches, and Purkinje fibers. In adults and adolescents, the SA node usually fires at a regular rate of 60 to 100 beats per minute (beats/min).

How Do I Recognize It?

ECG characteristics of a sinus rhythm include the following:

Rhythm:	R-R and P-P intervals are regular
Rate:	60 to 100 beats/min
P waves:	Positive (upright) in lead II; one precedes each QRS complex; P waves look alike
PR interval:	0.12 to 0.20 second and constant from beat to beat
QRS duration:	0.11 second or less unless abnormally conducted

ECG Pearl

Be sure to commit the ECG characteristics of sinus rhythm to memory because the dysrhythmias discussed in this text relate to their similarities and differences compared with sinus rhythm.

Fig. 3.2 shows an example of a sinus rhythm recorded simultaneously in three leads: V_1, II, and V_5. As you look at this figure from left to right, note the 10-mm calibration marker that appears at the far left of each lead. Although we will focus on lead II as we examine this rhythm strip, you will find that it helps to view waveforms, segments, and intervals in more than one lead.

A sinus rhythm has a regular atrial and ventricular rhythm. Find the QRS complexes on the rhythm strip. Place one point of your calipers or make a mark on a piece of paper at the beginning of an R wave. Place the other point of the calipers or make a second mark on the paper at the beginning of the R wave of the next QRS complex. Without adjusting the calipers, evaluate each succeeding R-R interval. If you are using paper, lift the paper and move it across the rhythm strip. The R-R intervals in this example are regular. Because you have already identified the R waves, determine the ventricular rate. Because the rhythm is regular, calculate the rate using the small box method. There are 19 small boxes between R waves; therefore, the ventricular rate is about 79 beats/min. Remember, the built-in (i.e., intrinsic) rate for a rhythm that begins in the SA node is 60 to 100 beats/min; therefore, the rate of the rhythm in our example fits within the criteria for a sinus rhythm.

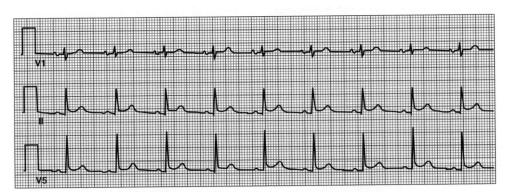

Fig. 3.2 Sinus rhythm at 79 beats/min with ST-segment elevation.

Now look to the left of the QRS complexes to find the P waves on the rhythm strip. A rhythm that begins in the SA node should have a positive (i.e., upright) P wave in lead II before each QRS complex (i.e., there should be a 1:1 relationship between P waves and QRS complexes). When you look at this rhythm strip, you can see one upright P wave before each QRS complex. Every P wave looks alike. Measure the P-P interval to see if the P waves occur regularly and then determine the atrial rate. You will find that the P waves occur regularly at a rate of 79 beats/min.

Now measure the PR interval and QRS duration. In a sinus rhythm, the PR interval measures 0.12 to 0.20 second and is constant from beat to beat. In this example, the PR interval is 0.16 second. The QRS complex usually measures 0.11 second or less. If there is a delay in conduction through the bundle branches, the QRS may be wide (i.e., greater than 0.11 second). In our example, the QRS measures between 0.04 and 0.08 second depending on the lead and complex selected for the measurement. Next, determine the QT interval by counting the number of small boxes between the beginning of the QRS complex and the end of the T wave and multiplying that number by 0.04 second. In our example, the QT interval measures about 8.5 boxes (0.34 second). This value is slightly less (shorter) than the normal value of 0.40 to 0.44 second.

Next, locate the TP segment and then the J point. Remember that deviation is measured as the number of millimeters of vertical ST-segment displacement from the J point (O'Gara et al., 2013). You will see that the ST segments in leads II and III of this rhythm strip are elevated. Now interpret the rhythm, specifying the origin (pacemaker site) of the rhythm and the ventricular rate. Because the rhythm shown in Fig. 3.2 fits the ECG criteria for a sinus rhythm, your interpretation should be sinus rhythm at 79 beats/min with ST-segment elevation (STE).

SINUS BRADYCARDIA

If the SA node fires at a rate slower than expected for the patient's age, the rhythm is called **sinus bradycardia**. The rhythm starts in the SA node and then travels the normal conduction pathway, resulting in atrial and ventricular depolarization. In adults and adolescents, sinus bradycardia has a heart rate of less than 60 beats/min. When seen in heart transplant recipients, bradycardia is sometimes defined as a heart rate that is persistently slower than 70 or 80 beats/min (Kusumoto et al., 2018). The term *severe sinus bradycardia* is sometimes used to describe sinus bradycardia with a rate of less than 40 beats/min. There is no set rate at which sinus bradycardia can be labeled pathologic (Berger et al., 2016).

How Do I Recognize It?

ECG characteristics of sinus bradycardia include the following:

Rhythm:	R-R and P-P intervals are regular
Rate:	Less than 60 beats/min
P waves:	Positive (upright) in lead II; one precedes each QRS complex; P waves look alike
PR interval:	0.12 to 0.20 second and constant from beat to beat
QRS duration:	0.11 second or less unless abnormally conducted

Fig. 3.3 is an example of sinus bradycardia. This rhythm's characteristics are the same as those of a sinus rhythm with one exception—the rate. A sinus rhythm rate is 60 to 100 beats/min; the sinus bradycardia rate is less than 60 beats/min.

Let's look at this rhythm strip using the same systematic format that you previously used. Begin by locating the QRS complexes on the rhythm strip. Evaluate each succeeding R-R interval. The R-R intervals in this example are regular. Now determine the ventricular rate. In this rhythm strip, the ventricular rate is 40 beats/min. Next, find the P waves on the rhythm strip. Remember that a rhythm that begins in the SA node should have a positive P wave (in lead II) before each QRS complex. In our example, you can see that there is a 1:1 relationship between P waves and QRS complexes, and every P wave looks alike. Now measure the P-to-P interval to see if the P waves occur regularly and determine the atrial rate. The P waves occur regularly at a rate of 40 beats/min. Next, measure the PR interval, QRS duration, and QT interval. In this example, the PR interval is 0.16 second, the QRS complex measures 0.08 second, and the QT interval is 0.40 second. ST-segment depression is present, and negative (i.e., inverted) T waves appear after each QRS complex. These findings must be noted in your final description of the rhythm. Therefore,

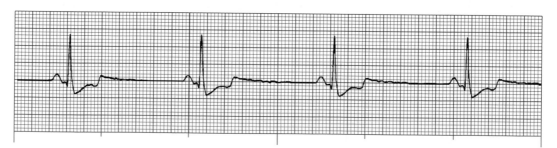

Fig. 3.3 Sinus bradycardia at 40 beats/min with ST-segment depression and inverted T waves.

the correct interpretation of this rhythm would be sinus bradycardia at 40 beats/min with ST-segment depression and inverted T waves.

⊙ ECG Pearl

In sinus bradycardia, the QT interval may be longer than expected because of the slower heart rate.

What Causes It?

Sinus bradycardia is the most common bradydysrhythmia encountered during sleep (Kusumoto et al., 2018). It is also common in well-conditioned athletes. Prolonged standing and stimulation of the vagus nerve can also result in heart rate slowing. For example, coughing, vomiting, straining to have a bowel movement, or sudden exposure of the face to cold water can slow the heart rate. In people who have a sensitive carotid sinus, heart rate slowing can occur when a tight collar is worn or with the impact of the stream of water on the neck while in the shower. Sinus bradycardia can also occur because of one or more medications a patient is taking. For example, a patient prescribed a beta-blocker for their hypertension may experience bradycardia. Other causes of sinus bradycardia include the following:

- Disease of the SA node
- Hyperkalemia
- Hypokalemia
- Hypothermia
- Hypothyroidism
- Hypoxia
- Increased intracranial pressure
- Inferior myocardial infarction (MI)
- Medications such as calcium blockers, digitalis, beta-blockers, amiodarone, and sotalol
- Obstructive sleep apnea
- Post heart transplant
- Posterior MI
- Tracheal suctioning
- Vagal stimulation

What Do I Do About It?

Remember that cardiac output equals stroke volume × heart rate. Therefore, a decrease in either stroke volume or heart rate may decrease cardiac output. Many patients tolerate a heart rate of 50 to 60 beats/min but become symptomatic when the rate drops below 50 beats/min. A patient with an unusually slow heart rate may complain of dizziness or lightheadedness, fatigue, weakness, or confusion resulting from decreased cerebral blood flow (Sidhu & Marine, 2020). Decreasing cardiac output will eventually produce hemodynamic compromise (Box 3.1).

⊙ ECG Pearl

Interventions and treatments discussed in this text assume that an assessment has been performed, the patient's clinical problem identified, and a physician order has been obtained when indicated. In the out-of-hospital setting, paramedics and nurses typically operate under standing physician orders, local

| Box **3.1** | Signs and Symptoms of Hemodynamic Compromise |

- Acute changes in mental status
- Chest pain or discomfort
- Cold, clammy skin
- Fall in urine output
- Heart failure
- Hypotension
- Pulmonary congestion
- Shortness of breath
- Signs of shock

protocols, or both. In the hospital setting, agency policy may permit standing orders to direct patient care when a patient's condition changes rapidly and requires immediate intervention. When performed by a clinician with appropriate training per that institution's policy, these orders may include routine therapies, monitoring guidelines, diagnostic procedures, and medication administration. Physician contact is necessary when standing orders or local protocols are unavailable.

If a patient presents with a bradycardia, assess how they are tolerating the rhythm. If the patient has no symptoms, no treatment is necessary. The term *symptomatic bradycardia* refers to signs and symptoms of hemodynamic compromise related to a slow heart rate. Treatment of symptomatic bradycardia should include assessing the patient's oxygen saturation level and determining if signs of increased breathing effort are present (e.g., retractions, tachypnea). Give supplemental oxygen if oxygenation is inadequate and assist breathing if ventilation is inadequate. Establish intravenous (IV) access and obtain a 12-lead ECG. Atropine, administered intravenously, is the drug of choice for symptomatic bradycardia. Reassess the patient's response and continue monitoring the patient.

Suppose symptomatic bradycardia develops because of one or more medications that a patient is taking. In that case, their provider may discontinue the drug and substitute another or reduce the dosage, reevaluate the patient's symptoms and rhythm, and decide the next steps based on their response. In the setting of an MI, sinus bradycardia is often transient. If the patient has no symptoms, a slow heart rate can be beneficial in a patient who has had an MI because the heart's demand for oxygen is less when the heart rate is slow.

⊙ ECG Pearl

Atropine is a drug used to increase the heart rate in a patient with symptomatic bradycardia. It works by blocking acetylcholine at the endings of the vagus nerves. The vagus nerves innervate the heart at the SA and AV nodes. Thus, atropine is most effective for narrow-QRS bradycardias. Atropine allows increased activity from the autonomic nervous system's sympathetic division by blocking acetylcholine's effects. As a result, the rate at which the SA node can fire is increased. Atropine also increases the rate at which an impulse is conducted through the AV node. Areas of the heart that are not innervated or minimally innervated by the vagus nerves (e.g., the ventricles) will not respond to atropine. Transplanted hearts do not usually respond to atropine because they lack vagal nerve innervation.

SINUS TACHYCARDIA

If the SA node fires at a rate faster than normal for the patient's age, the rhythm is called **sinus tachycardia**. Sinus tachycardia begins and ends gradually. The rhythm starts in the SA node and travels the normal pathway of conduction through the heart, resulting in atrial and ventricular depolarization.

How Do I Recognize It?

ECG characteristics of sinus tachycardia include the following:

Rhythm:	R-R and P-P intervals are regular
Rate:	Ventricular rate faster than 100 beats/ min with the maximum rate about 220 beats/min, minus the patient's age in years
P waves:	Positive (upright) in lead II; one precedes each QRS complex; P waves look alike
PR interval:	0.12 to 0.20 second and constant from beat to beat
QRS duration:	0.11 second or less unless abnormally conducted

Sinus tachycardia looks much like a sinus rhythm, except that it is faster. It may be hard to tell the difference between a P wave and a T wave at very fast rates. In adults, the ventricular rate associated with sinus tachycardia is faster than 100 beats/min, with the maximum rate of about 220 beats/ min, minus the patient's age in years. The ventricular rate is usually less than 220 beats/min in infants or 180 beats/min in children.

Fig. 3.4 is an example of sinus tachycardia. Let's look at this rhythm strip more closely. By glancing at the strip from left to right, you can see that the rate is faster than that of a sinus rhythm. Locate the QRS complexes, evaluate the R-R intervals, and then determine the ventricular rate. The R-R intervals in this example are regular, and the ventricular rate is 125 beats/min. The ventricular rate fits within the parameters of sinus tachycardia.

Look at the P waves on the rhythm strip, evaluate the P-P intervals for regularity, and determine the atrial rate.

One upright P wave appears before each QRS complex, every P wave looks alike, and the P waves occur regularly at a rate of 125 beats/min. Now measure the PR interval, QRS duration, and QT interval. In this example, the PR interval is 0.16 second, the QRS complex measures 0.06 second, and the QT interval is 0.32 second. (Remember that it is normal for the QT interval to shorten as the heart rate increases). Now interpret the rhythm, noting the ST-segment depression that is present. The correct interpretation is sinus tachycardia at 125 beats/min with ST-segment depression.

What Causes It?

Physiologic sinus tachycardia is a normal and transient response to the body's demand for increased oxygen. The patient is often aware of an increase in heart rate. Some patients complain of palpitations, a racing heart, or a feeling of pounding in their chests. Examples of conditions that can cause sinus tachycardia include the following:

- Acute myocardial infarction
- Anemia
- Anxiety, fear
- Caffeine-containing beverages
- Dehydration, hypovolemia
- Drugs such as cocaine, amphetamines, ecstasy, and cannabis
- Exercise
- Fever
- Heart failure
- Hyperthyroidism
- Hypoglycemia
- Hypoxia
- Infection
- Medications (e.g., epinephrine, atropine, dopamine)
- Nicotine
- Pain
- Panic attack
- Pericarditis
- Pneumothorax
- Postural changes
- Pregnancy
- Pulmonary edema
- Pulmonary embolism
- Sepsis
- Shock
- Sympathetic stimulation

In a patient with coronary artery disease (CAD), sinus tachycardia can cause problems. The heart's demand for oxygen increases as the heart rate increases. As the heart rate increases, there is less time for the ventricles to fill and less

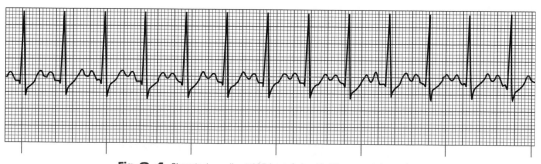

Fig. 3.4 Sinus tachycardia at 125 beats/min with ST-segment depression.

blood for the ventricles to pump out with each contraction, which can lead to decreased cardiac output. Recall that the coronary arteries fill when the ventricles are at rest. Therefore, rapid heart rates decrease the time available for coronary artery filling, decreasing the heart's blood supply. Chest discomfort can result if the supplies of blood and oxygen to the heart are inadequate. In a patient experiencing an acute MI, sinus tachycardia may be an early warning signal for heart failure, cardiogenic shock, and more serious dysrhythmias.

Whereas sinus tachycardia is an expected physiologic response to increased oxygen demand, inappropriate sinus tachycardia (IST) describes a sinus tachycardia that occurs for no apparent physiologic cause. For example, a person's heart rate may rapidly increase to more than 100 beats/min with minimal exertion, at rest, or both. Accompanying symptoms are usually nonspecific and include weakness, dizziness, fatigue, headache, shortness of breath, exercise intolerance, lightheadedness, chest discomfort, a racing heart, or palpitations. The mechanisms responsible for IST are not entirely understood, and a diagnosis is made only after other causes for the tachycardia have been ruled out (Yasin et al., 2018).

What Do I Do About It?

Treatment for physiologic sinus tachycardia is directed at correcting the underlying cause (i.e., fluid replacement, relief of pain, removal of offending medications or substances, reducing fever or anxiety). In a patient experiencing an acute MI, sinus tachycardia may be treated with medications to slow the heart rate and decrease myocardial oxygen demand (e.g., beta-blockers), provided there are no signs of heart failure or other contraindications.

Treatment of IST can be tricky. Lifestyle modifications are usually recommended, including decreasing caffeine and other stimulant intake, exercising regularly, and maintaining adequate hydration. Pharmacologic treatment with beta-blockers or calcium blockers, either alone or in combination, may be tried but are often ineffective, and symptoms can persist despite heart rate control. Ivabradine (Corlanor), a medication usually used to treat heart failure, has proved helpful in treating some IST patients. Surgical ablation may be performed in severe cases.

Some dysrhythmias with very rapid ventricular rates (i.e., above 150 beats/min) require the delivery of medications or a shock to stop the rhythm. However, it is essential to remember that shocking a sinus tachycardia is inappropriate; instead, treat the cause of the tachycardia.

SINUS ARRHYTHMIA

As you have seen so far, the SA node fires quite regularly most of the time. When it fires irregularly, the resulting rhythm is called **sinus arrhythmia**. Sinus arrhythmia begins in the SA node and follows the heart's normal conduction pathway, resulting in atrial and ventricular depolarization. A sinus arrhythmia usually occurs at a rate of 60 to 100 beats/min. Sinus arrhythmia associated with the phases of breathing and changes in intrathoracic pressure is called *respiratory sinus arrhythmia*. Sinus arrhythmia unrelated to the ventilatory cycle is called *nonrespiratory sinus arrhythmia*.

How Do I Recognize It?

Characteristics of sinus arrhythmia include the following:

Rhythm:	Irregular and often phasic with breathing; heart rate increases gradually during inspiration (R-R intervals shorten) and decreases with expiration (R-R intervals lengthen)
Rate:	Usually 60 to 100 beats/min
P waves:	Positive (upright) in lead II; one precedes each QRS complex; P waves look alike
PR interval:	0.12 to 0.20 second and constant from beat to beat
QRS duration:	0.11 second or less unless abnormally conducted

Let's look at the rhythm strip in Fig. 3.5. How does this rhythm differ from the others we have discussed so far? Without using calipers or a piece of paper, you can see that it is irregular. Recognizing that, the rhythm cannot be a sinus rhythm because a sinus rhythm is regular. Because the rhythm is irregular, we will use the 6-second method to calculate the rate, which is 70 beats/min. Looking closely at the rest of the rhythm strip, you can see one upright P wave

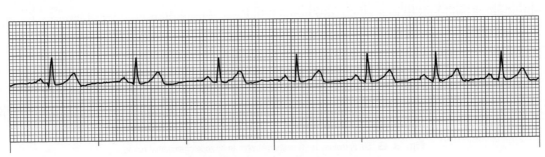

Fig. 3.5 Sinus arrhythmia at 70 beats/min.

before each QRS complex. Upon measuring the PR interval, the QRS duration, and the QT interval, you will find that they are within normal limits.

This rhythm strip was obtained from a 39-year-old man who was complaining of "feeling faint." If we were able to see the patient and watch his ventilatory rate and ECG at the same time, you would see a pattern. The patient's heart rate increases gradually during inspiration (i.e., the R-R intervals shorten) and decreases with expiration (i.e., the R-R intervals lengthen). We will identify this rhythm as a sinus arrhythmia at 70 beats/min.

What Causes It?

Respiratory sinus arrhythmia, which is the most common type of sinus arrhythmia, is a normal phenomenon that occurs with phases of breathing and changes in intrathoracic pressure. The heart rate increases with inspiration (i.e., the R-R intervals shorten) and decreases with expiration (i.e., the R-R intervals lengthen). The changes in rhythm disappear when patients hold their breath. Sinus arrhythmia is most commonly observed in children and young adults.

Nonrespiratory sinus arrhythmia can be seen in people with normal hearts, but it is more likely to be found in older individuals and those with heart disease. It is common after acute inferior wall MI, and it may be seen with increased intracranial pressure. Nonrespiratory sinus arrhythmia may result from the effects of medications (e.g., digitalis, morphine) or carotid sinus pressure.

What Do I Do About It?

Sinus arrhythmia usually does not require treatment unless accompanied by a slow heart rate that causes hemodynamic compromise. IV atropine may be indicated to treat the bradycardia if hemodynamic compromise is present because of the slow rate.

SINOATRIAL BLOCK

With SA block, also called sinus exit block, the SA node's pacemaker cells initiate an impulse, but it is blocked as it

exits the SA node, resulting in periodically absent PQRST complexes. SA block is thought to occur because of the failure of the transitional cells in the SA node to conduct the impulse from the pacemaker cells to the surrounding atrium. Thus, SA block is a disorder of impulse conduction.

How Do I Recognize It?

When an impulse is blocked as it exits the SA node, the atria are not activated. The lack of atrial activation appears on the ECG as a single missed beat (i.e., a P wave, QRS complex, and T wave are missing). The pause caused by the missed beat is the same as, or an exact multiple of, the distance between two P-P intervals of the underlying rhythm. ECG characteristics of SA block include the following:

Rhythm:	Irregular because of the pause(s) caused by the SA block—the pause is the same as, or an exact multiple of, the distance between two other P-P intervals
Rate:	Usually normal but varies because of the pause
P waves:	When present, positive (upright) in lead II; one precedes each QRS complex; P waves look alike
PR interval:	When present, 0.12 to 0.20 second and constant from beat to beat
QRS duration:	0.11 second or less unless abnormally conducted

Let's look at the example of SA block in Fig. 3.6. As you quickly scan the rhythm strip from left to right, the pause between the third and fourth beats is easily seen. The atrial and ventricular rhythm is irregular because of the pause. The rate is about 60 beats/min using the 6-second method of rate calculation. A positive P wave appears before each QRS complex, and the P waves look alike. The PR interval is 0.16 second and constant from beat to beat. The QRS complex measures 0.06 to 0.08 second, and the QT interval measures 0.32 to 0.36 second, which is within normal limits. Because the P waves are upright and each P wave is associated with a QRS complex, we know that the underlying rhythm came from the SA node. So far, we can identify

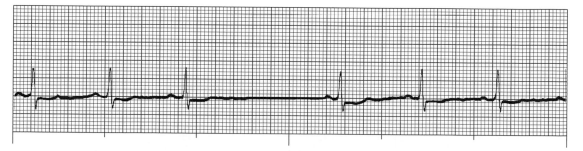

Fig. 3.6 Sinus rhythm at 60 beats/min with an episode of sinoatrial block.

this rhythm as a sinus rhythm with a ventricular rate of 60 beats/min.

Now we need to figure out what caused the pause between beats 3 and 4. First, look to the left of the pause and examine the waveforms of the beat that comes before the pause. Compare these waveforms with the others in the rhythm strip. It is essential to do this because sometimes waveforms hide on top of other waveforms, distorting their shape. In our example, nothing seems to be amiss. Now use your calipers or paper and plot P waves and R waves from left to right across the strip. When you do this, mark the rhythm strip where the next PQRST cycle should have occurred. You will find that precisely one PQRST cycle is missing. The P-P interval is an exact multiple of the distance between two P-P intervals of the underlying sinus rhythm. Although the SA node's pacemaking cells generated impulses regularly, the SA node's transitional cells failed to transmit the impulse (as seen between beats 3 and 4). To complete our interpretation of this rhythm, we will explain the pause as an SA block. Putting it all together, we have a sinus rhythm at a rate of 60 beats/min with an episode of SA block.

What Causes It?

SA block is rather uncommon. Possible causes of SA block include hypoxia, damage or disease to the SA node from CAD, myocarditis, or acute MI; carotid sinus sensitivity; increased vagal tone on the SA node; and medications (e.g., digitalis, quinidine, procainamide, salicylates). If episodes of SA block are frequent and accompanied by a slow heart rate, the patient may show signs of hemodynamic compromise.

What Do I Do About It?

Signs and symptoms associated with SA block depend on the number of sinus beats blocked. If the SA block episodes are transient and there are no significant signs or symptoms, the patient is observed. If signs of hemodynamic compromise are present and result from medication toxicity, the offending agents should be withheld. If the SA block episodes are frequent, IV atropine, temporary pacing, or insertion of a permanent pacemaker may be needed.

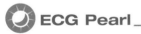 **ECG Pearl** _____

Sick sinus syndrome (SSS), also called sinus node dysfunction, is a dysrhythmia that most commonly affects adults over age 70 years and is usually related to degenerative SA node tissue changes. The effects of medications, inflammatory diseases of the heart, muscular dystrophy, and heart disease are possible causes. On the ECG, SSS can appear as alternating patterns of bradycardia and tachycardia (bradycardia-tachycardia syndrome) or skipped beats caused by episodes of SA block or sinus arrest. Patients may be asymptomatic, have

subtle or nonspecific symptoms, or experience syncope, dizziness or lightheadedness, palpitations, or confusion. Chest discomfort, shortness of breath, or fatigue may occur during exercise. Diagnosis of SSS usually requires Holter monitoring or the use of an event recorder. Electrophysiologic testing may be performed if SSS is suspected, and monitoring devices do not capture ECG evidence of it.

Placement of a permanent dual-chamber pacemaker may be necessary to relieve symptoms and restore a regular cardiac rhythm.

SINUS ARREST

Sinus arrest, also called sinus pause or SA arrest, is a disorder of impulse formation. With sinus arrest, the SA node's pacemaker cells do not initiate an electrical impulse for one or more beats, resulting in absent PQRST complexes on the ECG.

When the SA node fails to initiate an impulse, an escape pacemaker site (i.e., the AV junction or the Purkinje fibers) should kick in and assume responsibility for pacing the heart. The term *junctional* denotes a beat or rhythm originating at the AV junction. Therefore, when the SA node does not fire and an escape pacemaker kicks in, the pause associated with a sinus arrest may be terminated by a junctional or ventricular escape beat. If an escape pacemaker site does not fire, you will see absent PQRST complexes on the ECG.

How Do I Recognize It?

ECG characteristics of sinus arrest include the following:

Rhythm:	Irregular; the pause is of undetermined length, more than one PQRST complex is missing, and it is not the same distance as other P-P intervals
Rate:	Usually normal but varies because of the pause
P waves:	When present, positive (upright) in lead II; one precedes each QRS complex; P waves look alike
PR interval:	When present, 0.12 to 0.20 second and constant from beat to beat
QRS duration:	0.11 second or less unless abnormally conducted

An example of sinus arrest is shown in Fig. 3.7. Looking at the rhythm strip from left to right, you can see a period of no electrical activity between the third and fourth beats. Begin analyzing the rhythm strip by determining the atrial and ventricular rhythmicity and rate. The rate is about 60 beats/min using the 6-second rate calculation method because the rhythm is irregular.

You can see a positive P wave in front of each QRS complex. The P waves look alike. The PR interval is 0.20 second and constant from beat to beat. The QRS complex is 0.10 second,

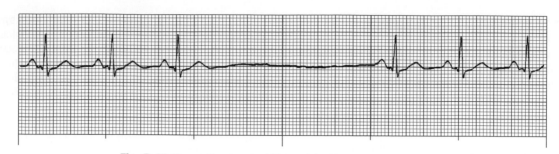

Fig. 3.7 Sinus rhythm at a rate of 60 beats/min with an episode of sinus arrest.

and the QT interval is 0.36 second. Because the P waves are upright and each P wave is associated with a QRS complex, we know that the underlying rhythm came from the SA node.

Now let's try to explain what caused the pause between beats 3 and 4. Look to the left of the pause and examine the waveforms of the beat that comes before the pause. Compare these waveforms with the others in the rhythm strip. There does not appear to be any distortion of the waveforms. Plot P waves and R waves from left to right across the strip using your calipers or paper. When you do this, mark the rhythm strip where the next PQRST cycles should have occurred. You will find that more than one PQRST cycle is missing. Because the SA node periodically failed to produce impulses, the P-P intervals are not exact multiples of other P-P intervals, characteristic of a sinus arrest. To complete our interpretation of this rhythm strip, we must add this explanation for the pause we saw; therefore, our final interpretation is a sinus rhythm at a rate of 60 beats/min with an episode of sinus arrest.

What Causes It?

Causes of sinus arrest include damage to or disease of the SA node from CAD, acute MI, or rheumatic disease; carotid sinus pressure, a sudden increase in parasympathetic activity on the SA node, stimulation of the pharynx, obstructive sleep apnea, hypothermia, and effects of medications such as beta-blockers and calcium blockers. Studies have shown that 2-second periods of sinus arrest have been seen during 24-hour ambulatory ECG monitoring in healthy older adults and 3-second periods in long-distance runners (Kusumoto et al., 2018). In addition to sinus bradycardia, SA block and sinus arrest may occasionally occur during sleep (particularly in the young and in conditioned athletes), are usually asymptomatic events, and generally require no intervention (Kusumoto et al., 2018).

What Do I Do About It?

Signs and symptoms associated with sinus arrest depend on the number of absent sinus beats and the length of the sinus arrest because there is no cardiac output during the period of arrest. Symptoms may occur abruptly and include weakness, lightheadedness, dizziness, or syncope. If the episodes of sinus arrest are transient and there are no significant signs or symptoms, observe the patient. If signs and symptoms result from carotid sinus sensitivity and resultant vagal stimulation, remove tight clothing, if applicable. If hemodynamic compromise is present, IV atropine, temporary pacing, or both may be indicated. If the episodes of sinus arrest are frequent and prolonged (i.e., more than 3 seconds) or a result of SA node disease, permanent pacemaker insertion is generally warranted. A summary of the characteristics of sinus mechanisms can be found in Table 3.1.

TABLE **3.1**	Sinus Mechanisms: Summary of Characteristics				
Dysrhythmia	Rhythm	Rate (beats/min)	P Waves (Lead II)	PR Interval	QRS Duration
Sinus rhythm	R-R and P-P intervals are regular	60 to 100	Positive; one precedes each QRS; P waves look alike	0.12 to 0.20 sec and constant from beat to beat	0.11 sec or less unless abnormally conducted
Sinus bradycardia	R-R and P-P intervals are regular	Less than 60	Positive; one precedes each QRS; P waves look alike	0.12 to 0.20 sec and constant from beat to beat	0.11 sec or less unless abnormally conducted
Sinus tachycardia	R-R and P-P intervals are regular	Faster than 100; maximum rate about 220 minus the patient's age in years	Positive; one precedes each QRS; P waves look alike	0.12 to 0.20 sec and constant from beat to beat	0.11 sec or less unless abnormally conducted
Sinus arrhythmia	Irregular and often phasic with breathing	Usually 60 to 100	Positive; one precedes each QRS; P waves look alike	0.12 to 0.20 sec and constant from beat to beat	0.11 sec or less unless abnormally conducted
Sinoatrial (SA) block	Irregular; the pause is the same as, or an exact multiple of, the distance between two other P-P intervals	Usually normal but varies because of the pause	When present, positive in lead II; one precedes each QRS complex; P waves look alike	When present, 0.12 to 0.20 sec and constant from beat to beat	0.11 sec or less unless abnormally conducted
Sinus arrest	Irregular; the pause is of undetermined length, more than one PQRST complex is missing, and it is not the same distance as other P-P intervals	Usually normal but varies because of the pause	When present, positive in lead II; one precedes each QRS complex; P waves look alike	When present, 0.12 to 0.20 sec and constant from beat to beat	0.11 sec or less unless abnormally conducted

REFERENCES

Berger, M. G., Rubenstein, J. C., & Roth, J. A. (2016). Cardiac arrhythmias. In I. J. Benjamin, R. C. Griggs, E. J. Wing, & J. G. Fitz (Eds.), *Andreoli & Carpenter's Cecil essentials of medicine* (9th ed.) (pp. 110–135). Philadelphia, PA: Saunders.

Kusumoto, F. M., Schoenfeld, M. H., Barrett, C., Edgerton, J. R., Ellenbogen, K. A., Gold, M. R., . . . Varosy, P. D. (2018). 2018 ACC/AHA/HRS guideline on the evaluation and management of patients with bradycardia and cardiac conduction delay. *Circulation, 140*(8), e382–e482.

O'Gara, P. T., Kushner, F. G., Ascheim, D. D., Casey Jr., D. E., Chung, M. K., de Lemos, J. A., ... Zhao, D. X. (2013). 2013 ACCF/AHA guideline for the management of ST-elevation myocardial infarction. *J Am Coll Cardiol, 61*(4), e78–e140.

Olshansky, B., & Sullivan, R. M. (2019). Inappropriate sinus tachycardia. *Europace, 21*(2), 194–207.

Sidhu, S., & Marine, J. E. (2020). Evaluating and managing bradycardia. *Trends Cardiovasc Med, 30*(5), 265–272.

Yasin, O. Z., Vaidya, V. R., Chacko, S. R., & Asirvatham, S. J. (2018). Inappropriate sinus tachycardia: current challenges and future directions. *J Innov Cardiac Rhythm Manage, 9*(7), 3239–3243.

STOP & REVIEW

Identify one or more choices that best complete the statement or answer the question.

1. Characteristics of rhythms that begin in the SA node include which of the following?
   a. P waves that look alike
   b. A constant PR interval
   c. A QRS duration of 0.10 second or longer
   d. A positive P wave before each QRS complex
   e. A regular atrial and ventricular rhythm (usually)

2. Which of the following are possible causes of sinus tachycardia?
   a. Pain
   b. Fever
   c. Exercise
   d. Beta-blockers, digitalis
   e. Obstructive sleep apnea
   f. Increased intracranial pressure

3. A lead II rhythm strip obtained from a 38-year-old woman with difficulty breathing reveals a regular atrial and ventricular rhythm, a ventricular rate of 120 beats/min, an upright P wave before each QRS complex, and a normal PR interval and QRS duration. This rhythm is
   a. sinus rhythm.
   b. sinus arrhythmia.
   c. sinus tachycardia.
   d. sinoatrial (SA) block.

4. Which of the following dysrhythmias is/are associated with one or more absent PQRST complexes?
   a. SA block
   b. Sinus arrest
   c. Sinus rhythm
   d. Sinus arrhythmia
   e. Sinus tachycardia
   f. Sinus bradycardia

5. Which of the following is true regarding respiratory sinus arrhythmia?
   a. Every other electrical impulse is blocked as it leaves the SA node.
   b. This rhythm is often associated with heart failure symptoms and dizziness.
   c. This rhythm is typically the result of degenerative changes in SA node tissue.
   d. The rhythm is irregular because the heart rate increases with inspiration and decreases with expiration.

6. A 35-year-old man has been experiencing nausea, vomiting, and diarrhea for the past 48 hours. His blood pressure is 112/70 mm Hg. The cardiac monitor reveals a sinus tachycardia at 124 beats/min. Management of this patient's dysrhythmia should include
   a. administering atropine.
   b. preparing for temporary pacing.
   c. replacing fluids and electrolytes.
   d. scheduling the patient for surgical ablation.

7. A lead II rhythm strip reveals a regular atrial and ventricular rhythm, a ventricular rate of 46 beats/min, an upright P wave before each QRS complex, a PR interval of 0.16 second, and a QRS duration of 0.08 second. This rhythm is
   a. sinus rhythm.
   b. sinoatrial block.
   c. sinus arrhythmia.
   d. sinus bradycardia.

8. SA block is a disorder of ____, whereas sinus arrest is a disorder of ____.
   a. impulse formation, impulse conduction
   b. impulse conduction, impulse formation

9. Differentiating between a P wave and T wave is most likely to be difficult with which of the following rhythms?
   a. SA block
   b. Sinus arrest
   c. Sinus tachycardia
   d. Sinus bradycardia

Questions 10 Through 17 Pertain to the Following Scenario

A 75-year-old man presents with weakness and "feeling lightheaded." His symptoms began about 30 minutes ago.

10. The patient's blood pressure is 75/40 mm Hg, pulse 44 beats/min, and ventilations 16. A bradycardia is present when the heart rate is less than
    a. 60 beats/min.
    b. 75 beats/min.
    c. 85 beats/min.
    d. 100 beats/min.

11. You prepare to apply electrodes and lead wires to the patient for continuous ECG monitoring in lead II. Lead II views the
    a. lateral surface of the left ventricle.
    b. inferior surface of the left ventricle.
    c. anterior surface of the left ventricle.
    d. posterior surface of the right ventricle.

12. You are examining the waveforms on this patient's ECG. What is the name given to the first negative deflection observed after the P wave?
    a. Q wave
    b. R wave
    c. S wave
    d. T wave

13. As you measure the intervals on this patient's rhythm strip, you recall that the PR interval's normal duration is _____ second.
    a. 0.04 to 0.10
    b. 0.06 to 0.14
    c. 0.12 to 0.20
    d. 0.16 to 0.24

14. Analysis of the patient's ECG reveals ST-segment depression in lead II. The presence of ST-segment depression suggests
    a. myocardial injury.
    b. myocardial ischemia.
    c. death of a portion of the left ventricular tissue.
    d. death of a portion of the cardiac conduction system.

15. For the ST-segment depression seen in lead II to be considered clinically significant, this finding would also need to be seen in which of the following anatomically contiguous leads?
    a. I or III
    b. I or aVL
    c. V_3 or V_4
    d. III or aVF

16. Supplemental oxygen is being administered because the patient's oxygen saturation level was 89% on room air. The patient reports that he continues to feel weak and lightheaded. The cardiac monitor continues to display sinus bradycardia and a second set of vital signs are essentially unchanged. Which of the following statements is true about this patient situation?
    a. The patient is asymptomatic.
    b. A 12-lead ECG should be obtained.
    c. Vascular access should be established.
    d. The patient is showing signs of hemodynamic compromise.
    e. Continuous observation is the only intervention necessary at this time.

17. The patient's symptoms persist, and his vital signs are essentially unchanged. The cardiac monitor shows a sinus bradycardia with ST-segment depression. You should prepare to administer
    a. atropine.
    b. atenolol.
    c. adenosine.
    d. amiodarone.

Short Answer

18. Fill in the blank areas in the following table.

Dysrhythmia	Rhythm	Rate (beats/min)	P waves
Sinus bradycardia	Regular		Positive; one precedes each QRS; P waves look alike
Sinus tachycardia			
Sinus arrhythmia			Positive; one precedes each QRS; P waves look alike
SA block			
Sinus arrest			

Sinus Mechanisms—Practice Rhythm Strips

Use the five steps of rhythm interpretation discussed in Chapter 2 to interpret each of the following rhythm strips. All rhythms were recorded in lead II unless otherwise noted.

19. Identify the rhythm.

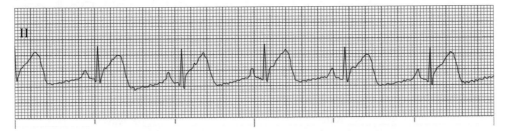

Fig. 3.8 (From Aehlert, B. (2004). *ECG study cards.* St. Louis: Mosby.)

Rhythm: _____ Rate: _____ P waves: _____
PR interval: _____ QRS duration: _____ QT interval: _____
Interpretation: _____

20. Identify the rhythm.

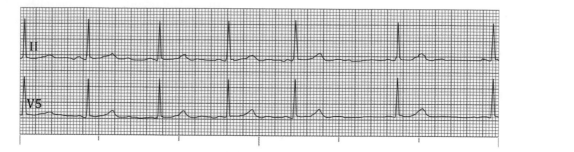

Fig. 3.9

Rhythm: _____ Rate: _____ P waves: _____
PR interval: _____ QRS duration: _____ QT interval: _____
Interpretation: _____

21. Lead I.

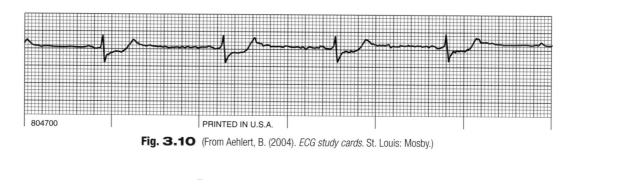

804700   PRINTED IN U.S.A.

Fig. 3.10 (From Aehlert, B. (2004). *ECG study cards.* St. Louis: Mosby.)

Rhythm: _____ Rate: _____ P waves: _____
PR interval: _____ QRS duration: _____ QT interval: _____
Interpretation: _____

22. This rhythm strip is from a 90-year-old woman with difficulty breathing.

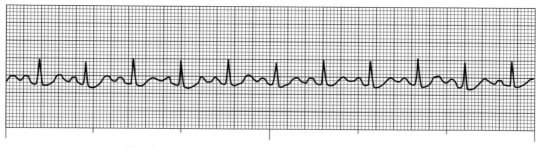

Fig. 3.11 (From Aehlert, B. (2004). *ECG study cards.* St. Louis: Mosby.)

Rhythm: _____ Rate: _____ P waves: _____
PR interval: _____ QRS duration: _____ QT interval: _____
Interpretation: _____

23. This rhythm strip is from a 73-year-old man complaining of chest pain. He has a history of hypertension and lung disease.

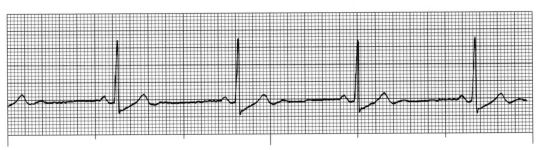

Fig. 3.12 (From Aehlert, B. (2004). *ECG study cards.* St. Louis: Mosby.)

Rhythm: _____ Rate: _____ P waves: _____
PR interval: _____ QRS duration: _____ QT interval: _____
Interpretation: _____

24. Identify the rhythm.

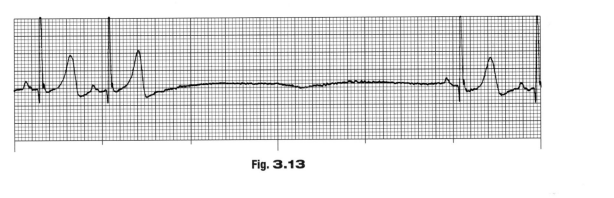

Fig. 3.13

Rhythm: _____ Rate: _____ P waves: _____
PR interval: _____ QRS duration: _____ QT interval: _____
Interpretation: _____

25. This rhythm strip is from a 57-year-old man with chest pain.

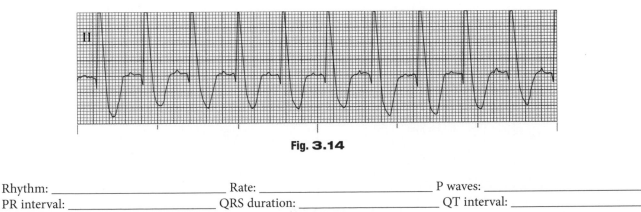

Fig. 3.14

Rhythm: _____ Rate: _____ P waves: _____
PR interval: _____ QRS duration: _____ QT interval: _____
Interpretation: _____

26. Identify the rhythm.

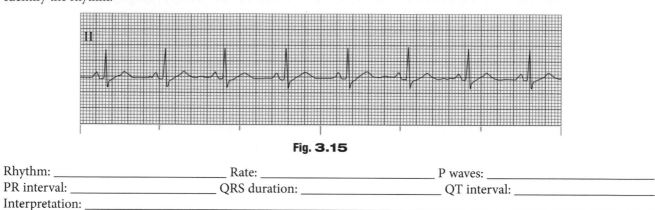

Fig. 3.15

Rhythm: _____ Rate: _____ P waves: _____
PR interval: _____ QRS duration: _____ QT interval: _____
Interpretation: _____

27. This rhythm strip is from a 4-month-old infant who reportedly ingested an oral pain reliever.

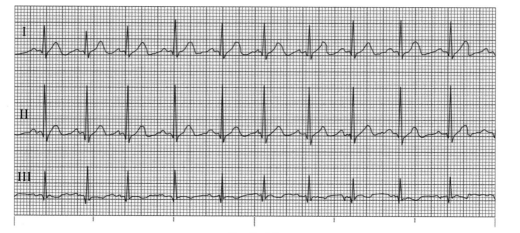

Fig. 3.16

Rhythm: _____ Rate: _____ P waves: _____
PR interval: _____ QRS duration: _____ QT interval: _____
Interpretation: _____

28. Identify the rhythm.

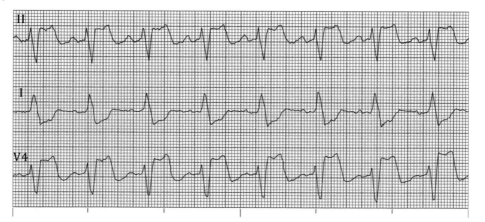

Fig. 3.17

Rhythm: _____ Rate: _____ P waves: _____
PR interval: _____ QRS duration: _____ QT interval: _____
Interpretation: _____

29. This rhythm strip is from a 40-year-old man complaining of back pain after jumping from a burning second-floor balcony.

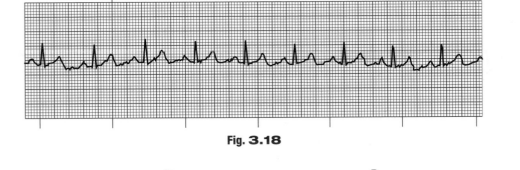

Fig. 3.18

Rhythm: _____ Rate: _____ P waves: _____
PR interval: _____ QRS duration: _____ QT interval: _____
Interpretation: _____

30. These rhythm strips are from a 44-year-old woman with chest pain.

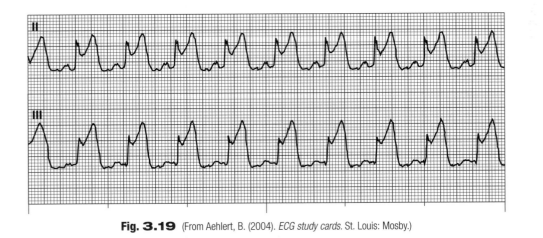

Fig. 3.19 (From Aehlert, B. (2004). *ECG study cards.* St. Louis: Mosby.)

Rhythm: _____ Rate: _____ P waves: _____
PR interval: _____ QRS duration: _____ QT interval: _____
Interpretation: _____

31. This rhythm strip is from a 6-year-old girl complaining of abdominal pain.

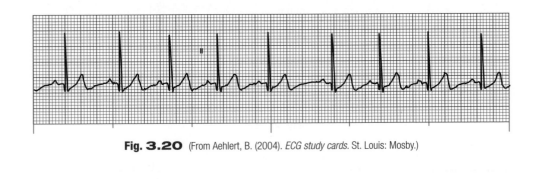

Fig. 3.20 (From Aehlert, B. (2004). *ECG study cards.* St. Louis: Mosby.)

Rhythm: _____ Rate: _____ P waves: _____
PR interval: _____ QRS duration: _____ QT interval: _____
Interpretation: _____

32. Identify the rhythm.

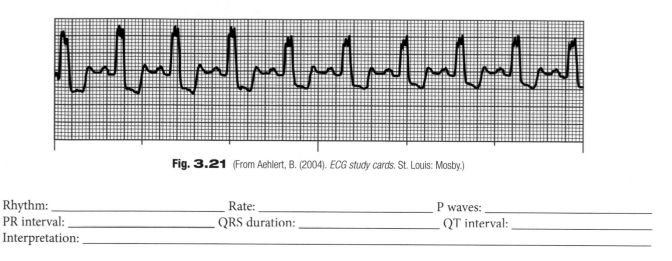

Fig. 3.21 (From Aehlert, B. (2004). *ECG study cards.* St. Louis: Mosby.)

Rhythm: _____ Rate: _____ P waves: _____
PR interval: _____ QRS duration: _____ QT interval: _____
Interpretation: _____

33. This rhythm strip is from a 24-year-old woman complaining of weakness and fatigue.

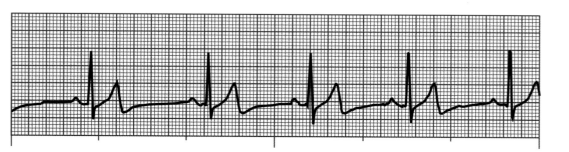

Fig. 3.22 (From Aehlert, B. (2004). *ECG study cards.* St. Louis: Mosby.)

Rhythm: _____ Rate: _____ P waves: _____
PR interval: _____ QRS duration: _____ QT interval: _____
Interpretation: _____

34. Identify the rhythm.

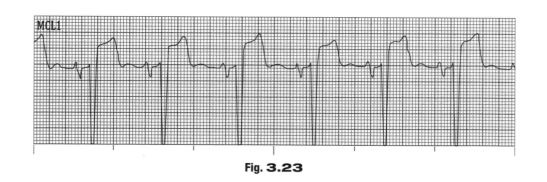

Fig. 3.23

Rhythm: _____ Rate: _____ P waves: _____
PR interval: _____ QRS duration: _____ QT interval: _____
Interpretation: _____

35. This rhythm strip is from a 29-year-old woman with a kidney stone.

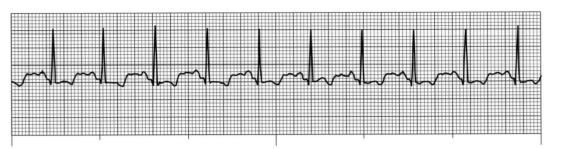

Fig. 3.24 (From Aehlert, B. (2004). *ECG study cards.* St. Louis: Mosby.)

Rhythm: _____ Rate: _____ P waves: _____
PR interval: _____ QRS duration: _____ QT interval: _____
Interpretation: _____

36. Identify the rhythm.

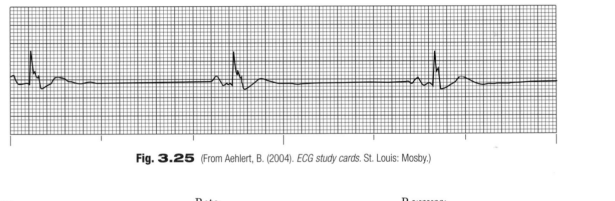

Fig. 3.25 (From Aehlert, B. (2004). *ECG study cards.* St. Louis: Mosby.)

Rhythm: _____ Rate: _____ P waves: _____
PR interval: _____ QRS duration: _____ QT interval: _____
Interpretation: _____

37. This rhythm strip is from a 53-year-old man with chest pain.

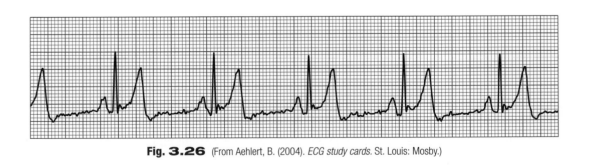

Fig. 3.26 (From Aehlert, B. (2004). *ECG study cards.* St. Louis: Mosby.)

Rhythm: _____ Rate: _____ P waves: _____
PR interval: _____ QRS duration: _____ QT interval: _____
Interpretation: _____

38. This rhythm strip is from a 62-year-old man complaining of chest pain.

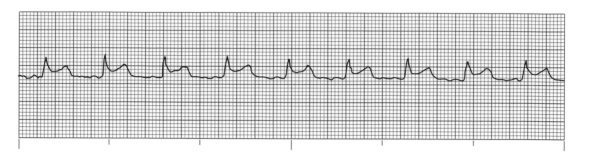

Fig. 3.27 (From Aehlert, B. (2004). *ECG study cards.* St. Louis: Mosby.)

Rhythm: _____ Rate: _____ P waves: _____
PR interval: _____ QRS duration: _____ QT interval: _____
Interpretation: _____

39. This rhythm strip is from an 8-month-old infant after a seizure.

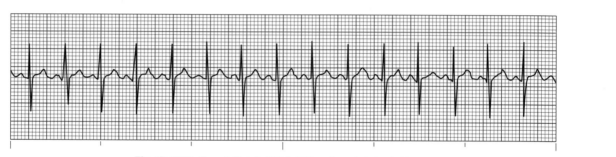

Fig. 3.28 (From Aehlert, B. (2004). *ECG study cards.* St. Louis: Mosby.)

Rhythm: _____ Rate: _____ P waves: _____
PR interval: _____ QRS duration: _____ QT interval: _____
Interpretation: _____

40. This rhythm strip is from a 33-year-old woman complaining of abdominal pain.

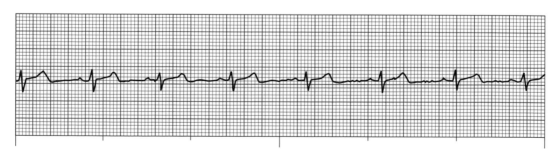

Fig. 3.29 (From Aehlert, B. (2004). *ECG study cards.* St. Louis: Mosby.)

Rhythm: _____ Rate: _____ P waves: _____
PR interval: _____ QRS duration: _____ QT interval: _____
Interpretation: _____

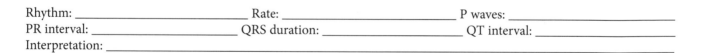
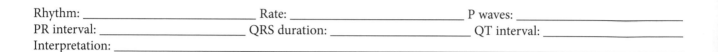

41. Identify the rhythm.

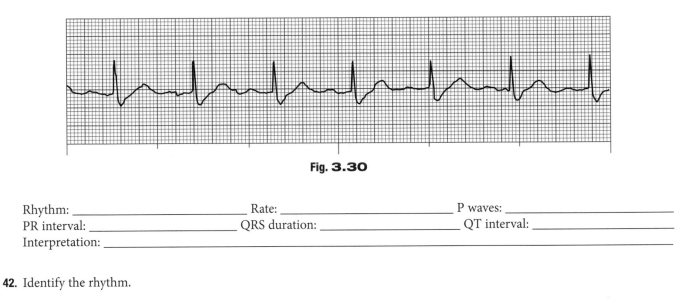

Fig. 3.30

Rhythm: _____ Rate: _____ P waves: _____
PR interval: _____ QRS duration: _____ QT interval: _____
Interpretation: _____

42. Identify the rhythm.

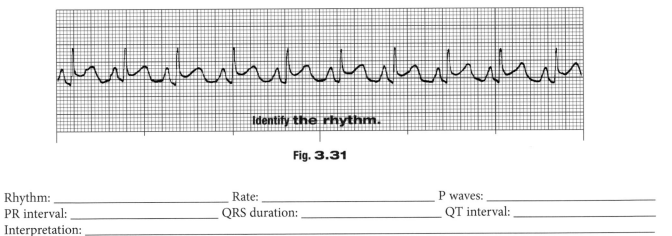

Identify the rhythm.

Fig. 3.31

Rhythm: _____ Rate: _____ P waves: _____
PR interval: _____ QRS duration: _____ QT interval: _____
Interpretation: _____

43. This rhythm strip is from a 37-year-old asymptomatic man.

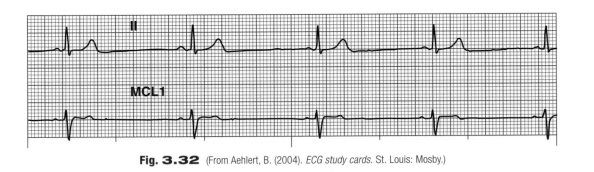

Fig. 3.32 (From Aehlert, B. (2004). *ECG study cards.* St. Louis: Mosby.)

Rhythm: _____ Rate: _____ P waves: _____
PR interval: _____ QRS duration: _____ QT interval: _____
Interpretation: _____

44. Identify the rhythm.

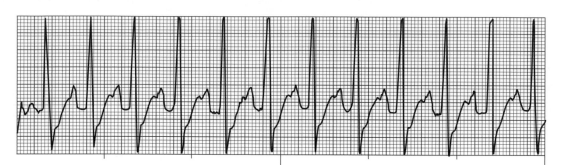

Fig. 3.33 (From Aehlert, B. (2004). *ECG study cards.* St. Louis: Mosby.

Rhythm: _____ Rate: _____ P waves: _____
PR interval: _____ QRS duration: _____ QT interval: _____
Interpretation: _____

45. This rhythm strip is from a 44-year-old construction worker with a sudden onset of chest pressure.

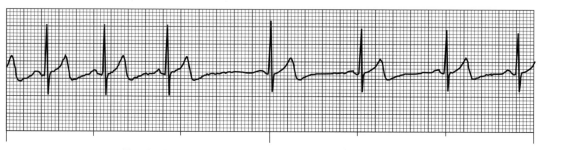

Fig. 3.34 (From Aehlert, B. (2004). *ECG study cards.* St. Louis: Mosby.)

Rhythm: _____ Rate: _____ P waves: _____
PR interval: _____ QRS duration: _____ QT interval: _____
Interpretation: _____

46. This rhythm strip is from an 85-year-old woman complaining of numbness in her legs.

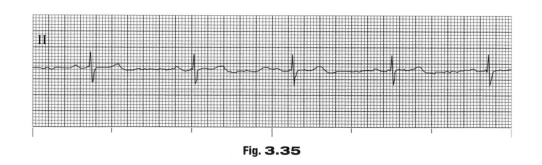

Fig. 3.35

Rhythm: _____ Rate: _____ P waves: _____
PR interval: _____ QRS duration: _____ QT interval: _____
Interpretation: _____

STOP & REVIEW ANSWERS

Multiple Choice Response

1. **A, B, D, E.** A rhythm that begins in the SA node has the following characteristics:
   - A positive (i.e., upright) P wave before each QRS complex
   - P waves that look alike
   - A constant PR interval
   - A regular atrial and ventricular rhythm (usually)

2. **A, B, C.** There are many causes of sinus tachycardia including pain, fever, and exercise. Medications such as calcium blockers, digitalis, beta-blockers, amiodarone, and sotalol, obstructive sleep apnea, and increased intracranial pressure are possible causes of sinus bradycardia.

3. **C.** A sinus tachycardia is differentiated from other rhythms that originate in the SA node by its rate (faster than 100 beats/min; maximum rate about 220 minus the patient's age in years).

4. **A, B.** Sinus arrest and SA block are associated with one or more absent PQRST complexes.

5. **D.** Respiratory sinus arrhythmia, which is the most common type of sinus arrhythmia, is a normal phenomenon that occurs with phases of breathing and changes in intrathoracic pressure. The heart rate increases with inspiration (i.e., the R-R intervals shorten) and decreases with expiration (i.e., the R-R intervals lengthen). Sinus arrhythmia is most commonly observed in children and young adults.

6. **C.** Based on the information provided, the most likely cause of the patient's sinus tachycardia is dehydration/hypovolemia, which is best managed by replacing fluids and electrolytes.

7. **D.** A sinus bradycardia's characteristics are the same as those of a sinus rhythm with one exception—the rate. A sinus rhythm rate is 60 to 100 beats/min; the sinus bradycardia rate is less than 60 beats/min.

8. **B.** With SA block, the SA node's pacemaker cells initiate an impulse, but it is blocked as it exits the SA node, resulting in periodically absent PQRST complexes. SA block is thought to occur because of the failure of the transitional cells in the SA node to conduct the impulse from the pacemaker cells to the surrounding atrium. Thus, SA block is a disorder of impulse *conduction*. With sinus arrest, the SA node's pacemaker cells fail to initiate an electrical impulse for one or more beats, resulting in absent PQRST complexes on the ECG. Thus, sinus arrest is a disorder of impulse *formation*.

9. **C.** With sinus tachycardia, it may be hard to tell the difference between a P wave and a T wave at very fast rates.

10. **A.** In adults, a bradycardia exists if the rate is less than 60 beats/min.

11. **B.** Lead II views the inferior surface of the left ventricle.

12. **A.** A QRS complex normally follows each P wave. The QRS complex begins as a downward deflection, the *Q wave*, and represents depolarization of the interventricular septum.

13. **C.** The PR interval changes with heart rate but typically measures 0.12 to 0.20 second in adults. As the heart rate increases, the duration of the PR interval shortens. A PR interval is considered *short* if it is less than 0.12 second and *long* if it is more than 0.20 second.

14. **B.** ST-segment depression of 0.5 mm or more in a patient experiencing an acute coronary syndrome is suggestive of myocardial ischemia.

15. **D.** For the ST-segment depression seen in lead II to be considered clinically significant, this finding would also need to be seen in lead III or aVF. Leads II, III, and aVF view the inferior wall of the left ventricle.

16. **B, C, D.** The term *symptomatic bradycardia* is used to describe a patient who experiences signs and symptoms of hemodynamic compromise related to a slow heart rate. Because this patient is complaining of weakness and lightheadedness and is hypotensive, he is clearly symptomatic with his slow heart rate. Treatment of symptomatic bradycardia should include applying a pulse oximeter and administering supplemental oxygen if indicated, which have already been done. Next, establish IV access and obtain a 12-lead ECG.

17. **A.** Atropine, administered intravenously, is the drug of choice for symptomatic bradycardia. Reassess the patient's response to the therapeutic interventions provided and continue monitoring the patient. Adenosine is used to slow the ventricular rate. Atenolol, a beta-blocker, would further slow the heart rate. Although amiodarone is an antiarrhythmic used to treat many atrial and ventricular dysrhythmias, it is not used to treat a sinus bradycardia.

Short Answer

18.

Dysrhythmia	Rhythm	Rate (beats/min)	P Waves
Sinus bradycardia	Regular	Less than 60	Positive; one precedes each QRS; P waves look alike
Sinus tachycardia	Regular	Faster than 100; maximum rate about 220 minus the patient's age in years	Positive; one precedes each QRS; P waves look alike
Sinus arrhythmia	Irregular and often phasic with breathing	Usually 60 to 100	Positive; one precedes each QRS; P waves look alike
SA block	Irregular; the pause is the same as, or an exact multiple of, the distance between two other P-P intervals	Usually normal but varies because of the pause	When present, positive in lead II; one precedes each QRS complex; P waves look alike
Sinus arrest	Irregular; the pause is of undetermined length, more than one PQRST complex is missing, and it is not the same distance as other P-P intervals	Usually normal but varies because of the pause	When present, positive in lead II; one precedes each QRS complex; P waves look alike

Sinus Mechanisms—Practice Rhythm Strip Answers

Note: The rate and interval measurements provided here were obtained using electronic calipers.

19. Fig. 3.8
Rhythm: Regular
Rate: 58 beats/min
P waves: Positive; one precedes each QRS
PR interval: 0.17 second
QRS duration: 0.06 second
QT interval: 0.38 second
Interpretation: Sinus bradycardia at 58 beats/min with ST-segment elevation (STE), baseline artifact is present

20. Fig. 3.9
Rhythm: Irregular
Rate: 70 beats/min
P waves: Positive; one precedes each QRS
PR interval: 0.12 to 0.14 second
QRS duration: 0.04 to 0.06 second
QT interval: 0.37 second
Interpretation: Sinus arrhythmia at 70 beats/min

21. Fig. 3.10
Rhythm: Irregular
Rate: 43 to 47 beats/min
P waves: Positive; one precedes each QRS
PR interval: 0.16 second
QRS duration: 0.06 second
QT interval: 0.40 to 0.42 second
Interpretation: Sinus bradydysrhythmia at 43 to 47 beats/min with ST-segment depression, baseline artifact is present

22. Fig. 3.11
Rhythm: Regular
Rate 112 beats/min
P waves: Positive; one precedes each QRS
PR interval: 0.16 second
QRS duration: 0.06 second
QT interval: 0.30 to 0.34 second
Interpretation: Sinus tachycardia at 112 beats/min with ST-segment depression

23. Fig. 3.12
Rhythm: Regular
Rate: 44 beats/min
P waves: Positive; one precedes each QRS
PR interval: 0.16 second
QRS duration: 0.06 second
QT interval: 0.38 to 0.40 second
Interpretation: Sinus bradycardia at 44 beats/min, ST-segment depression, baseline artifact is present. Note the upright U waves after each T wave.

24. Fig. 3.13
Rhythm: Irregular
Rate: 68 to 76 beats/min
P waves: When present, positive; one precedes each QRS
PR interval: 0.16 second
QRS duration: 0.08 second
QT interval: 0.44 second
Interpretation: Sinus rhythm at 76 beats/min with an episode of sinus arrest and return to sinus rhythm at 68 beats/min; tall T waves

25. Fig. 3.14
Rhythm: Regular
Rate: 104 beats/min
P waves: Positive but small; one precedes each QRS
PR interval: 0.16 second
QRS duration: 0.15 second
QT interval: 0.32 second
Interpretation: Sinus tachycardia at 104 beats/min with a wide QRS and deeply inverted T waves

26. Fig. 3.15
Rhythm: Regular
Rate: 78 beats/min
P waves: Positive; one precedes each QRS
PR interval: 0.14 second
QRS duration: 0.06 second
QT interval: 0.32 second
Interpretation: Sinus rhythm at 78 beats/min, ST-segment depression

27. Fig. 3.16
Rhythm: Irregular
Rate: 102 beats/min (within normal limits for age)
P waves: Positive; one precedes each QRS
PR interval: 0.16 second
QRS duration: 0.08 second
QT interval: 0.28 second
Interpretation: Sinus arrhythmia at 102 beats/min

28. Fig. 3.17
Rhythm: Regular
Rate: 79 beats/min
P waves: Positive; one precedes each QRS
PR interval: 0.22 second
QRS duration: 0.13 second
QT interval: 0.36 second
Interpretation: Sinus rhythm at 79 beats/min with a prolonged PR interval, wide QRS, STE in leads II and V$_4$, and ST-segment depression in lead I

29. Fig. 3.18
Rhythm: Regular
Rate: 86 beats/min
P waves: Positive; one precedes each QRS
PR interval: 0.16 second
QRS duration: 0.06 second
QT interval: 0.32 second
Interpretation: Sinus rhythm at 86 beats/min

30. Fig. 3.19
Rhythm: Regular
Rate: 94 beats/min
P waves: Positive; one precedes each QRS
PR interval: 0.16 second
QRS duration: 0.06 second
QT interval: 0.26 second
Interpretation: Sinus rhythm at 94 beats/min with STE

31. Fig. 3.20
Rhythm: Irregular
Rate: 86 beats/min
P waves: Positive; one precedes each QRS
PR interval: 0.12 to 0.14 second
QRS duration: 0.07 second
QT interval: 0.28 second
Interpretation: Sinus arrhythmia at 86 beats/min

32. Fig. 3.21
Rhythm: Regular
Rate: 94 beats/min
P waves: Positive; one precedes each QRS
PR interval: 0.16 to 0.18 second
QRS duration: 0.12 second
QT interval: 0.36 to 0.40 second
Interpretation: Sinus rhythm at 94 beats/min with a wide QRS and ST-segment depression

33. Fig. 3.22
Rhythm: Irregular
Rate: 50 beats/min
P waves: Positive; one precedes each QRS
PR interval 0.20 second
QRS duration: 0.09 second
QT interval: 0.38 second
Interpretation: Sinus bradyarrhythmia at 50 beats/min (the interpretation reflects that the rhythm is slow and irregular)

34. Fig. 3.23
Rhythm: Regular
Rate: 65 beats/min
P waves: Biphasic P waves before each QRS (a normal finding in leads MCL$_1$ and V$_1$)
PR interval: 0.20 second
QRS duration: 0.10 second
QT interval: 0.35 second
Interpretation: Sinus rhythm at 65 beats/min with biphasic P waves and STE

35. Fig. 3.24
Rhythm: Regular
Rate: 103 beats/min
P waves: Positive; one precedes each QRS
PR interval: 0.14 second
QRS duration: 0.08 second
QT interval: 0.30 second
Interpretation: Sinus tachycardia at 103 beats/min; inverted T waves

36. Fig. 3.25
Rhythm: Regular
Rate: 27 beats/min
P waves: Positive; one precedes each QRS
PR interval: 0.24 second
QRS duration: 0.10 to 0.12 second
QT interval: 0.40 second
Interpretation: Sinus bradycardia at 27 beats/min with a prolonged PR interval and ST-segment depression; notched QRS

37. Fig. 3.26
Rhythm: Regular
Rate: 53 beats/min
P waves: Positive; one precedes each QRS
PR interval: 0.17 second
QRS duration: 0.08 second
QT interval: 0.36 second
Interpretation: Sinus bradycardia at 53 beats/min with STE, hyperacute T waves, and baseline artifact

38. Fig. 3.27
Rhythm: Regular
Rate: 90 beats/min
P waves: Positive; a low amplitude P wave precedes each QRS
PR interval: 0.13 second
QRS duration: 0.04 to 0.06 second
QT interval: 0.31 second
Interpretation: Sinus rhythm at 90 beats/min with STE

39. Fig. 3.28
Rhythm: Regular
Rate: 150 beats/min
P waves: Positive; one precedes each QRS
PR interval: 0.12 second
QRS duration: 0.06 second
QT interval: 0.20 to 0.24 second
Interpretation: Sinus rhythm at 150 beats/min (rate within normal limits for age)

40. Fig. 3.29
Rhythm: Slightly irregular
Rate: 80 beats/min
P waves: Positive; one precedes each QRS
PR interval: 0.14 second
QRS duration: 0.08 second
QT interval: 0.33 second
Interpretation: Sinus arrhythmia at 80 beats/min

41. Fig. 3.30
Rhythm: Regular
Rate: 68 beats/min
P waves: Positive; one precedes each QRS
PR interval: 0.28 to 0.30 second
QRS duration: 0.06 to 0.08 second
QT interval: 0.41 second
Interpretation: Sinus rhythm at 68 beats/min with a prolonged PR interval and ST-segment depression; some baseline artifact is present

42. Fig. 3.31
Rhythm: Regular
Rate: 97 beats/min
P waves: Positive; one precedes each QRS
PR interval: 0.17 second
QRS duration: 0.05 second
QT interval: 0.32 second
Interpretation: Sinus rhythm at 97 beats/min with STE

43. Fig. 3.32
Rhythm: Irregular
Rate: 50 beats/min
P waves: Positive; one precedes each QRS
PR interval: 0.12 to 0.16 second
QRS duration: 0.08 second
QT interval: 0.36 to 0.40 second
Interpretation: Sinus bradyarrhythmia at 50 beats/min

44. Fig. 3.33
Rhythm: Regular
Rate: 115 beats/min
P waves: Positive; one precedes each QRS
PR interval: 0.20 second
QRS duration: 0.10 to 0.12 second
QT interval: Unable to determine because T waves are not clearly visible
Interpretation: Sinus tachycardia at 115 beats/min with ST-segment depression

45. Fig. 3.34
Rhythm: Irregular
Rate: 70 beats/min
P waves: Positive; one precedes each QRS
PR interval: 0.12 to 0.16 second
QRS duration: 0.06 to 0.08 second
QT interval: 0.28 to 0.32 second
Interpretation: Sinus arrhythmia at 70 beats/min with STE and baseline artifact

46. Fig. 3.35
Rhythm: Irregular
Rate: 50 beats/min
P waves: Positive; one precedes each QRS
PR interval: 0.20 to 0.22 second
QRS duration: 0.06 second
QT interval: 0.42 second
Interpretation: Sinus bradyarrhythmia at 50 beats/min with a prolonged PR interval, baseline artifact is present

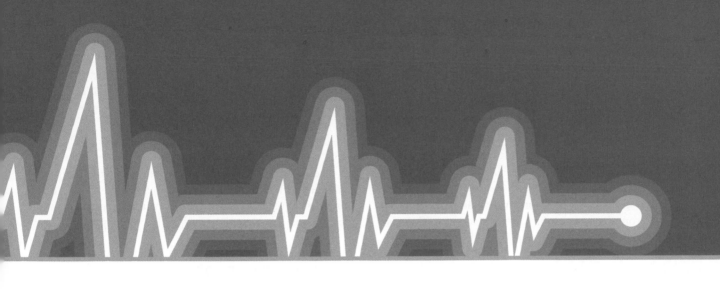

Atrial Rhythms

4

LEARNING OBJECTIVES

After reading this chapter, you should be able to:

1. Explain the concepts of altered automaticity, triggered activity, and reentry.
2. Explain the terms *bigeminy*, *trigeminy*, and *quadrigeminy* and *run* when describing premature complexes.
3. Describe the electrocardiogram (ECG) characteristics, possible causes, signs and symptoms, and initial emergency care for premature atrial complexes (PACs).
4. Explain the difference between a compensatory and noncompensatory pause.
5. Explain the terms *wandering atrial pacemaker* and *multifocal atrial tachycardia*.
6. Describe the ECG characteristics, possible causes, signs and symptoms, and initial emergency care for wandering atrial pacemaker (multiform atrial rhythm).
7. Describe the ECG characteristics, possible causes, signs and symptoms, and initial emergency care for MAT.

8. Describe the ECG characteristics, possible causes, signs and symptoms, and initial emergency care for atrial tachycardia (AT).
9. Explain the terms *paroxysmal atrial tachycardia* and *paroxysmal supraventricular tachycardia* (PSVT).
10. List examples of vagal maneuvers.
11. Discuss the indications for synchronized cardioversion.
12. Describe the ECG characteristics, possible causes, signs and symptoms, and initial emergency care for atrioventricular nodal reentrant tachycardia (AVNRT).
13. Describe the ECG characteristics, possible causes, signs and symptoms, and initial emergency care for atrioventricular reentrant tachycardia (AVRT)
14. Describe the ECG characteristics, possible causes, signs and symptoms, and initial emergency care for atrial flutter.
15. Describe the ECG characteristics, possible causes, signs and symptoms, and initial emergency care for atrial fibrillation (AFib).

KEY TERMS

atrial tachycardia (AT): A regular rhythm that arises from an ectopic focus in the atria at a rate faster than 100 beats per minute (beats/min) and does not require the participation of the AV node to maintain the dysrhythmia.

bigeminy: Dysrhythmia in which every other beat is a premature ectopic beat.

blocked (nonconducted) PAC: PAC not followed by a QRS complex.

bursts: Three or more sequential ectopic beats; also referred to as a "salvo" or "run."

compensatory pause: Pause for which the normal beat after a premature complex occurs when expected; also called a complete pause.

couplet: Two consecutive premature complexes.

delta wave: Slurring of the beginning portion of the QRS complex, caused by preexcitation.

focal atrial tachycardia: AT that begins in a small area (focus) within the atria.

multiform atrial rhythm: Dysrhythmia that occurs because of impulses originating from various sites, including the SA node, the atria, and/or

the AV junction; requires at least three different P waves, seen in the same lead, for proper diagnosis.

multifocal atrial tachycardia (MAT): An irregular rhythm at a rate faster than 100 beats/min with three or more P waves of differing shapes observed in the same lead.

nonconducted (blocked) PAC: PAC that is not followed by a QRS complex.

noncompensatory pause: A pause that often follows a premature atrial complex that represents the delay during which the SA node resets its rhythm for the next beat; the pause is noncompensatory if the normal beat after the premature complex occurs before it was expected (i.e., the period between the complex before and after the premature beat is less than two normal R-R intervals).

paroxysmal supraventricular tachycardia (PSVT): A regular supraventricular tachycardia that starts and ends suddenly.

preexcitation: premature activation of the ventricles by a supraventricular impulse arising from an accessory pathway.

premature complex: Early beat occurring before the next expected beat; can be atrial, junctional, or ventricular.

Continued

KEY TERMS—cont'd

quadrigeminy: Dysrhythmia in which every fourth beat is a premature ectopic beat.

supraventricular: Originating from a site above the bifurcation of the bundle of His, such as the SA node, atria, or AV junction.

synchronized cardioversion: A type of electrical therapy during which a shock is timed or programmed for delivery during ventricular depolarization (i.e., the QRS complex).

trigeminy: Dysrhythmia in which every third beat is a premature ectopic beat

vagal maneuvers: Methods used to stimulate the vagus nerve in an attempt to slow conduction through the AV node, thereby slowing the heart rate.

wandering atrial pacemaker (multiform atrial rhythm): Cardiac dysrhythmia that occurs because of impulses originating from various sites, including the SA node, the atria, and/or the AV junction; requires at least three different P waves, seen in the same lead, for proper diagnosis.

INTRODUCTION

The atria are thin-walled, low-pressure chambers that receive blood from the systemic circulation and lungs. There is usually a continuous flow of blood from the superior and inferior vena cavae into the atria. About 70% of this blood flows directly through the atria and into the ventricles before the atria contract. When the atria contract, an additional 30% is added to the filling of the ventricles. This additional contribution of blood because of atrial contraction is called atrial kick.

P waves reflect atrial depolarization. A rhythm that begins in the SA node has one positive (i.e., upright) P wave before each QRS complex. A rhythm that begins in the atria will have a positive P wave that is shaped differently from P waves that begin in the SA node. This difference in P wave configuration occurs because the impulse begins in the atria and follows a different conduction pathway to the AV node.

ATRIAL DYSRHYTHMIAS: MECHANISMS

Atrial dysrhythmias reflect abnormal electrical impulse formation and conduction in the atria. They result from altered automaticity, triggered activity, or reentry. Recall from Chapter 2 that altered automaticity and triggered activity are disorders in impulse *formation*. Reentry is a disorder in impulse *conduction*. Dysrhythmias caused by impulse formation disorders are often referred to as *automatic*, and those caused by a disorder in impulse conduction are referred to as *reentrant*.

Atrial dysrhythmias associated with altered automaticity include PACs, multifocal atrial tachycardia (MAT), and atrial fibrillation (AFib). Atrial rhythms associated with reentry include atrial flutter, AVNRT, and AVRT.

Most atrial dysrhythmias are not life threatening, but some may be associated with extremely fast ventricular rates. Increases in heart rate shorten all phases of the cardiac cycle, but the most important is a decrease in the length of time spent in diastole. Remember that as the heart rate increases, there is less time for the ventricles to fill and less blood for the ventricles to pump out with each contraction; therefore, an excessively fast heart rate can decrease cardiac output. Examples of factors that influence heart rate include hormone levels (e.g., thyroxin, epinephrine, norepinephrine), medications, stress, anxiety, fear, and body temperature.

PREMATURE ATRIAL COMPLEXES

Premature beats appear early; that is, they occur before the next expected beat. Premature beats are identified by their site of origin:

- Premature atrial complexes (PACs)
- Premature junctional complexes (PJCs)
- Premature ventricular complexes (PVCs)

The term *complex* is used instead of *contraction* to correctly identify an early beat because the electrocardiogram (ECG) depicts electrical activity, not the heart's mechanical function. Some practitioners prefer the term *conduction* instead of complex.

Premature beats may occur in patterns:

- Paired beats (**couplet**): Two premature beats in a row
- Runs or **bursts**: Three or more premature beats in a row
- **Bigeminy**: Every other beat is a premature beat
- **Trigeminy**: Every third beat is a premature beat
- **Quadrigeminy**: Every fourth beat is a premature beat

How Do I Recognize It?

A PAC occurs when an irritable site (i.e., focus) within the atria fires before the next SA node impulse is expected to fire, interrupting the sinus rhythm. If the irritable site is close to the SA node, the atrial P wave will look very similar to the P waves initiated by the SA node. The P wave of a PAC may be biphasic (i.e., partly positive, partly negative), flattened, notched, pointed, or lost in the preceding T wave.

When compared with the P-P intervals of the underlying rhythm, a PAC is premature—occurring before the next expected sinus P wave. PACs are identified by the following:

- Early (premature) P waves
- Positive (upright) P waves (in lead II) that differ in shape from sinus P waves
- Early P waves that may or may not be followed by a QRS complex

⊙ ECG Pearl _____

A PAC has a positive P wave before the QRS complex. Sometimes the P waves are clearly seen, and sometimes they are not. If the P wave of an early beat isn't obvious, look for it in the T wave of the preceding beat. The T wave of the preceding beat may be of higher amplitude than other T waves or have an extra "hump," suggesting a hidden P wave.

___

ECG characteristics of PACs include the following:

Rhythm:	Irregular because of the early beat(s)
Rate:	Usually within normal range but depends on the underlying rhythm
P waves:	Premature (occurring earlier than the next expected sinus P wave), positive (upright) in lead II, one before each QRS complex, often differ in shape from sinus P waves—may be flattened, notched, pointed, biphasic, or lost in the preceding T wave
PR interval:	May be normal or prolonged depending on the prematurity of the beat
QRS duration:	Usually 0.11 second or less but may be wide (aberrant) or absent, depending on the prematurity of the beat; the QRS of the PAC is similar in shape to those of the underlying rhythm unless the PAC is abnormally conducted

Look at the rhythm strip in Fig. 4.1. At a glance, you can see that the ventricular rhythm is irregular and that the rate is about 110 beats per minute (beats/min). Now let's look more closely. Begin by locating the QRS complexes on the rhythm strip. Evaluate each succeeding R-R interval. The R-R intervals in this example occur regularly except for three beats.

Now find the P waves on the rhythm strip. Remember that P waves that begin in the SA node are ordinarily smooth and rounded. Atrial P waves will look different. Using a pen or pencil, mark an "S," for SA node, above each normal looking P wave. Mark an "A," for atrial, above those P waves that look different. When you are finished, you should have an

"A" marked over the P waves in beats 2, 7, and 10. The rest of the P waves should be marked with an "S." Notice that the waveforms marked with an "S" above them occur regularly except when they are interrupted by the three atrial beats.

With the use of your calipers or a piece of paper, find two sinus beats that appear next to each other, such as beats 4 and 5. Using the sinus beats as your guide, determine the atrial rate. The distance between the sinus beats is about 13.5 boxes, or 111 beats/min, which is close to our initial estimated rate of 110 beats/min. Based on the rate (i.e., faster than 100 beats/min) and an upright P wave before each QRS, we know that the underlying rhythm is sinus tachycardia. Now move your calipers or paper to the right. If beat 6 occurred on time, it will line up with your calipers or paper. It is on time. Now move your calipers to the right again. The right point of your calipers shows where the next sinus beat should have occurred. You can see that beat 7 occurred earlier than expected. When you continue this process, you will find that beat 10 is also early. Working backward and without adjusting your calipers, if you place your calipers' left point on beat 1 in the rhythm strip, you will see that beat 2 is also early. So far, we can identify this rhythm as a sinus tachycardia at 111 beats/min with three premature beats.

Next, measure the PR interval, QRS duration, and QT interval. The PR interval is 0.16 second, and the QRS is 0.08 second in duration. Accurate determination of the QT interval is not possible because the T waves in this rhythm strip are difficult to identify.

We must pinpoint where the premature beats came from because premature beats can start from more than one area of the heart. To do this, we must examine the premature beats more closely. Look carefully at beats 2, 7, and 10. The QRS complexes look the same as those of the underlying rhythm because the impulse journeyed normally through the conduction system. Now look to the left of the QRS complex in each early beat and inspect the P waves. Each P wave is positive (i.e., upright) but looks different from the P waves of the sinus beats, which tells you that the P waves came from the atria. The early beats are PACs. A PAC is not an entire rhythm—it is a single beat; therefore, you must identify the underlying rhythm and the ectopic beat(s). To complete our identification of this rhythm, we have a sinus tachycardia at 111 beats/min with three PACs.

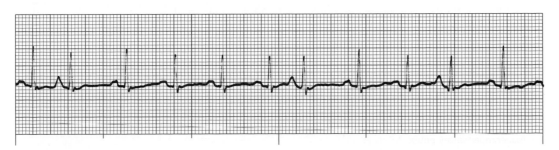

Fig. 4.1 Sinus tachycardia at 111 beats/min with three premature atrial complexes (PACs). From the left, beats 2, 7, and 10 are PACs.

Noncompensatory Versus Compensatory Pause

A **noncompensatory** (i.e., incomplete) **pause** often follows a PAC, representing the delay during which the SA node resets its rhythm for the next beat. A **compensatory** (i.e., complete) **pause** often follows PVCs (Fig. 4.2).

To find out whether the pause after a **premature complex** is compensatory or noncompensatory, measure the distance between the R-R intervals of three normal beats. Then compare that measurement with the distance between the R-R intervals of three beats, one of which includes the premature complex. The pause is *noncompensatory* if the period between the complex before and after a premature beat is less than two normal R-R intervals (Fig. 4.3). The pause is *compensatory* if the period between the complex before and after a premature beat is the same as two normal R-R intervals.

Aberrantly Conducted Premature Atrial Complexes

If a PAC occurs very early, the right bundle branch can be slow to respond to the impulse (i.e., refractory). The impulse travels down the left bundle branch with no problem. Stimulation of the left bundle branch subsequently results in stimulation of the right bundle branch. The QRS will appear wide (i.e., greater than 0.11 second) because of this delay in ventricular depolarization. PACs associated with a wide QRS complex are called aberrantly conducted PACs, indicating that conduction through the ventricles is abnormal. Fig. 4.4 shows a rhythm strip with two PACs. The first PAC (*arrow* in Fig. 4.4) was conducted abnormally, producing a wide QRS complex. The second PAC (*arrow* in Fig. 4.4) was conducted normally. Compare the T waves before each PAC with those of the underlying sinus bradycardia.

Nonconducted Premature Atrial Complexes

Sometimes when a PAC occurs very early and close to the T wave of the preceding beat, only a P wave may be seen with no QRS after it, appearing as a pause (Fig. 4.5). This type of PAC is called a **nonconducted** or **blocked PAC** because the P wave occurred too early to be conducted. Nonconducted PACs occur because the AV junction is still refractory to stimulation and cannot conduct the impulse to the ventricles (thus no QRS complex). Look for the early P wave in the T wave of the preceding beat.

WHAT CAUSES THEM?

PACs may be the result of altered automaticity or reentry. PACs are very common and can occur at any age but are

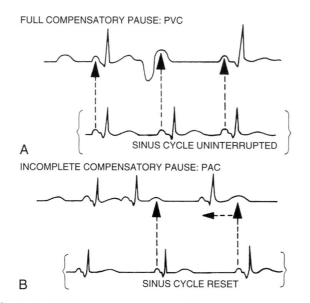

Fig. 4.2 A, A full compensatory pause often follows a premature ventricular complex *(PVC)*. B, A premature atrial complex *(PAC)* is often followed by a noncompensatory (incomplete) pause. (From Crawford, M. V., & Spence, M. I. (1994). *Commonsense approach to coronary care* (rev ed 6). St Louis: Mosby.)

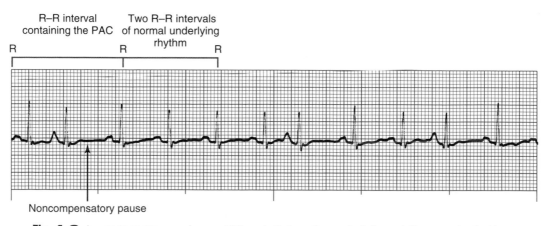

Fig. 4.3 A noncompensatory pause is present if the period between the complex before and after a premature beat is less than two normal R-R intervals. *PAC,* Premature atrial complex.

PAC conducted normally

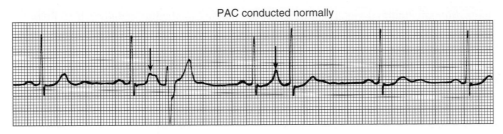

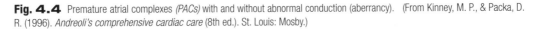

Aberrantly conducted PAC

Fig. 4.4 Premature atrial complexes *(PACs)* with and without abnormal conduction (aberrancy).   (From Kinney, M. P., & Packa, D. R. (1996). *Andreoli's comprehensive cardiac care* (8th ed.). St. Louis: Mosby.)

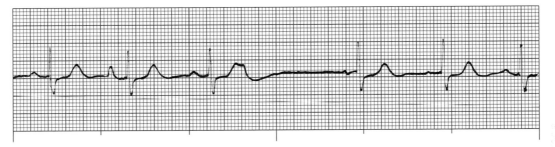

Fig. 4.5 Sinus rhythm with a nonconducted (blocked) premature atrial complex. Note the distorted T wave of the third QRS complex from the left.

particularly frequent in older adults. Their presence does not necessarily imply underlying cardiac disease. Possible causes of PACs include the following:

- Acute coronary syndromes
- Atrial enlargement
- Digitalis toxicity
- Electrolyte imbalance
- Emotional stress
- Heart failure
- Hyperthyroidism

- Mental and physical fatigue
- Stimulants: caffeine, tobacco, cocaine
- Sympathomimetic medications, such as epinephrine
- Valvular heart disease

WHAT DO I DO ABOUT THEM?

PACs usually do not require treatment if they are infrequent. If PACs are frequent, the patient may notice a skipped beat or occasional palpitations (i.e., the sensation of a racing heart, skipped beats, or flip-flops). Some patients are unaware of their occurrence. In susceptible individuals, frequent PACs may induce episodes of AFib or PSVT. Frequent PACs are treated by correcting the underlying cause:
- Correcting electrolyte imbalances
- Reducing stress
- Reducing or eliminating stimulants
- Treating heart failure

If the patient is symptomatic, frequent PACs may be treated with beta-blockers, such as atenolol or metoprolol.

WANDERING ATRIAL PACEMAKER

How Do I Recognize It?

Multiform atrial rhythm is an updated term for the rhythm formerly known as **wandering atrial pacemaker.** With this rhythm, the P waves' size, shape, and direction vary, sometimes from beat to beat. The difference in the P waves' look results from the gradual shifting of the dominant pacemaker among the SA node, the atria, and/or the AV junction (Fig. 4.6). Wandering atrial pacemaker requires at least three different P waves, seen in the same lead, for proper diagnosis. ECG characteristics of wandering atrial pacemaker include the following:

Rhythm:	Usually irregular as the pacemaker site shifts from the SA node to ectopic atrial locations or AV junction
Rate:	Usually 60 to 100 beats/min but may be slower; if the rate is faster than 100 beats/min, the rhythm is termed *multifocal atrial tachycardia*
P waves:	Size, shape, and direction may change from beat to beat; may be upright, inverted, biphasic, rounded, flat, pointed, notched, or buried in the QRS complex
PR interval:	Varies as the pacemaker site shifts from the SA node to ectopic atrial locations or AV junction
QRS duration:	0.11 second or less unless abnormally conducted

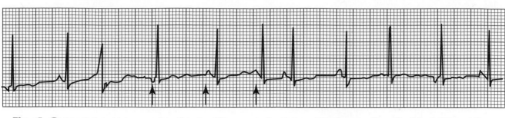

Fig. 4.6 Wandering atrial pacemaker. Note the differences in the shapes of the P waves. (From Paul, S., & Hebra, J. D. (1998). *The nurse's guide to cardiac rhythm interpretation: implications for patient care.* Philadelphia: Saunders.)

Wandering atrial pacemaker is associated with a normal or slow rate and irregular P-P, R-R, and PR intervals because of the different sites of impulse formation. The QRS duration usually is 0.11 second or less because conduction through the ventricles is typically normal.

ECG Pearl

At least three different P-wave configurations, seen in the same lead, are required to diagnose wandering atrial pacemaker or multifocal atrial tachycardia.

What Causes It?

Wandering atrial pacemaker may be observed in normal, healthy hearts (particularly in athletes) and during sleep. It may also occur with some types of underlying heart disease and with sinus node dysfunction. This dysrhythmia usually produces no signs and symptoms unless it is associated with a slow rate.

What Do I Do About It?

Wandering atrial pacemaker is usually a transient rhythm that resolves on its own when the firing rate of the SA node increases and the sinus resumes pacing responsibility.

MULTIFOCAL ATRIAL TACHYCARDIA

How Do I Recognize It?

When the wandering atrial pacemaker rhythm is associated with a ventricular rate of more than 100 beats/min, the dysrhythmia is called **multifocal atrial tachycardia (MAT)** (Fig. 4.7). As evidenced by its name, MAT results from the random and chaotic firing of multiple ectopic sites in the atria. ECG characteristics of MAT include the following:

Rhythm:	Ventricular rhythm is always irregular as the pacemaker site shifts from the SA node to ectopic atrial locations or AV junction
Rate:	Faster than 100 beats/min
P waves:	One P wave before each QRS but the size, shape, and direction of the P wave may change from beat to beat; may be upright, inverted, biphasic, rounded, flat, pointed, notched, or buried in the QRS complex; at least three different P-wave configurations (seen in the same lead) are required for a diagnosis of MAT.
PR interval:	Varies as the pacemaker site shifts from the SA node to ectopic atrial locations or the AV junction
QRS duration:	0.11 second or less unless abnormally conducted

What Causes It?

The exact mechanism of MAT is unknown but may involve altered automaticity or triggered activity. MAT is most often seen in older adults with severe chronic obstructive pulmonary disease (COPD), but it is also seen in the setting of acute coronary syndromes, heart failure, pneumonia, hypoxia, valvular heart disease, hypokalemia, hypomagnesemia, or theophylline or digoxin toxicity. The average age of onset of MAT in adults is 72 years. Adults with MAT have a high mortality rate, with estimates around 45%, but this is generally attributed to the presence of underlying conditions (Virani et al., 2021).

What Do I Do About It?

Common symptoms associated with MAT include palpitations, lightheadedness, anxiety, dyspnea, chest discomfort,

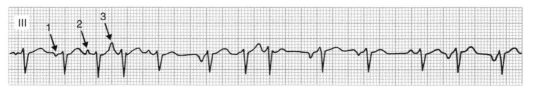

Fig. 4.7 Multifocal atrial tachycardia. Note the rapidly occurring P waves showing variable shapes and PR intervals. This fast, irregular rhythm may be mistaken for atrial fibrillation. Arrows with numbers (1–3) above show a segment with multiple consecutive different P waves. (From Goldberger, A. L., & Goldberger, Z. D. (2018). *Goldberger's clinical electrocardiography: a simplified approach* (9th ed.). Philadelphia: Elsevier.)

and syncope. Because MAT is challenging to treat, it is best to consult a cardiologist before starting treatment. Efforts are focused on managing the underlying cause. If the patient is symptomatic, a beta-blocker (e.g., metoprolol) is typically the drug of choice; however, because MAT is often associated with chronic lung disease, a calcium blocker may be used if a beta-blocker is contraindicated or not tolerated. Patients with MAT who do not respond to medical therapy may require AV nodal ablation with subsequent cardiac pacemaker implantation.

SUPRAVENTRICULAR TACHYCARDIA

Supraventricular arrhythmias begin above the bundle of His; this means that supraventricular arrhythmias include rhythms that begin in the SA node, atrial tissue, or the AV junction. The term *supraventricular tachycardia* (SVT) includes supraventricular rhythms with a ventricular rate faster than 100 beats/min at rest (Page et al., 2016). Three examples of SVTs are shown in Fig. 4.8. Sinus tachycardia, which is technically an SVT, is not shown.

⊙ ECG Pearl _____

Some SVTs need the AV node to sustain the rhythm, and some do not. For example, AVNRT and AVRT require the AV node as part of the reentry circuit to continue the tachycardia. Other SVTs use the AV node only to conduct the rhythm to the ventricles. For example, atrial tachycardia, atrial flutter, and AFib arise from a site (or sites) within the atria; they do not need the AV node to sustain the rhythm.

The onset of SVT symptoms often begins in adulthood and can affect the quality of life depending on the frequency and duration of episodes and whether symptoms occur with exercise and at rest (Page et al., 2016). Complaints of light-headedness are common. A drop in blood pressure typically occurs during SVT and is greatest in the first 10 to 30 seconds, normalizing within 30 to 60 seconds despite minimal heart rate changes (Page et al., 2016).

⊙ ECG Pearl _____

It is essential to look closely for P waves in all dysrhythmias, but it is crucial when trying to figure out the origin of a tachycardia. If P waves are not visible in one lead, try looking in another before finalizing your rhythm diagnosis.

Atrial Tachycardias

Atrial tachycardia (AT) is the third most common type of SVT (Virani et al., 2021). It is a regular rhythm that arises from an ectopic focus in the atria at a rate faster than 100 beats/min and does not require the AV node's participation to maintain the dysrhythmia (Ellenbogen & Koneru, 2018) (Fig. 4.9). This rapid atrial rate overrides the SA node and becomes the pacemaker. AT is often precipitated by a PAC. When three or more PACs occur in a row at a rate of more than 100 beats/min, AT is present.

HOW DO I RECOGNIZE IT?

There is often 1:1 conduction of the atrial impulse to the ventricles with AT, which means that every atrial impulse is conducted through the AV node to the ventricles, resulting in a P wave preceding each QRS complex. Although the P waves

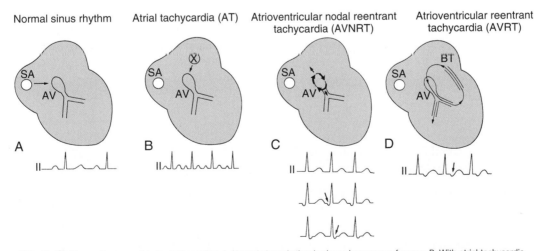

Fig. 4.8 Types of supraventricular tachycardias. A, Normal sinus rhythm is shown here as a reference. B, With atrial tachycardia *(AT)*, a focus *(X)* outside the sinoatrial *(SA)* node fires off automatically at a rapid rate. C, With atrioventricular *(AV)* nodal reentrant tachycardia *(AVNRT)*, the cardiac stimulus originates as a wave of excitation that spins around the AV junctional area. As a result, P waves may be buried in the QRS or appear immediately before or just after the QRS complex *(arrows)* because of nearly simultaneous activation of the atria and ventricles. D, A similar type of reentrant (circus movement) mechanism in Wolff-Parkinson-White syndrome. This mechanism is referred to as *atrioventricular reentrant tachycardia (AVRT)*. Note the P wave in lead II somewhat after the QRS complex. *BT,* Bypass tract. (From Goldberger, A. L., & Goldberger, Z. D. (2018). *Goldberger's clinical electrocardiography: a simplified approach* (9th ed.). Philadelphia: Elsevier.)

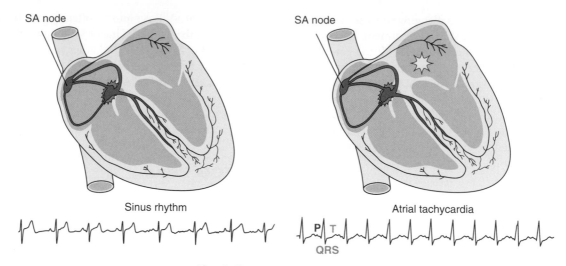

Fig. 4.9 Atrial tachycardia. *SA,* Sinoatrial.

appear upright, they tend to look different from those seen when the impulse is initiated from the SA node. AT can have negative P waves in the inferior leads if it arises from the lower part of the atrium. Because conducted travel through the ventricles in the usual manner, the QRS complexes appear normal. ECG characteristics of AT include the following:

Rhythm:	Regular
Rate:	101 to 250 beats/min
P waves:	One P wave precedes each QRS complex in lead II; these P waves differ in shape from sinus P waves; an isoelectric baseline is usually present between P waves; if the atrial rhythm originates in the low portion of the atrium, P waves will be negative in the inferior leads; with rapid rates, it may be challenging to distinguish P waves from T waves
PR interval:	May be shorter or longer than normal; may be difficult to measure because P waves may be hidden in the T waves of preceding beats
QRS duration:	0.11 second or less unless abnormally conducted

Paroxysmal supraventricular tachycardia (PSVT) is a term used to describe a rapid, regular SVT that starts and ends suddenly. These features are characteristic of AVNRT or AVRT, and, less frequently, AT (Page et al., 2016) (Fig. 4.10). PSVT may last for minutes, hours, or days. If the onset or end of PSVT is not observed on the ECG, the dysrhythmia is simply called *SVT.*

With very rapid atrial rates, the AV node begins to filter some of the impulses coming to it. By doing so, it protects the ventricles from excessively rapid rates. When the AV node selectively filters the conduction of some of these impulses, the rhythm is called paroxysmal supraventricular (or atrial) tachycardia with block. PSVT with block is often associated with AV node disease, medications that slow conduction through the AV node, or digitalis toxicity. When PSVT with block exists, more than one P wave is present before each QRS. PSVT with 2:1 block exists when the AV node blocks every other atrial impulse from traveling to the ventricles (Fig. 4.11).

There is more than one type of AT. ATs may be caused by an automatic, triggered, or reentrant mechanism (Zimetbaum, 2020). MAT has already been discussed. AT that begins in a small area (focus) within the atria is called *focal AT.* **Focal AT** often presents with PSVT. *Automatic AT,* also called *ectopic AT,* is a type of focal AT in which a small

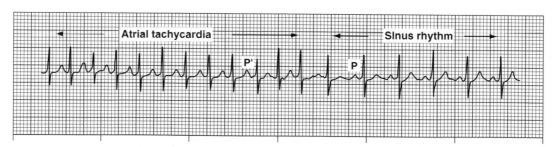

Fig. 4.10 Atrial tachycardia (AT) (a type of supraventricular tachycardia) that ends spontaneously with the abrupt resumption of sinus rhythm. AT that starts or ends suddenly is called *paroxysmal supraventricular tachycardia* (PSVT). The P' waves of the tachycardia (rate: about 150 beats/min) are superimposed on the preceding T waves. (From Goldberger, A. L., & Goldberger, Z. D. (2018). *Goldberger's clinical electrocardiography: a simplified approach* (9th ed.). Philadelphia: Elsevier.)

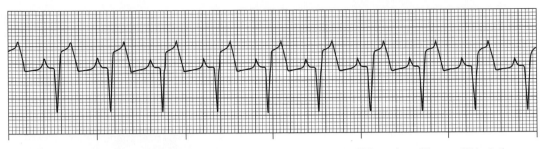

Fig. 4.11 Atrial tachycardia with 2:1 block. P waves are clearly seen before the QRS complexes. Others are hidden in the T waves. The atrial rate is 180 beats/min, and the ventricular rate is 90 beats/min. (From Andreoli T.E., Benjamin I., Griggs R.C., Wing E.J. (2011), *Andreoli and Carpenter's Cecil essentials of medicine.* Philadelphia: Saunders.)

cluster of cells with altered automaticity fire. The impulse is spread from the cluster of cells to the surrounding atrium and then to the ventricles via the AV node. P waves look different from sinus P waves, but they are still related to the QRS complex. Vagal maneuvers may slow the ventricular rate but do not usually stop the tachycardia.

ECG Pearl

Although correct use of the term *paroxysmal* requires observing the onset or cessation of the dysrhythmia and identifying the underlying rhythm that preceded it, some practitioners use the term to describe the sudden onset or cessation of a patient's *symptoms* associated with the dysrhythmia.

WHAT CAUSES IT?

AT can occur in people with normal hearts or those with organic heart disease. AT may be related to an acute event such as the following:

- Acute illness with excessive catecholamine release
- Digitalis toxicity
- Electrolyte imbalance
- Heart disease including coronary artery disease (CAD), valvular disease, cardiomyopathies, and congenital heart disease
- Infection
- Pulmonary embolism
- Stimulant use (e.g., caffeine, albuterol, theophylline, cocaine)

The autonomic nervous system is associated with initiating or triggering some ATs (Ellenbogen & Koneru, 2018). Reports of AT triggered by belching, changes in posture, and swallowing, and the termination of AT with a Valsalva maneuver or with the administration of beta-blockers support the probable association between autonomic nervous system activity and AT in some patients (Ellenbogen & Koneru, 2018).

ECG Pearl

The signs and symptoms experienced by a patient with a tachycardia depend on the ventricular rate, how long the tachycardia lasts, the patient's general health, and the presence of underlying heart disease. The faster the heart rate, the more likely the patient will have signs and symptoms resulting from the rapid rate.

WHAT DO I DO ABOUT IT?

Assessment findings and symptoms associated with AT vary widely and may include the following:

- Acute changes in mental status
- Asymptomatic
- Dizziness or lightheadedness
- Dyspnea
- Fatigue
- Fluttering sensation in the chest
- Hypotension
- Ischemic chest discomfort
- Palpitations
- Signs of shock
- Syncope or near syncope

When taking the patient's history, try to find out how often the episodes occur, how long they last, and possible triggers. If the patient complains of palpitations, find out if they are regular or irregular. Palpitations that occur regularly with a sudden onset and end usually are the result of AVNRT or AVRT. Irregular palpitations may be the result of premature complexes, AFib, or MAT. Tachycardias may cause syncope because the rapid ventricular rate decreases cardiac output and blood flow to the brain. Syncope is most likely to occur just after the onset of a rapid AT or when the rhythm stops abruptly. Predisposed individuals may experience angina or heart failure.

A rhythm that lasts from three beats up to 30 seconds is a *nonsustained rhythm*. A *sustained rhythm* lasts more than 30 seconds or requires pharmacologic or electrical intervention to terminate the rhythm because of hemodynamic instability.

If episodes of AT are short, the patient may be asymptomatic. If AT is sustained and the patient is symptomatic because of the rapid rate, treatment should include applying a pulse oximeter and administering oxygen (if indicated), obtaining the patient's vital signs, and establishing intravenous (IV) access. A 12-lead ECG should be obtained. If the patient is not hypotensive, vagal maneuvers may be tried. Vagal maneuvers are discussed later. Although vagal maneuvers are rarely successful, they may be attempted to terminate the rhythm or slow conduction through the AV node. If vagal maneuvers fail, antiarrhythmic medications should be tried if the patient is hemodynamically stable. Adenosine can help restore sinus rhythm or diagnose the tachycardia mechanism in patients with suspected focal AT (Page et al., 2016).

Beta-blockers or calcium blockers (e.g., diltiazem, verapamil) may be ordered to slow the ventricular rate (Page et al., 2016). If AT is sustained and causing persistent signs of hemodynamic compromise, IV adenosine may be ordered, and if it is ineffective or if administration is not feasible, synchronized cardioversion should be performed (Page et al., 2016). Synchronized cardioversion is discussed later in this chapter.

PSVT with AV block often occurs because of excess digitalis. In these cases, the patient's ventricular rate is not excessively fast. The drug should be withheld and serum digoxin levels obtained. Long-term medication therapy may include the use of calcium blockers or beta-blockers.

When AT is difficult to control and causes serious signs and symptoms, radiofrequency catheter ablation may be necessary. When catheter ablation is performed, electrophysiologic studies are done to locate the abnormal pathways and reentry circuits in the heart. Once localized, a special ablation catheter is placed at the site of the abnormal pathway. A low-energy, high-frequency current is delivered through this catheter. With each burst of energy from the catheter, an area of tissue is destroyed (ablated). The energy is applied in various areas until the unwanted pathway is no longer functional and the circuit is broken. ATs occasionally can recur at a different site after a successful ablation.

⊙ ECG Pearl

Adenosine slows the rate of the SA node, slows conduction time through the AV node, can interrupt reentry pathways that involve the AV node, and can restore sinus rhythm in SVT. Reentry circuits are the underlying mechanism for many episodes of SVT. Adenosine acts at specific receptors to cause a temporary block of conduction through the AV node, interrupting these reentry circuits. It is prudent to record a 12-lead ECG while administering adenosine. Adenosine has an onset of action of 10 to 40 seconds and a duration of 1 to 2 minutes. Because of its short half-life (i.e., 10 seconds), the medication is administered intravenously as rapidly as possible (i.e., over a period of seconds) and immediately followed with a saline flush.

Vagal Maneuvers

Vagal maneuvers are methods used to slow impulse conduction through the AV node and, subsequently, the ventricular rate in dysrhythmias that require the AV node to sustain the rhythm. Before performing a vagal maneuver, place the patient on a cardiac monitor, apply a pulse oximeter and blood pressure monitor, and establish IV access. Ensure that a defibrillator with pacing capability and antiarrhythmic medications are at the bedside.

Carotid sinus massage (CSM), also called carotid sinus pressure, is a vagal maneuver performed with the patient's neck extended. The carotid pulse is palpated, and then steady pressure is applied to the right or left carotid sinus just underneath the angle of the jaw for 5 to 10 seconds (Fig. 4.12).

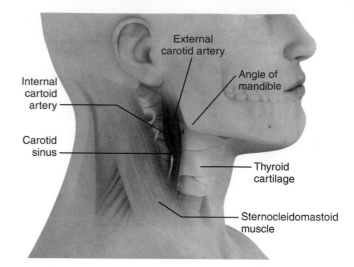

Fig. 4.12 Location of the carotid sinus. (From Roberts, J. R., Custalow, C. B., & Thomsen, T. W. (2019). *Roberts and Hedges' clinical procedures in emergency medicine and acute care* (7th ed.). Philadelphia: Elsevier.)

Avoid CSM in older adults and patients with a history of stroke, known carotid artery stenosis, or a carotid bruit on auscultation. Simultaneous, bilateral carotid pressure is not recommended. Because many organizations stipulate that CSM only be performed by a physician, it is prudent to check your agency's policy about this procedure.

Application of a cold stimulus (e.g., a washcloth soaked in iced water, a cold pack, or crushed ice mixed with water in a plastic bag or glove) to the face for up to 10 seconds is another type of vagal maneuver that is based on the classic diving reflex. When using this method, do not obstruct the patient's mouth or nose or apply pressure to the eyes. The use of a cold stimulus to the face is often effective in infants but seldom in adults.

The Valsalva maneuver is a type of vagal maneuver during which the patient is instructed to make a forced expiratory effort against a closed glottis for 15 seconds before resuming normal breathing. Examples include bearing down as though to have a bowel movement, taking a deep breath and then having patients put their thumb in their mouth with closed lips and attempting to exhale without expelling any air, or asking the patient to blow into a 10 mL syringe with enough force to move the plunger. Performing a Valsalva maneuver or CSM with postural modifications, such as supine positioning and passive leg raising during the procedure, may increase the probability of successful rhythm conversion (Appelboam et al., 2015; Minczak & Laub, 2019).

Valsalva maneuvers are contraindicated in patients with recent MI, aortic stenosis, carotid artery stenosis, glaucoma, or retinopathy.

Synchronized Cardioversion

Synchronized cardioversion is a type of electrical therapy during which a shock is timed or programmed for delivery during ventricular depolarization (i.e., the QRS complex).

When the "Sync" control is pressed on the defibrillator, the machine searches for the QRS complex. When a QRS complex is detected, the monitor places a flag or sync marker on that complex. It may appear as an oval, square, line, or highlighted triangle on the ECG display, depending on the machine used. Delivering a shock during the QRS complex reduces the potential for the delivery of current during ventricular repolarization, including the vulnerable period of the T wave (i.e., the relative refractory period). The shock control is pressed and held on the defibrillator until a message appears on the screen indicating that the shock has been delivered.

Indications

Synchronized cardioversion is used to treat rhythms with a clearly identifiable QRS complex and a rapid ventricular rate in a patient with a pulse and signs of hemodynamic compromise. Examples of rhythms treated with cardioversion include narrow-QRS tachycardias, AFib, atrial flutter, and monomorphic ventricular tachycardia.

ATRIOVENTRICULAR NODAL REENTRANT TACHYCARDIA

Atrioventricular nodal reentrant tachycardia (AVNRT) is the most common type of SVT. It results from a reentry circuit that uses two separate pathways leading into the AV node (Peterson, 2018). One pathway conducts impulses rapidly but has a long refractory period (i.e., slow recovery time). The other pathway conducts impulses slowly but has a short refractory period (i.e., fast recovery time). The pathways join into a final common pathway before impulses exit the AV node and continue to the bundle of His. Under the right conditions, these fast and slow pathways can form an electrical circuit or loop (i.e., a reentry circuit). As one side of the loop is recovering, the other is firing.

Typical AVNRT is the most common type of AVNRT and is usually caused by single or multiple PACs. A PAC, finding the fast pathway refractory, conducts the impulse to the ventricles using the slow pathway (Mani & Pavri, 2014). If the fast pathway has recovered, the impulse can rapidly conduct the fast pathway and depolarize the atria. The impulse can then reenter

the slow pathway to conduct again. If this pattern continues, AVNRT is initiated, resulting in a very rapid and regular ventricular rhythm ranging from 150 to 250 beats/min.

A less common type of AVNRT is called atypical AVNRT. It is often initiated by a premature complex that conducts down the fast pathway and returns using the slow pathway.

HOW DO I RECOGNIZE IT?

AVNRT has the following ECG characteristics:

Rhythm: Ventricular rhythm is usually very regular
Rate: 150 to 250 beats/min
P waves: Often hidden in the QRS complex; if the ventricles are stimulated first and then the atria, a negative P wave will appear after the QRS in leads II, III, and aVF; when the atria are depolarized after the ventricles, the P wave typically distorts the end of the QRS complex
PR interval: P waves are not seen before the QRS complex; therefore, the PR interval is not measurable
QRS duration: 0.11 second or less unless abnormally conducted

Let's look at the example of AVNRT in Fig. 4.13. You can see narrow-QRS complexes that occur at a regular rate of 168 beats/min. P waves are not clearly seen. Because AVNRT begins in the area of the AV node, the impulse spreads to the atria and ventricles at almost the same time, resulting in P waves that are usually hidden in the QRS complex. If the ventricles are stimulated first and then the atria, a negative (inverted) P wave will appear after the QRS in leads II, III, and aVF. When the atria are depolarized after the ventricles, the P wave typically distorts the end of the QRS complex. The PR interval is not measurable because P waves are not seen before the QRS complex.

In our example of AVNRT, you can see ST-segment depression. ST-segment changes (usually depression) are common in patients with SVTs. In most patients, these ST-segment changes are thought to be the result of repolarization changes. However, in older adults and those with a high likelihood of ischemic heart disease, ST-segment changes may represent ECG changes consistent with an acute coronary syndrome. The patient should be watched closely. Obtain appropriate laboratory tests and a 12-lead ECG to rule out infarction as needed.

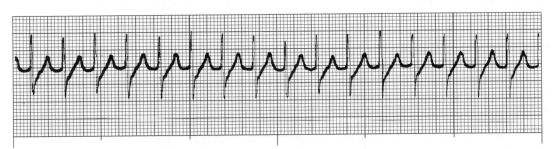

Fig. 4.13 Atrioventricular nodal reentrant tachycardia.

WHAT CAUSES IT?

AVNRT can occur at any age but is most often seen in young adults who have no structural heart disease or ischemic heart disease. Whether a person is born with a tendency to have AVNRT or whether it develops later in life for an unknown reason has not been clearly determined. It also occurs in patients with COPD, CAD, valvular heart disease, heart failure, and digitalis toxicity. AVNRT is more common in women than in men and may develop or be exacerbated by pregnancy or certain menstrual cycle phases (Zimetbaum, 2020). AVNRT can be triggered by hypoxia, stress, anxiety, caffeine, smoking, sleep deprivation, and many medications. AVNRT can cause angina or myocardial infarction (MI) in patients with CAD.

WHAT DO I DO ABOUT IT?

Because AVNRT may be short-lived or sustained, treatment depends on the tachycardia's duration and severity of the patient's signs and symptoms. Assessment findings and symptoms that may be associated with rapid ventricular rates may include the following:

- Chest pain or pressure
- Dizziness
- Dyspnea
- Lightheadedness
- Nausea
- Nervousness, anxiety

- Palpitations (common)
- Pounding sensation in the neck
- Polyuria
- Signs of shock
- Syncope
- Weakness

If the patient is stable but symptomatic and the symptoms result from the rapid heart rate, apply a pulse oximeter and administer supplemental oxygen, if indicated. Obtain the patient's vital signs, establish IV access, and obtain a 12-lead ECG. While continuously monitoring the patient's ECG, attempt a vagal maneuver if there are no contraindications. AVNRT is usually responsive to vagal maneuvers. If vagal maneuvers do not slow the rate or cause conversion of the tachycardia to a sinus rhythm, the first antiarrhythmic given is adenosine. The administration of calcium blockers or betablockers is indicated when AVNRT fails to convert to sinus rhythm or if it recurs. It has been estimated that 80% to 98% of stable patients with SVT respond to pharmacologic therapy with adenosine, diltiazem, or verapamil (Page et al., 2016).

An unstable patient has signs and symptoms of hemodynamic compromise. Examples of these signs and symptoms include acute mental status changes, chest pain or discomfort, hypotension, shortness of breath, pulmonary congestion, heart failure, acute MI, and signs of shock. If the patient is unstable, treatment should include applying a pulse oximeter and administering supplemental oxygen (if indicated), IV access, and sedation (if the patient is awake and time permits) followed by synchronized cardioversion.

Recurrent AVNRT may require treatment with a longacting calcium blocker or beta-blocker. Antiarrhythmics such as amiodarone may also be used. Recurrent episodes vary in frequency, duration, and severity from several times a day to every 2 to 3 years. Patients resistant to drug therapy or who do not wish to remain on lifelong medications for the dysrhythmia are candidates for radiofrequency catheter ablation. Catheter ablation has become the treatment of choice in managing patients with symptomatic recurrent episodes of AVNRT. It is successful in permanently interrupting the circuit and curing the dysrhythmia in most cases.

ATRIOVENTRICULAR REENTRANT TACHYCARDIA

AVRT is the most common type of SVT in children and the second most common in adults. Its prevalence decreases with age, whereas the prevalence of AVNRT and AT increases with advancing age (Virani et al., 2021).

Preexcitation refers to the premature activation of the ventricles by a supraventricular impulse arising from an accessory pathway. As a result, the impulse excites the ventricles earlier than would be expected if the impulse had traveled through the normal conduction system.

In patients with AVRT, a reentry circuit is formed that often involves four components—the atrium, the normal AV node, the ventricle, and an accessory pathway, also called a bypass tract (Saksena et al., 2012) (Fig. 4.14). Some people have more than one accessory pathway, and several types of accessory pathways have been described. The accessory pathway's location and the conductive properties of the pathway and AV node determine the extent of preexcitation. Unlike the AV node, an accessory pathway cannot slow or reduce the number of atrial impulses transmitted to the ventricles; therefore, patients with preexcitation syndromes are prone to tachydysrhythmias, including PSVT, AVRT, and AFib. The number of atrial impulses reaching the ventricles may approach 300 to 350 beats/min, significantly increasing the risk of development of ventricular fibrillation.

The most common form of preexcitation is the Wolff-Parkinson-White (WPW) pattern. This pattern includes a triad of findings that consists of the following: (1) a short PR interval, (2) a wide QRS complex, and (3) a delta wave (Fig. 4.15). A **delta wave** is an initial slurred deflection at the beginning of the QRS complex that may be positive or negative. It reflects the relatively slow ventricular depolarization over the accessory pathway (Mark et al., 2009). A patient is said to have a WPW *syndrome* when a WPW preexcitation pattern is present on the ECG, and a tachydysrhythmia occurs that is related to the accessory pathway (Virani et al., 2021).

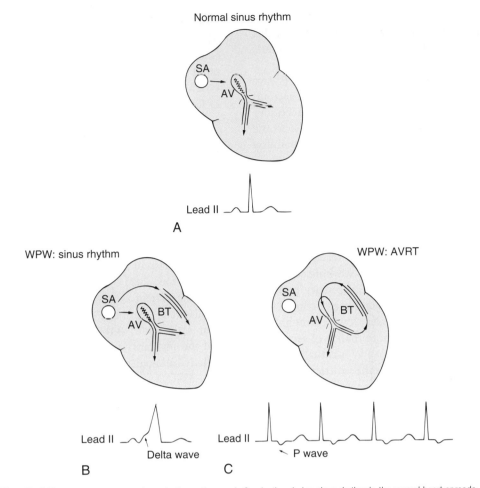

Fig. 4.14 Normal and abnormal conduction pathways. A, Conduction during sinus rhythm in the normal heart spreads from the sinoatrial *(SA)* node to the atrioventricular *(AV)* node and then down the bundle branches. The *jagged line* indicates physiologic slowing of conduction in the AV node. B, With Wolff-Parkinson-White *(WPW)* pattern, an abnormal accessory conduction pathway called a bypass tract *(BT)* connects the atria and ventricles. With WPW, during sinus rhythm, the electrical impulse is conducted quickly down the BT, preexciting the ventricles before the impulse arrives via the AV node. Consequently, the PR interval is short, and the QRS complex is wide, with slurring at its onset (delta wave). C, WPW predisposes patients to develop an atrioventricular reentrant tachycardia *(AVRT)*, in which a premature atrial beat may spread down the normal pathway to the ventricles, travel back up the BT, and recirculate down the AV node again. This reentrant loop can repeat itself over and over, resulting in a tachycardia. Notice the normal QRS complex and often negative P wave in lead II during this type of tachycardia. (From Goldberger, A. L., & Goldberger, Z. D. (2018). *Goldberger's clinical electrocardiography: a simplified approach* (9th ed.). Philadelphia: Elsevier.)

- Short PR
- Wide QRS
- Delta Wave (arrow)

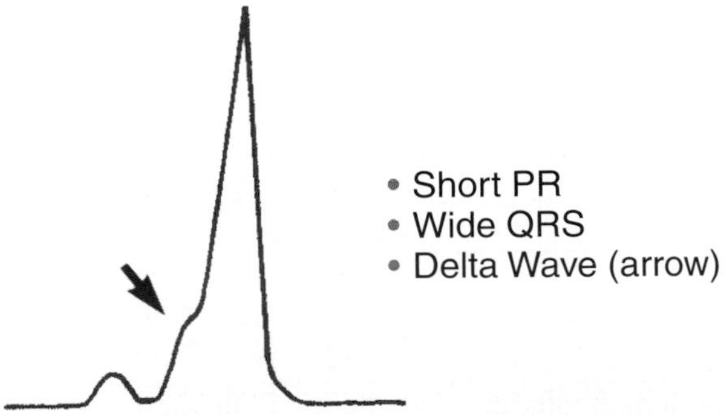

Fig. 4.15 Typical Wolff Parkinson White pattern showing a short PR interval, wide QRS complex, and a delta wave. (From Goldberger, A. L., & Goldberger, Z. D. (2018). *Goldberger's clinical electrocardiography: a simplified approach* (9th ed.). Philadelphia: Elsevier.)

HOW DO I RECOGNIZE IT?

ECG characteristics of the WPW pattern include the following:

Rhythm:	Regular, unless associated with AFib
Rate:	Usually 60 to 100 beats/min if the underlying rhythm is sinus in origin
P waves:	Normal and positive in lead II unless WPW is associated with AFib
PR interval:	0.12 second or less if P waves are observed because the impulse travels very quickly across the accessory pathway, bypassing the normal delay in the AV node
QRS duration:	Usually more than 0.12 second; slurred upstroke of the QRS complex (i.e., delta wave) may be seen in one or more leads

The ECG characteristics of WPW described here are usually seen when the patient is *not* experiencing a tachycardia. WPW syndrome usually goes undetected until it manifests in a patient as a tachycardia.

When WPW is associated with a sinus rhythm, the P wave looks normal. The PR interval is short (less than 0.12 second) because the impulse travels very quickly across the accessory pathway, bypassing the normal delay in the AV node. As the impulse crosses the insertion point of the accessory pathway in the ventricular muscle, that part of the ventricle is stimulated earlier (preexcited) than if the impulse had followed the normal conduction pathway through the bundle of His and Purkinje fibers. On the ECG, ventricular preexcitation can be seen as a delta wave in some leads (Fig. 4.16).

Conduction through the Purkinje fibers is usually very fast; however, with WPW, the impulse's spread is slow because it must spread from working cell to working cell in the ventricular muscle. This is because the accessory pathway bypasses the specialized cells of the heart's conduction system. Because the impulse spreads slowly through the working cells, the QRS is usually more than 0.12 second in duration. The QRS complex seen in WPW is actually a combination of the impulse that preexcites the ventricles through the accessory pathway and the impulse that follows the AV node's normal conduction pathway (Hamdan, 2010). As a result, the end (i.e., terminal) portion of the QRS usually looks normal. However, because the ventricles are activated abnormally, they repolarize abnormally. This is seen on the ECG as changes in the ST segment and T wave. The ST segment and T wave direction are usually opposite the direction of the delta wave and QRS complex, which can mimic ECG signs of myocardial ischemia or injury.

WHAT CAUSES IT?

Most people with WPW syndrome have no associated heart disease. WPW syndrome is one of the most common causes of tachydysrhythmias in infants and children. Although the accessory pathway in WPW syndrome is believed to be congenital in origin, symptoms associated with preexcitation often do not appear until the patient is a teenager or during young adulthood.

WHAT DO I DO ABOUT IT?

Although some people with AVRT never have symptoms, common signs and symptoms associated with AVRT and a rapid ventricular rate include the following:

- Anxiety
- Chest discomfort
- Dizziness
- Lightheadedness
- Palpitations (common)
- Shortness of breath during exercise
- Signs of shock
- Weakness

If a delta wave is noted on the ECG, but the patient is asymptomatic, no specific treatment is required. Asymptomatic adults with ventricular preexcitation appear to be at no increased risk of sudden death than the general population (Virani et al., 2021).

If the patient is symptomatic because of the rapid ventricular rate, treatment will depend on how unstable the patient is, the width of the QRS complex (i.e., wide or narrow), and the regularity of the ventricular rhythm. Consultation with a cardiologist is recommended when caring for a patient with AVRT.

Vagal maneuvers are recommended if the patient is stable and there are no contraindications (Page et al., 2016). Medications such as adenosine, digoxin, diltiazem, and verapamil should be avoided. These medications are contraindicated because they slow or block conduction across the AV node, but they may speed up conduction through the accessory pathway, thereby resulting in a further *increase* in the ventricular rate. If the patient is unstable, preparations should be made for synchronized cardioversion.

ATRIAL FLUTTER AND ATRIAL FIBRILLATION

Atrial flutter is a reentrant rhythm in which an irritable site within the atria fires regularly at a very rapid rate (Fig. 4.17). Typical atrial flutter, also known as common atrial flutter,

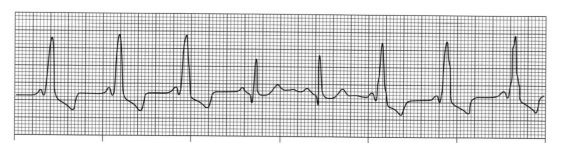

Fig. 4.16 This rhythm strip shows an example of intermittent preexcitation. The first three beats show preexcitation, followed by abrupt normalization of the QRS complex in the next two beats. The preexcitation pattern returns for the final three beats. (From Zipes, D. P., & Jalife, J. (2000). *Cardiac electrophysiology: from cell to bedside* (3rd ed.). Philadelphia: Saunders.)

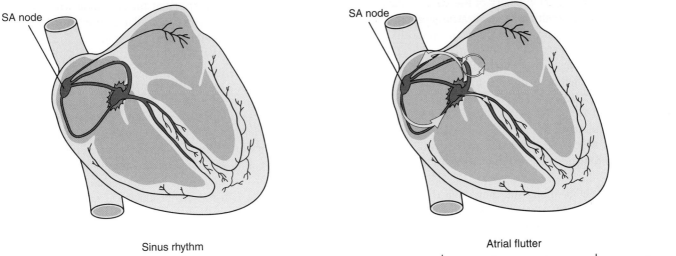

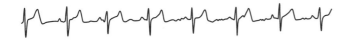

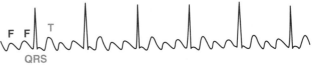

Fig. 4.17 Atrial flutter. *F* = flutter wave. *SA*, Sinoatrial.

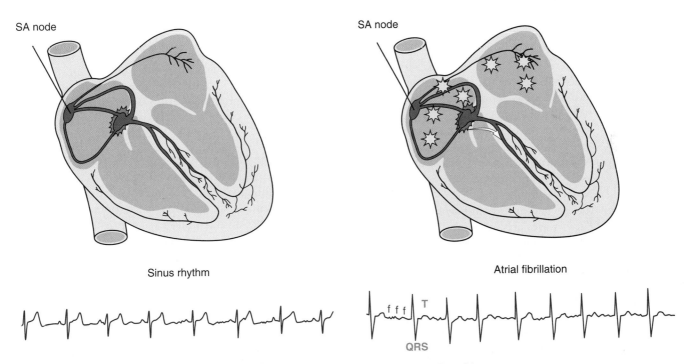

Fig. 4.18 Atrial fibrillation. *f* = fibrillatory wave. *SA*, Sinoatrial.

involves a reentry circuit around the right atrium's tricuspid valve. Atrial waveforms are produced that resemble the teeth of a saw or a picket fence; these are called flutter waves or F waves. Because P waves are not observed in atrial flutter, the PR interval is not measurable. The QRS complex is usually 0.11 second or less because atrial flutter is a supraventricular rhythm, and the impulse is conducted normally through the AV junction and Purkinje fibers. However, if flutter waves are buried in the QRS complex or if an intraventricular conduction delay exists, the QRS will appear wide (i.e., greater than 0.11 second).

AFib is the most common dysrhythmia worldwide (Kalstø et al., 2019). It occurs because of altered automaticity in one or several rapidly firing sites in the atria or reentry involving one or more circuits in the atria (Fig. 4.18). Irritable sites in the atria fire at a rate of 300 to 600 times per minute. These rapid impulses cause the muscles of the atria to quiver (i.e., fibrillate), thereby resulting in weak atrial contraction, decreased stroke volume, a subsequent decrease in cardiac output, and a loss of atrial kick. AFib may occur alone or in association with other atrial dysrhythmias.

AFib is classified according to the duration of episodes (January et al., 2014):

- Paroxysmal AFib—AFib that lasts 7 days or less with or without intervention
- Persistent AFib—AFib that lasts more than 7 days
- Long-standing persistent AFib—AFib that lasts 12 months or longer
- Permanent AFib—Long-standing AFib that is refractory to cardioversion; this term is also used when both the patient and his or her physician make a joint decision to stop further attempts to restore or maintain a sinus rhythm
- Nonvalvular AFib—AFib that occurs in the absence of rheumatic mitral stenosis, a mechanical or bioprosthetic heart valve, or mitral valve repair

How Do I Recognize It?

ECG characteristics of atrial flutter include the following:

Rhythm:	Atrial regular; ventricular regular or irregular depending on AV conduction and blockade
Rate:	Atrial rate typically ranges from 240 to 300 beats/min; ventricular rate varies and is determined by AV blockade; the ventricular rate will usually not exceed 180 beats/min as a result of the intrinsic conduction rate of the AV junction
P waves:	No identifiable P waves; saw-toothed "flutter" waves are present
PR interval:	Not measurable
QRS duration:	0.11 second or less but may be widened if flutter waves are buried in the QRS complex or if abnormally conducted

With atrial flutter, an irritable focus within the atrium typically depolarizes at a rate of 300 beats/min. If each impulse were transmitted to the ventricles, the ventricular rate would equal 300 beats/min. The healthy AV node protects the ventricles from these extremely fast atrial rates. Suppose an irritable site in the atria fires at a rate of 300 beats/min, but

every other impulse arrived at the AV node while it is still refractory. The resulting ventricular response of 150 beats/min is called 2:1 conduction. (The ratio of the atrial rate [300 beats/min] to the ventricular rate [150 beats/min] is 2 to 1) (Fig. 4.19). Atrial flutter with an atrial rate of 300 beats/min and a ventricular rate of 100 beats/min results in 3:1 conduction, 75 beats/min results in 4:1 conduction, 50 beats/min results in 6:1 conduction, and so on. Although conduction ratios in atrial flutter are often even (i.e., 2:1, 4:1, 6:1), variable conduction can also occur, which produces an irregular ventricular rhythm. In individuals with an accessory pathway, atrial flutter may be associated with 1:1 conduction because the AV node is bypassed, producing extremely rapid ventricular rates. When atrial flutter is present with 2:1 conduction, it may be difficult to tell the difference between atrial flutter and sinus tachycardia, AT, AVNRT, AVRT, or SVT.

With AFib, the AV node attempts to protect the ventricles from the hundreds of impulses bombarding it per minute. It does this by blocking many of the impulses generated by the irritable sites in the atria. The ventricular rate and rhythm are determined by the degree of blocking by the AV node of these rapid impulses. The ECG characteristics of AFib include the following:

Rhythm:	Ventricular rhythm usually irregularly irregular
Rate:	Atrial rate usually 300 to 600 beats/min; ventricular rate variable
P waves:	No identifiable P waves, fibrillatory waves present; erratic, wavy baseline
PR interval:	Not measurable
QRS duration:	0.11 second or less unless abnormally conducted

Let's take a look at the example of AFib in Fig. 4.20. One of the first things you notice is that the ventricular rhythm is irregular. With AFib, atrial depolarization occurs very irregularly, which results in an irregular ventricular rhythm. The ventricular rhythm associated with AFib is described as irregularly irregular because there is no pattern to the irregularity. Because the ventricular rhythm is irregular, we will use the 6-second rate calculation method to determine the ventricular rate, which is about 80 beats/min.

There is no P wave in AFib because of atrial muscle quivering and because there is no uniform wave of atrial depolarization. Instead, you see a baseline that looks erratic

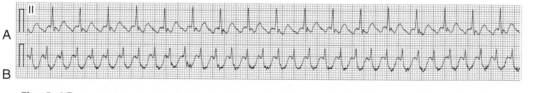

Fig. 4.19 Atrial flutter with 2:1 atrioventricular (AV) conduction (A) compared with 1:1 (one-to-one) AV conduction (B) in the same patient. In the latter case, the flutter waves are hard to see. Because of the very rapid ventricular response (about 300 beats/min), atrial flutter with 1:1 conduction is a medical emergency, often necessitating synchronized cardioversion. (From Goldberger, A. L., & Goldberger, Z. D. (2018). Goldberger's clinical electrocardiography: a simplified approach (9th ed.). Philadelphia: Elsevier.)

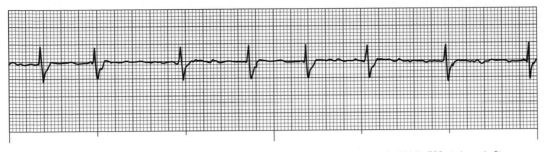

Fig. 4.20 Atrial fibrillation with a ventricular response of 80 beats/min. (From Aehlert, B. (2004). *ECG study cards.* St. Louis: Mosby.)

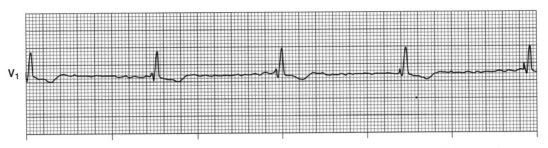

Fig. 4.21 Atrial fibrillation with third-degree atrioventricular block. The ventricular rate is slow and regular because of the block. (From Goldberger, A. L. (2006). *Clinical electrocardiography: a simplified approach* (7th ed.). St. Louis: Mosby.)

(i.e., wavy), which corresponds with the rapid atrial rate. These wavy deflections are called fibrillatory waves or f waves. Some clinicians refer to fibrillatory waves of large amplitude as coarse fibrillatory waves and those of small amplitude as fine fibrillatory waves. This distinction has no clinical relevance.

We cannot measure a PR interval because there is no P wave. The QRS complex is narrow (i.e., measuring 0.08 to 0.10 second) because the impulse started above the bifurcation of the bundle of His and was conducted normally through the AV node and bundle and Purkinje fibers. We cannot measure a QT interval because T waves are not clearly seen.

AFib may be confused with MAT because both rhythms are irregular. However, although varying in size, shape, and direction, P waves are clearly visible in MAT, and a distinct isoelectric period is seen between P waves (Page et al., 2016). If AFib occurs with a slow, regular ventricular rate, suspect toxicity caused by digitalis, beta-blockers, or calcium blockers. Toxicity can occur when a patient who has AFib is prescribed medications to slow the ventricular rate. Excess medication can cause third-degree AV block (Fig. 4.21). When AFib is present with a third-degree AV block, the diagnosis of AFib is made based on the presence of f waves (Morady & Zipes, 2019).

ECG Pearl

Atrial flutter or AFib that has a rapid ventricular rate is described as uncontrolled. Atrial flutter or AFib with a rapid ventricular response (RVR) is commonly called Aflutter with RVR or AFib with RVR.

Box 4.1 Conditions Associated With Atrial Flutter

- Cardiac surgery
- Cardiomyopathy
- Chronic lung disease
- Complication of myocardial infarction
- Digitalis or quinidine toxicity
- Hyperthyroidism
- Ischemic heart disease
- Mitral or tricuspid valve stenosis or regurgitation
- Pericarditis or myocarditis
- Pulmonary embolism

What Causes It?

Atrial flutter is often precipitated by a brief episode of AT or AFib (January et al., 2014). It may last for seconds to hours and occasionally persists for 24 hours or longer. Chronic atrial flutter is unusual because it usually converts to sinus rhythm or AFib, either on its own or with treatment. Conditions associated with atrial flutter are shown in Box 4.1.

Although most patients with AFib have some form of cardiovascular disease, AFib can occur in patients without detectable heart disease or related symptoms. "Lone AFib" is a phrase used to describe AFib that occurs with no known precipitating cause. AFib can be inherited; having a family member with AFib increases an individual's risk of the dysrhythmia by 40% (January et al., 2014).

Risk factors associated with AFib appear in Box 4.2, and possible causes of AFib appear in Table 4.1. The most significant risk factor for AFib is hypertension, followed by body

<table>
<tr><td>Box **4.2**</td><td>**Risks Factors Associated With Atrial Fibrillation**</td></tr>
</table>

- Age 75 and older
- Cardiac failure
- Cardiothoracic surgery
- Diabetes mellitus
- Hypertension
- Obesity
- Obstructive sleep apnea
- Smoking
- Stroke
- Thromboembolism
- Transient ischemic attack
- Vascular disease (e.g., myocardial infarction, peripheral artery disease, aortic plaque)
- Valvular heart disease

TABLE 4.1   **Causes of Atrial Fibrillation**

Cardiovascular Conditions	Potentially Reversible Causes
• Coronary artery disease • Dilated cardiomyopathy • Heart failure • Hypertension • Hypertrophic cardiomyopathy • Ischemic heart disease • Pericardial disease • Rheumatic heart disease • Stroke, transient ischemic attack, thromboembolism • Valvular disease (especially mitral valve disease) • Vascular disease (myocardial infarction, peripheral artery disease, aortic plaque)	• Electrocution • Excessive alcohol intake ("holiday heart") • Hyperthyroidism • Myocardial infarction • Myocarditis • Open heart or thoracic surgery • Pericarditis • Pneumonia • Pulmonary embolism

mass index, smoking, cardiac disease, and diabetes mellitus (Virani et al., 2021). Hypertension increases the risk of AFib by 40% in women and 50% in men, diabetes increases the risk by 60% in women and 40% in men, whereas a 10-year increase in age doubles the risk for AFib (Kalstø et al., 2019).

Because the atria do not contract effectively and expel all of the blood within them during episodes of AFib, blood may pool within these chambers and form clots. A clot may dislodge on its own or because of conversion of AFib to a sinus rhythm.

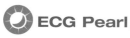 **ECG Pearl**

AFib is associated with a 10% higher risk of falls than among individuals without AFib and an increased risk of death in other conditions (e.g., diabetes mellitus, end-stage renal disease, sepsis, noncardiac surgery) (Virani et al., 2021). Heart failure

may cause and be caused by AFib (Kalstø et al., 2019). Because AFib and heart failure share many risk factors, about 40% of individuals with either AFib or heart failure will develop the other condition (Virani et al., 2021).

What Do I Do About It?

Patients with atrial flutter may be asymptomatic or present with complaints of palpitations, difficulty breathing, fatigue, lightheadedness, or chest discomfort. About 25% of patients who experience AFib are asymptomatic (Morady & Zipes, 2019). When symptoms are present, the severity of the signs and symptoms associated with AFib vary with the ventricular rate (either too fast or too slow), the loss of effective atrial contraction, sympathetic activation, and the beat-to-beat variability in ventricular filling (January et al., 2014). Examples of symptoms include fatigue (the most common symptom), palpitations, shortness of breath, chest discomfort or pain, exercise intolerance, dizziness/lightheadedness, and weakness.

Obtaining a thorough medical history and carrying out patient assessment are essential. When acquiring the patient's history, asking about the number of episodes of atrial flutter or AFib, their frequency, the nature of the patient's symptoms, and possible triggers may help determine the pattern of the dysrhythmia. The patient's provider may order ambulatory monitoring, exercise stress testing, or both to capture and identify the dysrhythmia and detect possible precipitating causes.

During episodes of AFib, anticipate that the patient's heart rate will be irregularly irregular. Irregular jugular venous pulsations, variable intensity of the first heart sound, and a pulse deficit (i.e., the apical pulse rate is faster than the peripheral pulse rate) may also be observed during the physical examination (Morady & Zipes, 2019).

Treatment decisions for AFib and atrial flutter are based on the ventricular rate, the duration of the rhythm, the patient's general health, and how they tolerate the rhythm. It is best to consult a cardiologist when considering specific therapies.

When vagal maneuvers are used in the management of atrial flutter, the response is usually slowing of AV conduction and the ventricular response, possibly revealing underlying flutter waves, and then returning to the former rate. Vagal maneuvers will not usually convert atrial flutter because the reentry circuit is located in the atria, not the AV node. Similarly, because the reentry circuit is located in the atria, not the AV node, vagal maneuvers will not usually convert AFib. Still, they may result in a brief slowing of AV conduction and the ventricular response, possibly revealing fibrillatory waves (Fig. 4.22).

Rate control and rhythm control are the two primary treatment strategies used to control AFib or atrial flutter symptoms. With rate control, the patient remains in atrial flutter or AFib, but the ventricular rate is controlled (i.e., slowed) to decrease acute symptoms, reduce signs of ischemia, and reduce or prevent signs of heart failure from developing. Rate control is achieved using medications that prolong the AV node's refractory period (e.g., beta-blockers, calcium blockers) or catheter ablation.

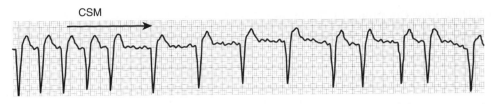

Fig. 4.22 Atrial fibrillation. Carotid sinus massage *(CSM)* results in transient slowing of the ventricular response, revealing the fibrillating baseline. The ventricular rate subsequently accelerates. (From Roberts, J. R., Custalow, C. B., & Thomsen, T. W. (2019). *Roberts and Hedges' clinical procedures in emergency medicine and acute care* (7th ed). Philadelphia: Elsevier.)

TABLE 4.2	Atrial Rhythms: Summary of Characteristics				
Dysrhythmia	**Rhythm**	**Rate (beats/min)**	**P waves (lead II)**	**PR interval**	**QRS duration**
PACs	Irregular because of the early beat(s)	Usually within normal range but depends on underlying rhythm	Premature, positive, one before each QRS, differ from sinus P waves, may be lost in preceding T wave	May be WNL or prolonged	0.11 sec or less unless abnormally conducted
Wandering atrial pacemaker	Usually irregular as pacemaker site shifts from SA node to ectopic atrial locations or AV junction	Usually 60 to 100; if rate greater than 100 beats/min, rhythm is called *multifocal atrial tachycardia*	Size, shape, and direction may change from beat to beat	Varies	0.11 sec or less unless abnormally conducted
Atrial tachycardia	Regular	101 to 250	One precedes each QRS; atrial P waves differ from sinus P waves; isoelectric baseline usually present between P waves	May be shorter or longer than normal	0.11 sec or less unless abnormally conducted
AVNRT	Ventricular rhythm is usually very regular	150 to 250	P waves often hidden in QRS complex	Not measurable	0.11 sec or less unless abnormally conducted
Wolff-Parkinson-White (WPW) Pattern	Regular, unless associated with AFib	60 to 100 if the underlying rhythm is sinus in origin	Positive, one before each QRS unless associated with AFib	0.12 sec or less if P waves are seen	Usually more than 0.12 sec; delta wave may be seen in one or more leads

AFib, Atrial fibrillation; *AV,* atrioventricular; *AVNRT,* atrioventricular nodal reentrant tachycardia; *PAC,* premature atrial complex; *SA,* sinoatrial; *WNL,* within normal limits.

With rhythm control, sinus rhythm is reestablished using approaches that may include pharmacologic cardioversion, electric cardioversion, or catheter ablation. Because pharmacologic or electric cardioversion carries a risk of thromboembolism, anticoagulation is recommended before attempting to convert AFib or atrial flutter to a sinus rhythm when the dysrhythmia duration exceeds 48 hours or when the duration is unknown (January et al., 2019). Synchronized cardioversion should be considered if the patient with AFib or atrial flutter is hemodynamically unstable. A summary of atrial rhythm characteristics can be found in Tables 4.2 and 4.3.

TABLE **4.3**	Atrial Rhythms: Summary of Characteristics				
Dysrhythmia	Rhythm	Rate (beats/min)	P waves (lead II)	PR interval	QRS duration
Atrial flutter	Atrial regular; ventricular regular or irregular	Atrial rate typically from 240 to 300; ventricular rate varies and is determined by AV blockade	No identifiable P waves; saw-toothed "flutter" waves present	Not measurable	0.11 sec or less unless abnormally conducted
Atrial fibrillation (AFib)	Ventricular rhythm usually irregularly irregular	Atrial rate usually 300 to 600; ventricular rate variable	No identifiable P waves; fibrillatory waves present; erratic, wavy baseline	Not measurable	0.11 sec or less unless abnormally conducted

AV, Atrioventricular.

REFERENCES

Appelboam, A., Reuben, A., Mann, C., Gagg, J., Ewings, P., Barton, A., REVERT trial collaborators. (2015). Postural modification to the standard Valsalva manoeuvre for emergency treatment of supraventricular tachycardias (REVERT): a randomised controlled trial. *Lancet, 386*(10005), 1747–1753.

Ellenbogen, K. A., & Koneru, J. N. (2018). Atrial tachycardia. In D. P. Zipes, J. Jalife, & W. G. Stevenson (Eds.), *Cardiac electrophysiology: From cell to bedside* (7th ed.) (pp. 681–699). Philadelphia, PA: Elsevier.

Hamdan, M. H. (2010). Cardiac arrhythmias. In T. E. Andreoli, I. J. Benjamin, R. C. Griggs, & E. J. Wing (Eds.), *Andreoli and Carpenter's Cecil essentials of medicine* (8th ed.) (pp. 118–144). Philadelphia, PA: Saunders.

January, C. T., Wann, L. S., Alpert, J. S., Calkins, H., Cigarroa, J. E., Cleveland, J. C., ... Yancy, C. W. (2014). 2014 AHA/ACC/HRS guideline for the management of patients with atrial fibrillation: a report of the American College of Cardiology/American Heart Association Task Force on Practice Guidelines and the Heart Rhythm Society. *Circulation, 130*(23), e199–e267.

January, C. T., Wann, L. S., Calkins, H., Chen, L. Y., Cigarroa, J. E., Cleveland, J. C., Yancy, C. W. (2019). 2019 AHA/ACC/HRS focused update of the 2014 AHA/ACC/HRS guideline for the management of patients with atrial fibrillation. *J Am Coll Cardiol, 74*(1), 104–132.

Kalstø, S. M., Siland, J. E., Rienstra, M., & Christophersen, I. E. (2019). Atrial fibrillation genetics update: toward clinical implementation. *Front Cardiovasc Med, 6*(127), 1–16.

Mani, B. C., & Pavri, B. B. (2014). Dual atrioventricular nodal pathways physiology: a review of relevant anatomy, electrophysiology, and electrocardiographic manifestations. *Indian Pacing Electrophysiol J, 14*(1), 12–25.

Mark, D. G., Brady, W. J., & Pines, J. M. (2009). Preexcitation syndromes: diagnostic consideration in the ED. *Am J Emerg Med, 27*(7), 878–888.

Minczak, B. M., & Laub, G. W. (2019). Techniques for supraventricular tachycardias. In J. R. Robert, C. B. Custalow, & T. W. Thomsen (Eds.), *Roberts and Hedges' clinical procedures in emergency medicine and acute care* (7th ed.) (pp. 221–237). Philadelphia, PA: Elsevier.

Morady, F., & Zipes, D. P. (2019). Atrial fibrillation: clinical features, mechanisms, and management. In D. P. Zipes, P. Libby, R. O. Bonow, D. L. Mann, G. F. Tomaselli, & E. Braunwald (Eds.), *Braunwald's heart disease: a textbook of cardiovascular medicine* (11th ed.) (pp. 730–752). Philadelphia, PA: Elsevier.

Page, R. L., Joglar, J. A., Caldwell, M. A., Calkins, H., Conti, J. B., Deal, B. J., ... Al-Khatib, S. M. (2016). 2015 ACC/AHA/HRS guideline for the management of adult patients with supraventricular tachycardia. *Circulation, 133*(14), e506–e574.

Peterson, K. (2018). Advanced dysrhythmias. In V. S. Good, & P. L. Kirkwood (Eds.), *Advanced critical care nursing* (2nd ed.) (pp. 12–33). St. Louis, MO: Elsevier.

Saksena, S., Bharati, S., Lindsay, B. D., & Levy, S. (2012). Paroxysmal supraventricular tachycardia and pre-excitation syndromes. In S. Saksena, & A. J. Camm (Eds.), *Electrophysiological disorders of the heart* (2nd ed.) (pp. 531–558). Philadelphia, PA: Saunders.

Virani, S. S., Alonso, A., Aparicio, H. J., Benjamin, E. J., Bittencourt, M. S., Callaway, C. W., ... Tsao, C. W. (2021). Heart disease and stroke statistics—2021 update: a report from the American Heart Association. *Circulation, 143*(8), e254–e743.

Zimetbaum, P. (2020). Supraventricular cardiac arrhythmias. In L. Goldman & A. I. Schafer (Eds.), *Goldman-Cecil medicine* (26th ed.) (pp. 331–343). Philadelphia, PA: Elsevier.

STOP & REVIEW

Identify one or more choices that best complete the statement or answer the question.

1. The most common type of supraventricular tachycardia (SVT) in adults is
   a. AT.
   b. AVRT.
   c. AVNRT.
   d. atrial flutter.

2. All supraventricular dysrhythmias
   a. involve accessory pathways.
   b. begin above the bifurcation of the bundle of His.
   c. begin below the bifurcation of the bundle of His.
   d. require the AV node's participation to sustain the dysrhythmia.

3. Which of the following dysrhythmias is most likely to be associated with a reduction in cardiac output and loss of atrial kick?
   a. AFib
   b. PACs
   c. Sinus tachycardia
   d. Wandering atrial pacemaker

4. Which of the following ECG characteristics distinguishes atrial flutter from other atrial dysrhythmias?
   a. The presence of fibrillatory waves
   b. P waves of varying size and amplitude
   c. The presence of delta waves before the QRS
   d. The "saw-tooth" or "picket-fence" appearance of waveforms before the QRS

5. The Wolff-Parkinson-White pattern is associated with
   a. a delta wave.
   b. flutter waves.
   c. fibrillatory waves.
   d. a long PR interval.
   e. a short PR interval.
   f. a wide QRS complex.
   g. a narrow QRS complex.

6. In AFib, the PR interval is usually
   a. not measurable.
   b. within normal limits.
   c. less than 0.20 second in duration.
   d. more than 0.20 second in duration.

7. Signs and symptoms experienced during a tachydysrhythmia are usually primarily related to
   a. atrial irritability.
   b. vasoconstriction.
   c. slowed conduction through the AV node.
   d. decreased ventricular filling time and stroke volume.

8. On the ECG, an impulse that begins in the atria and occurs earlier than the next expected sinus beat will appear as a
   a. P wave that appears after the QRS complex.
   b. QRS measuring more than 0.11 second in duration.
   c. P wave with a PR interval measuring more than 0.20 second.
   d. P wave that may appear in the T wave of the preceding beat.

9. A compensatory pause is a
   a. series of waveforms.
   b. delay that occurs following a premature beat that resets the SA node.
   c. period during the cardiac cycle during which cardiac cells cannot be stimulated to conduct an electrical impulse, no matter how strong the stimulus.
   d. period during the cardiac cycle during which cardiac cells can be stimulated to conduct an electrical impulse, if exposed to a stronger than normal stimulus.

10. Which of the following are typical ECG characteristics associated with wandering atrial pacemaker?
    a. Rhythm is usually irregular
    b. Rate is usually faster than 100 beats/min
    c. Delta waves are seen in one or more leads
    d. QRS is often more than 0.12 second in duration
    e. P waves differing in size, shape, and direction
    f. PR intervals vary because of shifting pacemaker sites

Questions 11 Through 14 Pertain to the Following Scenario

A 35-year-old woman is complaining of palpitations. She is alert and oriented to person, place, time, and event. Her blood pressure is 144/82 mm Hg, ventilations 18/min and unlabored. She appears anxious and states her "heart is racing."

11. Which of the following statements is correct concerning the assessment of this patient?
   a. Despite the patient's age, palpitations generally indicate the presence of cardiac disease.
   b. A complaint of palpitations is a cause for concern only if they are of sudden onset and their rhythm is irregular.
   c. A complaint of palpitations is always associated with evidence of a rhythm disturbance on the cardiac monitor.
   d. Information relayed by the patient can provide important clues about her cardiovascular status.

12. A pulse oximeter has been applied. The patient's oxygen saturation on room air is 97%. The cardiac monitor reveals the rhythm below. This rhythm (Fig. 4.23), recorded in lead II, is
   a. sinus tachycardia.
   b. AVNRT.
   c. AVRT.
   d. AFib.

13. The PR interval in Fig. 4.23
   a. is 0.06 second.
   b. is 0.12 second.
   c. is 0.20 second.
   d. cannot be measured.

14. Intravenous (IV) access has been established. A repeat set of vital signs reveals the following: blood pressure 140/82 mm Hg, pulse 188, ventilations 20. The patient's anxiety has increased. She denies chest discomfort and shortness of breath. Her skin is pink and warm, but moist. Which of the following interventions are likely to be ordered based on the information provided?
   a. Administer IV atropine.
   b. Attempt vagal maneuvers.
   c. Begin chest compressions.
   d. Administer supplemental oxygen.
   e. Administer sedation and perform synchronized cardioversion.

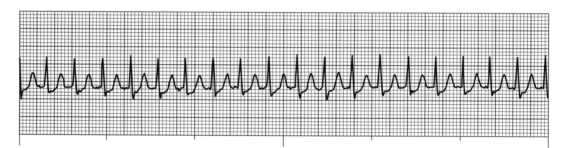

Fig. 4.23 (From Aehlert, B. (2004). *ECG study cards*. St. Louis: Mosby.)

Matching

Match the terms below with their descriptions by placing the letter of each correct answer in the space provided.

a. Atrial kick
b. Premature
c. Beta-blockers
d. Accessory pathway
e. Trigeminy
f. Bruit
g. Adenosine
h. Delta wave
i. Uncontrolled
j. Nonconducted PAC
k. Hypertension

l. Aberrantly conducted PAC
m. Anticoagulant
n. Erratic
o. Heart failure
p. Vagal maneuvers
q. Palpitations
r. Stroke
s. Preexcitation
t. Wolff-Parkinson-White (WPW) pattern
u. Bigeminy

_____ **15.** Most common form of preexcitation

_____ **16.** Common complaint in a patient with a rapid heart rate

_____ **17.** Term used to describe rhythms that originate from above the ventricles but in which the impulse travels by a pathway other than the AV node and bundle of His

_____ 18. Baseline appearance in atrial fibrillation

_____ 19. ECG finding associated with Wolff-Parkinson-White pattern

_____ 20. Patients who experience AFib are at increased risk of having this

_____ 21. Blood pushed into the ventricles because of atrial contraction

_____ 22. An extra bundle of working myocardial tissue that forms a connection between the atria and ventricles outside the normal conduction system

_____ 23. Methods used to stimulate the vagus nerve in an attempt to slow conduction through the AV node

_____ 24. This condition may cause or be caused by AFib

_____ 25. Atrial flutter or fibrillation with a rapid ventricular rate

_____ 26. Every other beat comes from somewhere other than the SA node

_____ 27. An early P wave with no QRS following it

_____ 28. Earlier than expected

_____ 29. These should be avoided in the presence of severe underlying pulmonary disease

_____ 30. Blowing or swishing sound within a vessel

_____ 31. The name given a PAC associated with a wide QRS complex

_____ 32. Drug of choice for AVNRT

_____ 33. The most significant risk factor for AFib

_____ 34. Every third beat comes from somewhere other than the SA node

_____ 35. Before elective cardioversion, prophylactic treatment with a(n) __ is recommended for the patient in atrial flutter or fibrillation.

Atrial Rhythms—Practice Rhythm Strips

Use the five steps of rhythm interpretation to interpret each of the following rhythm strips. All rhythms were recorded in lead II unless otherwise noted.

36. Identify the rhythm.

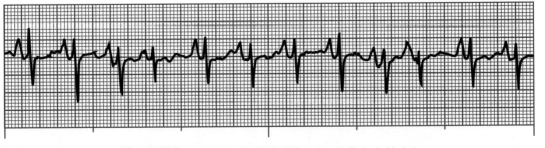

Fig. 4.24   (From Aehlert, B. (2004). _ECG study cards._ St. Louis: Mosby.)

Rhythm: _____   Rate: _____   P waves: _____
PR interval: _____   QRS duration: _____   QT interval: _____
Interpretation: _____

37. This rhythm strip is from an 85-year-old man experiencing chest pain and shortness of breath.

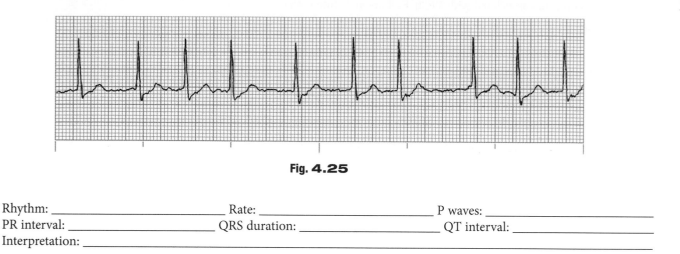

Fig. 4.25

Rhythm: _____ Rate: _____ P waves: _____
PR interval: _____ QRS duration: _____ QT interval: _____
Interpretation: _____

38. This rhythm strip is from a 53-year-old woman with an altered level of responsiveness.

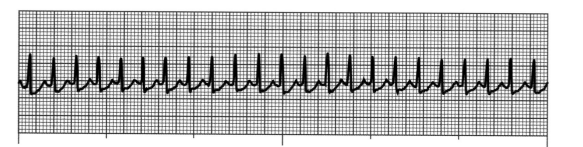

Fig. 4.26 (From Aehlert, B. (2004). *ECG study cards.* St. Louis: Mosby.)

Rhythm: _____ Rate: _____ P waves: _____
PR interval: _____ QRS duration: _____ QT interval: _____
Interpretation: _____

39. These rhythm strips are from an 82-year-old man experiencing back pain.

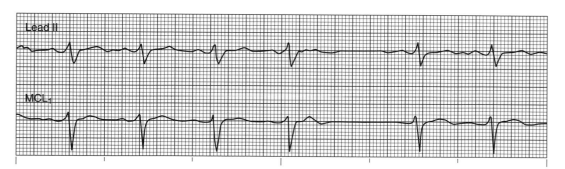
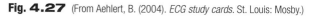

Fig. 4.27 (From Aehlert, B. (2004). *ECG study cards.* St. Louis: Mosby.)

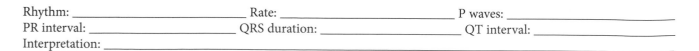

Rhythm: _____ Rate: _____ P waves: _____
PR interval: _____ QRS duration: _____ QT interval: _____
Interpretation: _____

40. Identify the rhythm.

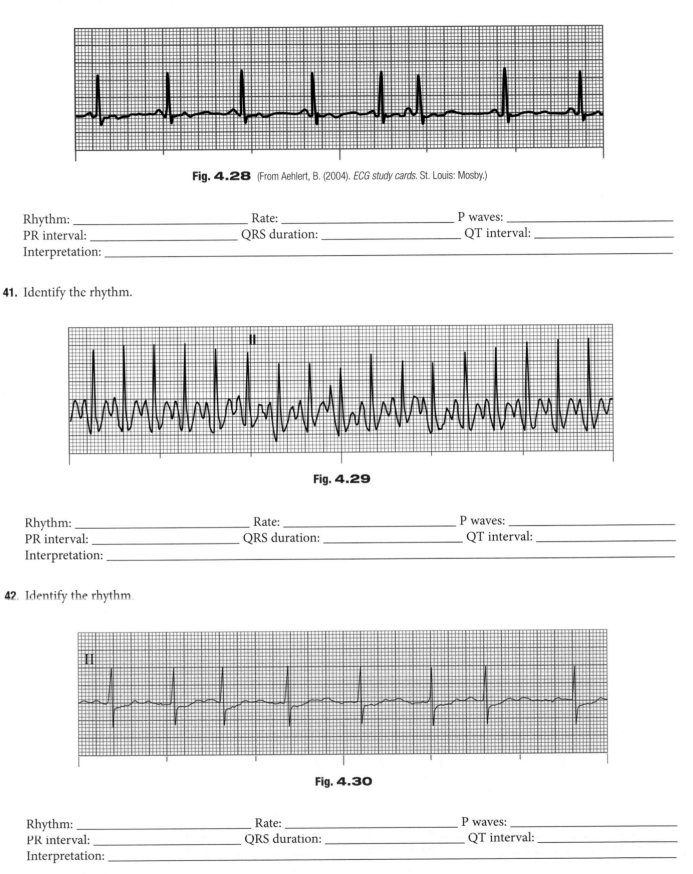

Fig. 4.28 (From Aehlert, B. (2004). *ECG study cards.* St. Louis: Mosby.)

Rhythm: _____ Rate: _____ P waves: _____
PR interval: _____ QRS duration: _____ QT interval: _____
Interpretation: _____

41. Identify the rhythm.

Fig. 4.29

Rhythm: _____ Rate: _____ P waves: _____
PR interval: _____ QRS duration: _____ QT interval: _____
Interpretation: _____

42. Identify the rhythm.

Fig. 4.30

Rhythm: _____ Rate: _____ P waves: _____
PR interval: _____ QRS duration: _____ QT interval: _____
Interpretation: _____

43. Identify the rhythm.

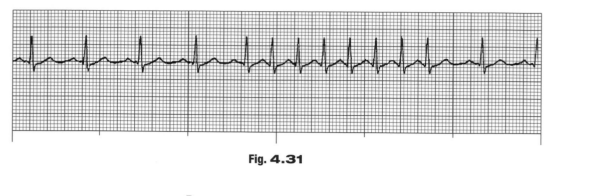

Fig. 4.31

Rhythm: _____ Rate: _____ P waves: _____
PR interval: _____ QRS duration: _____ QT interval: _____
Interpretation: _____

44. These rhythm strips are from a 74-year-old woman with difficulty breathing.

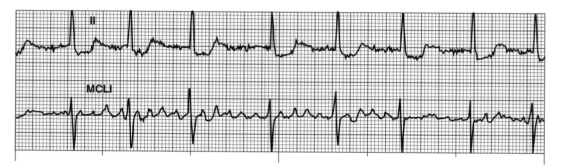

Fig. 4.32 (From Aehlert, B. (2004). *ECG study cards.* St. Louis: Mosby.)

Rhythm: _____ Rate: _____ P waves: _____
PR interval: _____ QRS duration: _____ QT interval: _____
Interpretation: _____

45. These rhythm strips are from a 78-year-old man complaining of shortness of breath.

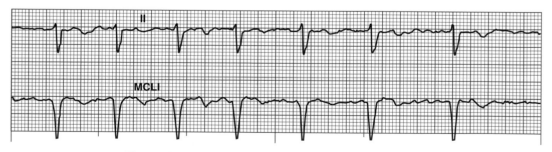

Fig. 4.33 (From Aehlert, B. (2004). *ECG study cards.* St. Louis: Mosby.)

Rhythm: _____ Rate: _____ P waves: _____
PR interval: _____ QRS duration: _____ QT interval: _____
Interpretation: _____

46. Identify the rhythm.

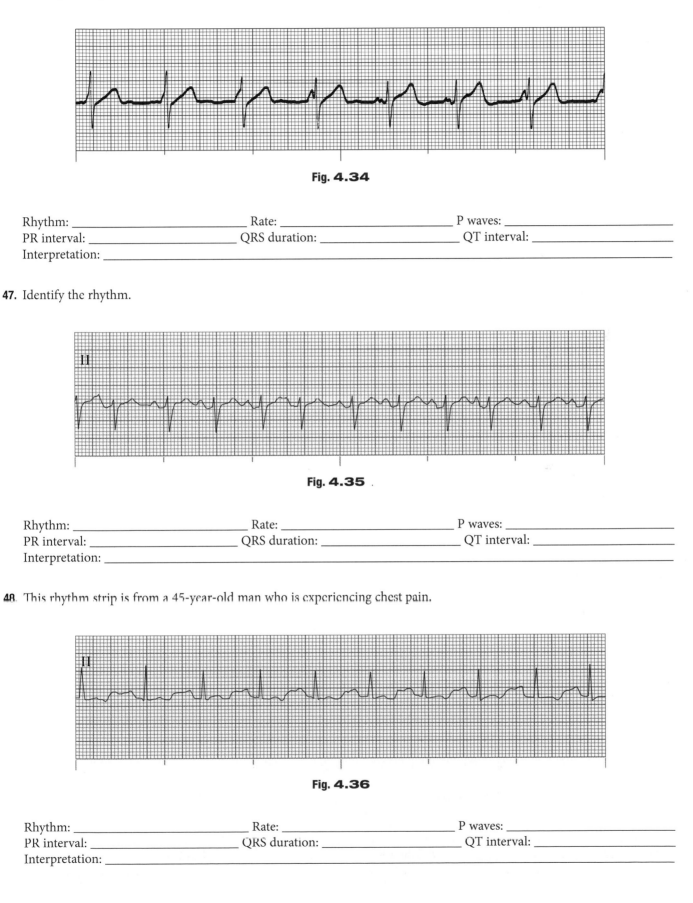

Fig. 4.34

Rhythm: _____ Rate: _____ P waves: _____
PR interval: _____ QRS duration: _____ QT interval: _____
Interpretation: _____

47. Identify the rhythm.

Fig. 4.35 .

Rhythm: _____ Rate: _____ P waves: _____
PR interval: _____ QRS duration: _____ QT interval: _____
Interpretation: _____

48. This rhythm strip is from a 45-year-old man who is experiencing chest pain.

Fig. 4.36

Rhythm: _____ Rate: _____ P waves: _____
PR interval: _____ QRS duration: _____ QT interval: _____
Interpretation: _____

49. This rhythm strip is from a 14-year-old adolescent with chest pain.

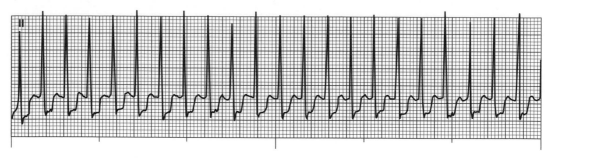

Fig. 4.37 (From Aehlert, B. (2004). *ECG study cards.* St. Louis: Mosby.)

Rhythm: _____ Rate: _____ P waves: _____

PR interval: _____ QRS duration: _____ QT interval: _____

Interpretation: _____

50. The following rhythm strip is from the same 14-year-old patient as in Fig. 4.37. This rhythm was seen after 6 mg of intravenous adenosine.

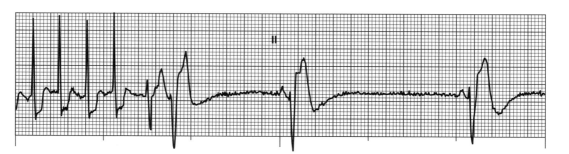

Fig. 4.38 (From Aehlert, B. (2004). *ECG study cards.* St. Louis: Mosby.)

Rhythm: _____ Rate: _____ P waves: _____

PR interval: _____ QRS duration: _____ QT interval: _____

Interpretation: _____

51. Identify the rhythm.

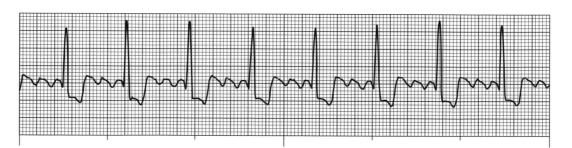

Fig. 4.39 (From Aehlert, B. (2004). *ECG study cards.* St. Louis: Mosby.)

Rhythm: _____ Rate: _____ P waves: _____

PR interval: _____ QRS duration: _____ QT interval: _____

Interpretation: _____

52. Identify the rhythm.

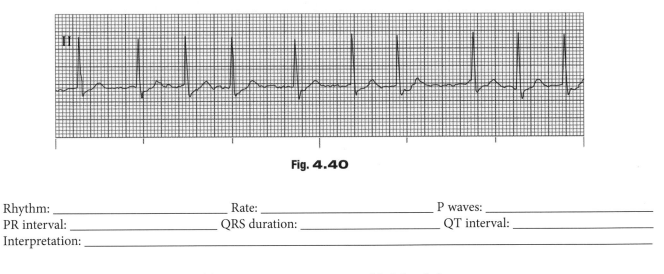

Fig. 4.40

Rhythm: _____ Rate: _____ P waves: _____
PR interval: _____ QRS duration: _____ QT interval: _____
Interpretation: _____

53. This rhythm strip is from a 72-year-old man experiencing nausea and lightheadedness.

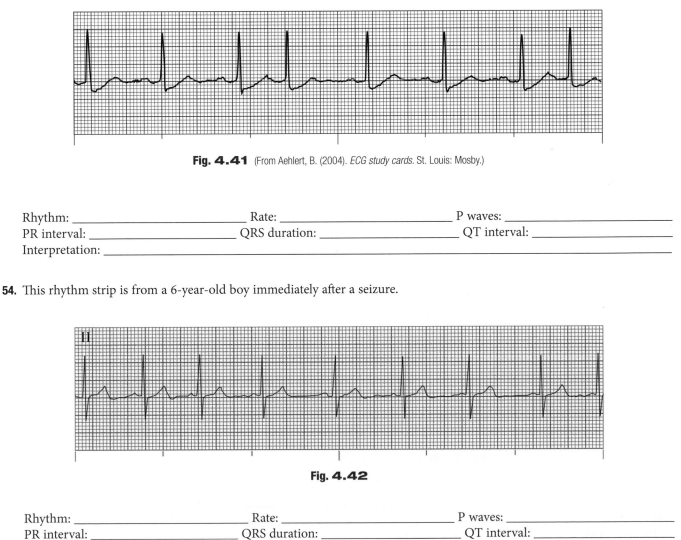

Fig. 4.41 (From Aehlert, B. (2004). *ECG study cards.* St. Louis: Mosby.)

Rhythm: _____ Rate: _____ P waves: _____
PR interval: _____ QRS duration: _____ QT interval: _____
Interpretation: _____

54. This rhythm strip is from a 6-year-old boy immediately after a seizure.

Fig. 4.42

Rhythm: _____ Rate: _____ P waves: _____
PR interval: _____ QRS duration: _____ QT interval: _____
Interpretation: _____

55. Identify the rhythm.

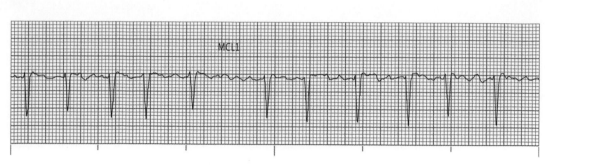

Fig. 4.43

Rhythm: _____ Rate: _____ P waves: _____
PR interval: _____ QRS duration: _____ QT interval: _____
Interpretation: _____

56. Identify the rhythm.

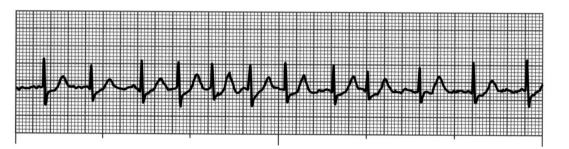

Fig. 4.44 (From Aehlert, B. (2004). *ECG study cards.* St. Louis: Mosby.)

Rhythm: _____ Rate: _____ P waves: _____
PR interval: _____ QRS duration: _____ QT interval: _____
Interpretation: _____

57. This rhythm strip is from a 54-year-old man who had a syncopal episode.

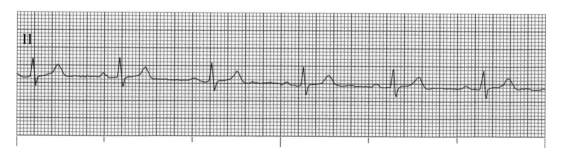

Fig. 4.45 (From Aehlert, B. (2004). *ECG study cards.* St. Louis: Mosby.)

Rhythm: _____ Rate: _____ P waves: _____
PR interval: _____ QRS duration: _____ QT interval: _____
Interpretation: _____

58. This rhythm strip is from a 57-year-old man with no cardiac history.

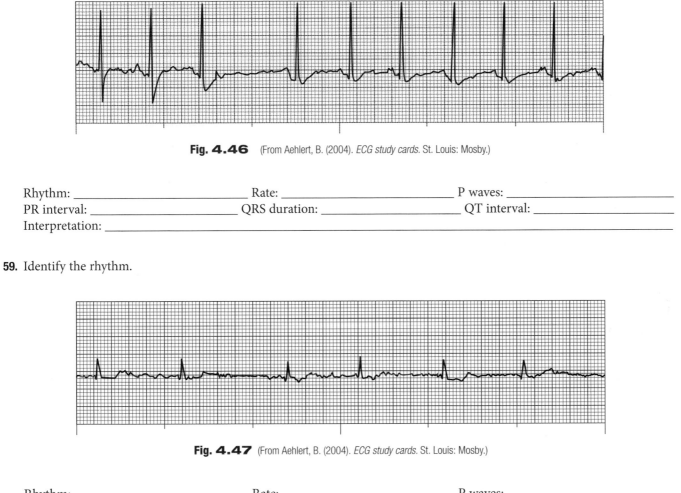

Fig. 4.46   (From Aehlert, B. (2004). *ECG study cards.* St. Louis: Mosby.)

Rhythm: _____ Rate: _____ P waves: _____
PR interval: _____ QRS duration: _____ QT interval: _____
Interpretation: _____

59. Identify the rhythm.

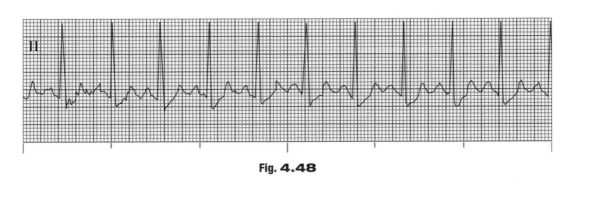

Fig. 4.47   (From Aehlert, B. (2004). *ECG study cards.* St. Louis: Mosby.)

Rhythm: _____ Rate: _____ P waves: _____
PR interval: _____ QRS duration: _____ QT interval: _____
Interpretation: _____

60. This rhythm strip is from a 67-year-old woman found unresponsive on the side of the road. Outdoor temperature was 112° F. Her blood pressure was 238/110 mm Hg, and her ventilatory rate was 60 breaths/min.

Fig. 4.48

Rhythm: _____ Rate: _____ P waves: _____
PR interval: _____ QRS duration: _____ QT interval: _____
Interpretation: _____

61. This rhythm strip is from a 67-year-old woman experiencing dizziness and a "funny feeling" in her chest.

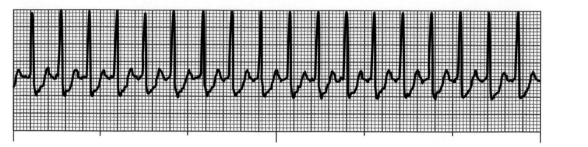

Fig. 4.49 (From Aehlert, B. (2004). *ECG study cards.* St. Louis: Mosby.)

Rhythm: _____ Rate: _____ P waves: _____
PR interval: _____ QRS duration: _____ QT interval: _____
Interpretation: _____

62. Identify the rhythm.

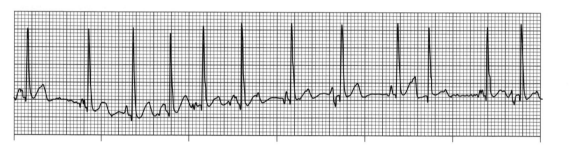

Fig. 4.50 (From Zipes, D. P., Libby, P., Bonow, R. O., Mann, D. L., Tomaselli, G. F., & Braunwald, E. (2019). *Braunwald's heart disease: a textbook of cardiovascular medicine* (11th ed.). Philadelphia: Elsevier.)

Rhythm: _____ Rate: _____ P waves: _____
PR interval: _____ QRS duration: _____ QT interval: _____
Interpretation: _____

63. This rhythm strip is from an 81-year-old woman who experienced a massive myocardial infarction.

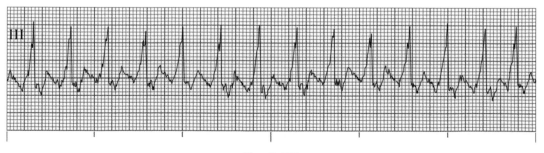

Fig. 4.51

Rhythm: _____ Rate: _____ P waves: _____
PR interval: _____ QRS duration: _____ QT interval: _____
Interpretation: _____

64. Identify the rhythm.

Lead II (continuous)

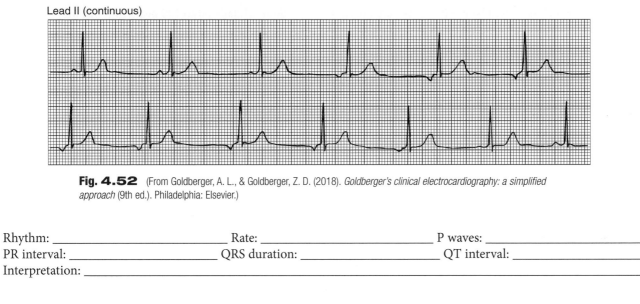

Fig. 4.52 (From Goldberger, A. L., & Goldberger, Z. D. (2018). *Goldberger's clinical electrocardiography: a simplified approach* (9th ed.). Philadelphia: Elsevier.)

Rhythm: _____ Rate: _____ P waves: _____
PR interval: _____ QRS duration: _____ QT interval: _____
Interpretation: _____

65. This rhythm strip is from a 62-year-old woman experiencing chest pain. She has a history of three previous heart attacks and underwent a three-vessel coronary artery bypass graft 10 years ago.

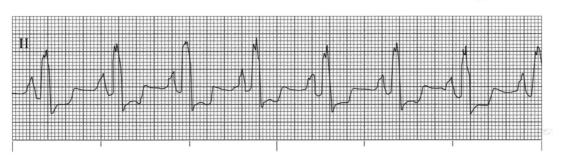

Fig. 4.53

Rhythm: _____ Rate: _____ P waves: _____
PR interval: _____ QRS duration: _____ QT interval: _____
Interpretation: _____

66. Identify the rhythm.

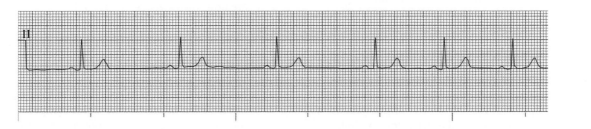

Fig. 4.54

Rhythm: _____ Rate: _____ P waves: _____
PR interval: _____ QRS duration: _____ QT interval: _____
Interpretation: _____

1. **C.** AVNRT, which is caused by reentry in the area of the AV node, is the most common type of SVT in adults.

2. **B.** A supraventricular rhythm originates from a site above the bifurcation of the bundle of His, such as the SA node, atria, or AV junction.

3. **A.** With AFib, rapid impulses cause the muscles of the atria to quiver (fibrillate), resulting in ineffective atrial contraction, decreased stroke volume, a subsequent decrease in cardiac output, and loss of atrial kick.

4. **D**. With atrial flutter, atrial waveforms are produced that resemble the teeth of a saw or a picket fence; these are called *flutter waves* or *F waves.*

5. **A, E, F**. The WPW pattern includes a triad (meaning three) of ECG findings that consist of the following: (1) a short PR interval, (2) a delta wave, and (3) a wide QRS complex. In addition, secondary ST- and T-wave changes are often present.

6. **A.** A PR interval cannot be measured with AFib because there are no P waves associated with this dysrhythmia.

7. **D**. Signs and symptoms experienced during a tachydysrhythmia are usually primarily related to a decrease in the length of time spent in diastole. Remember that as the heart rate increases, there is less time for the ventricles to fill and less blood for the ventricles to pump out with each contraction. Thus, an excessively fast heart rate can lead to decreased cardiac output.

8. **D.** When compared with the P-P intervals of the underlying rhythm, a PAC is premature—occurring before the next expected sinus P wave. PACs are identified by early (premature) P waves, positive (upright) P waves (in lead II) that differ in shape from sinus P waves (atrial P waves may be flattened, notched, pointed, biphasic, or lost in the preceding T wave), and early P waves that may or may not be followed by a QRS complex.

9. **B.** A compensatory pause is a delay that occurs following a premature beat that resets the SA node. A series of waveforms is called a complex. The cardiac cycle period during which cardiac cells cannot be stimulated to conduct an electrical impulse, no matter how strong the stimulus, describes the effective (absolute) refractory period. The period during the cardiac cycle during which cardiac cells can be stimulated to conduct an electrical impulse, if exposed to a stronger than normal stimulus, describes the relative refractory period.

10. **A, F**. ECG characteristics of wandering atrial pacemaker include the following:
Rhythm: Usually irregular as the pacemaker site shifts from the SA node to ectopic atrial locations or AV junction

Rate: Usually 60 to 100 beats/min but may be slower; if the rate is faster than 100 beats/min, the rhythm is termed *multifocal atrial tachycardia*
P waves: Size, shape, and direction may change from beat to beat; may be upright, inverted, biphasic, rounded, flat, pointed, notched, or buried in the QRS complex
PR interval: Varies as the pacemaker site shifts from the SA node to ectopic atrial locations or AV junction
QRS duration: 0.11 second or less unless abnormally conducted

11. **D.** Information relayed by the patient as part of the history can provide important clues to her cardiovascular (and pulmonary) status. Ask questions to determine the patient's description of her symptoms, when and how often they occur, how long they last, possible triggers, and what measures she has taken to relieve them. A complaint of palpitations warrants timely assessment and intervention, whether or not their rhythm is regular. It is essential to determine if chest pain or discomfort, difficulty breathing, or shortness of breath accompany her palpitations. Some practitioners recommend having the patient "tap out" the rhythm of the palpitations to help determine rhythmicity. Palpitations that occur regularly with a sudden onset and end usually are caused by AVNRT or AVRT. Irregular palpitations may be the result of premature complexes, AFib, or multifocal atrial tachycardia. Patients may report palpitations even when there is no evidence of a rhythm disturbance on the cardiac monitor. This occurs most often in patients with anxiety disorders. Although symptoms such as chest pain or discomfort, dyspnea, palpitations, edema, and syncope are classic cardiac disease symptoms, they may also occur because of other organ system diseases (such as musculoskeletal, pulmonary, renal, and gastrointestinal).

12. **B.** The rhythm shown is AVNRT at 188 beats/min.

13. **D.** The PR interval cannot be measured because there are no P waves visible in Fig. 4.23.

14. **B.** The patient is symptomatic but *stable*. Because atropine is administered to increase heart rate and this patient is already tachycardic, it is contraindicated in this situation. Vagal maneuvers may be tried. If vagal maneuvers were unsuccessful, anticipate orders for IV administration of adenosine. Chest compressions are not indicated (the patient is responsive, breathing, and has a pulse). Oxygen administration is not indicated because the patient's oxygen saturation is 97% on room air. Sedation and cardioversion would be appropriate if the patient were *unstable* (showing signs of hemodynamic compromise).

Matching

Practice Rhythm Strip Answers

Note: The rate and interval measurements provided here were obtained using electronic calipers.

36. Fig. 4.24

Rhythm: Irregular

Rate: 120 beats/min

P waves: Positive, one precedes each QRS, P waves of beats 4 and 10 are early and differ from sinus P waves

PR interval: 0.16 second

QRS duration: 0.09 second

QT interval: 0.20 second (T-wave end is not clearly visible with all beats)

Interpretation: Sinus tachycardia at 120 beats/min with PACs (beats 4 and 10)

37. Fig. 4.25

Rhythm: Irregular

Rate: 100 beats/min

P waves: Fibrillatory waves present

PR interval: None

QRS duration: 0.08 second

QT interval: 0.32 second

Interpretation: AFib at 100 beats/min

38. Fig. 4.26

Rhythm: Regular

Rate: 235 beats/min

P waves: None visible; hidden in T waves

PR interval: None

QRS duration: 0.08 second

QT interval: 0.22 second

Interpretation: AVNRT at 235 beats/min with ST-segment depression

39. Fig. 4.27

Rhythm: Irregular

Rate: 60 beats/min

P waves: Positive, one precedes each QRS, one early P wave distorts the T wave of beat 4 (most clearly seen in lead MCL$_1$)

PR interval: 0.20 second (lead II)

QRS duration: 0.14 second (lead II)

QT interval: 0.42 second (lead II)

Interpretation: Sinus rhythm at 60 beats/min with a wide QRS and a nonconducted PAC

40. Fig. 4.28

Rhythm: Irregular

Rate: 80 beats/min

P waves: Positive, one precedes each QRS; an early P wave appears with beat 6 and differs from the sinus P waves

PR interval: 0.12 second (sinus beats)

QRS duration: 0.08 second (sinus beats)

QT interval: 0.26 second (sinus beats)

Interpretation: Sinus rhythm at 80 beats/min with a PAC (beat 6)

41. Fig. 4.29

Rhythm: Regular

Rate: 177 beats/min

P waves: Positive, one precedes each QRS

PR interval: 0.13 second

QRS duration: 0.08 second

QT interval: 0.22 second

Interpretation: Sinus tachycardia at 177 beats/min

42. Fig. 4.30

Rhythm: Irregular

Rate: 80 beats/min

P waves: Fibrillatory waves present

PR interval: None

QRS duration: 0.08 second

QT interval: Unable to determine; T waves are not consistently visible

Interpretation: AFib at 80 beats/min

43. Fig. 4.31

Rhythm: Irregular

Rate: 97 beats/min (sinus beats), 203 beats/min (PSVT)

P waves: Positive, one precedes each QRS (sinus beats), hidden in T waves (PSVT)

PR interval: 0.16 second (sinus beats)

QRS duration: 0.08 second

QT interval: 0.26 to 0.30 second

Interpretation: Sinus rhythm at 97 beats/min with a PAC precipitating a run of PSVT at 203 beats/min, back to a sinus rhythm at 97 beats/min

44. Fig. 4.32

Rhythm: Irregular

Rate: 80 beats/min

P waves: Flutter waves of varying ratios present

PR interval: None

QRS duration: 0.06 to 0.09 second

QT interval: Unable to determine

Interpretation: Atrial flutter at 80 beats/min

45. Fig. 4.33

Rhythm: Irregular

Rate: 70 beats/min

P waves: Fibrillatory waves present

PR interval: None

QRS duration: 0.11 second

QT interval: 0.34 second

Interpretation: AFib at 70 beats/min

46. Fig. 4.34

Rhythm: Regular

Rate: 70 beats/min

P waves: Positive, one precedes each QRS but vary in shape

PR interval: Varies

QRS duration: Varies

QT interval: 0.37 second

Interpretation: Underlying rhythm is sinus, but pacemaker site varies; ventricular rate about 70 beats/min; patient with known WPW syndrome; note the delta waves

47. Fig. 4.35

Rhythm: Irregular

Rate: 120 beats/min

P waves: Positive, one precedes each QRS, sinus P waves look alike; early P waves of beats 2 and 6 distort the T waves of the preceding beats

PR interval: 0.18 second (sinus beats)

QRS duration 0.10 second

QT interval 0.31 second

Interpretation: Sinus tachycardia at 120 beats/min with two PACs (beats 2 and 6)

48. Fig. 4.36

Rhythm: Irregular (all beats but the first are regular)

Rate: 94 beats/min

P waves: Positive, one precedes each QRS

PR interval: 0.20 to 0.22 second

QRS duration: 0.06 second

QT interval: 0.24 second

Interpretation: Sinus rhythm at 94 beats/min with inverted T waves (because the rhythm is technically irregular, the rhythm could be interpreted as sinus arrhythmia)

49. Fig. 4.37

Rhythm: Regular

Rate: 226 beats/min

P waves: None visible; hidden in T waves

PR interval: None

QRS duration: 0.07 second

QT interval: 0.23 second

Interpretation: AVNRT at 226 beats/min with ST-segment depression

50. Fig. 4.38

Rhythm: Regular to irregular as rhythm conversion occurs

Rate: 202 beats/min (AVNRT) to about 30 beats/min (sinus beats)

P waves: None visible with AVNRT; positive before each QRS with sinus beats

PR interval: 0.13 second (sinus beats)

QRS duration: 0.08 to 0.10 second (AVNRT, last sinus beat)

QT interval: 0.24 second (sinus beats)

Interpretation: AVNRT at 202 beats/min with ST-segment depression; rhythm conversion evidenced by a sinus beat, a possible PAC, and then sinus bradycardia at about 30 beats/min

51. Fig. 4.39

Rhythm: Regular

Rate: 85 beats/min

P waves: Flutter waves present

PR interval: None

QRS duration: 0.06 second

QT interval: Unable to determine

Interpretation: Atrial flutter at 85 beats/min with ST-segment depression

52. Fig. 4.40

Rhythm: Irregular

Rate: 100 beats/min

P waves: Fibrillatory waves present

PR interval: None

QRS duration: 0.08 second

QT interval: 0.31 second

Interpretation: AFib at 100 beats/min

53. Fig. 4.41

Rhythm: Irregular

Rate: 80 beats/min

P waves: Positive, one precedes each QRS, sinus P waves look alike, early P waves of beats 4 and 8 distort the T waves of the preceding beats

PR interval: 0.23 second (sinus beats)

QRS duration: 0.08 second

QT interval: 0.40 second

Interpretation: Sinus rhythm at 80 beats/min with a prolonged PR interval, two PACs (beats 4 and 8), and ST-segment depression

54. Fig. 4.42
Rhythm: Irregular
Rate: 90 beats/min (within normal limits for age)
P waves: Positive, one precedes each QRS, P wave amplitude varies among beats
PR interval: 0.12 second
QRS duration: 0.08 second
QT interval: 0.32 second
Interpretation: Sinus arrhythmia at 90 beats/min

55. Fig. 4.43
Rhythm: Irregular
Rate: 110 beats/min
P waves: Flutter waves present
PR interval: None
QRS duration: 0.08 to 0.10 second
QT interval: Unable to determine
Interpretation: Atrial flutter at 110 beats/min

56. Fig. 4.44
Rhythm: Irregular
Rate: 120 beats/min
P waves: Fibrillatory waves present
PR interval: None
QRS duration: 0.08 second
QT interval: 0.28 to 0.32 second
Interpretation: AFib at 120 beats/min

57. Fig. 4.45
Rhythm: Regular
Rate: 60 beats/min
P waves: Positive, one precedes each QRS
PR interval: 0.20 second
QRS duration: 0.08 second
QT interval: 036 second
Interpretation: Sinus rhythm at 60 beats/min

58. Fig. 4.46
Rhythm: Irregular
Rate: 90 beats/min
P waves: Positive, one precedes each QRS, but some vary in shape and amplitude; an early P wave appears after beat 3
PR interval: 0.12 to 0.18 second
QRS duration: 0.08 second
QT interval: 0.28 to 0.30 second; unable to clearly determine because of artifact
Interpretation: Sinus rhythm at 90 beats/min with a nonconducted PAC; baseline artifact is present

59. Fig. 4.47
Rhythm: Irregular
Rate: 60 beats/min
P waves: Fibrillatory waves present
PR interval: None
QRS duration: 0.06 to 0.08 second
QT interval: Unable to determine
Interpretation: AFib at 60 beats/min

60. Fig. 4.48
Rhythm: Regular
Rate: 109 beats/min
P waves: Positive, one precedes each QRS, artifact present
PR interval: 0.18 to 0.20 second
QRS duration: 0.08 to 0.10 second
QT interval: 0.28 to 0.32 second; artifact present
Interpretation: Sinus tachycardia at 109 beats/min with ST-segment depression; baseline artifact is present

61. Fig. 4.49
Rhythm: Regular
Rate: 180 beats/min
P waves: None visible; hidden in T waves
PR interval: None
QRS duration: 0.04 to 0.06 second
QT interval: 0.24 second
Interpretation: AVNRT at 180 beats/min with ST-segment depression

62. Fig. 4.50
Rhythm: Irregular
Rate: 120 beats/min
P waves: Vary in size, shape, and direction
PR interval: Varies
QRS duration: 0.06 to 0.08 second
QT interval: 0.24 to 0.28 second
Interpretation: MAT at 120 beats/min

63. Fig. 4.51
Rhythm: Irregular
Rate: 140 beats/min
P waves: Flutter waves visible despite artifact
PR interval: None
QRS duration: 0.12 to 0.16 second
QT interval: Unable to determine
Interpretation: Atrial flutter with a ventricular response of 140 beats/min; artifact is present

64. Fig. 4.52
Rhythm: Irregular
Rate: 50 beats/min (top strip)
P waves: Vary in size, shape, and direction
PR interval: Varies
QRS duration: 0.06 to 0.08 second
QT interval: 0.40 to 0.44 second
Interpretation: Wandering atrial pacemaker at 50 beats/min

65. Fig. 4.53
Rhythm: Regular
Rate: 75 beats/min
P waves: Positive, one precedes each QRS but vary in size and shape
PR interval: 0.16 to 0.18 second
QRS duration: 0.12 to 0.14 second
QT interval: 0.36 second

Interpretation: Sinus rhythm at 75 beats/min with wide, notched QRS complexes, ST-segment depression, and inverted T waves

66. Fig. 4.54
   Rhythm: Irregular
   Rate: 60 beats/min

P waves: Positive, one precedes each QRS, but some vary in amplitude
PR interval: 0.15 second
QRS duration: 0.06 second
QT interval: 0.40 second
Interpretation: Sinus arrhythmia at 60 beats/min

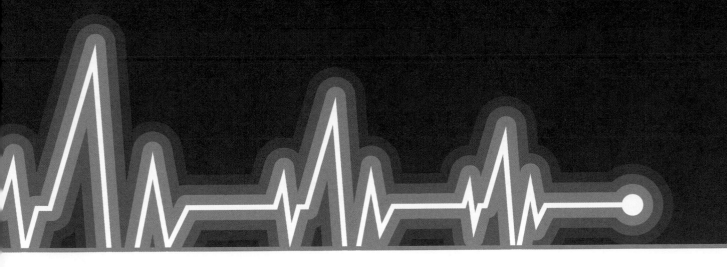

Junctional Rhythms 5

LEARNING OBJECTIVES

After reading this chapter, you should be able to:

1. Describe the electrocardiogram (ECG) characteristics, possible causes, signs and symptoms, and initial emergency care for premature junctional complexes (PJCs).
2. Describe the ECG characteristics and possible causes for junctional escape beats.
3. Explain the difference between PJCs and junctional escape beats.
4. Describe the ECG characteristics, possible causes, signs and symptoms, and initial emergency care for a junctional escape rhythm.
5. Describe the ECG characteristics, possible causes, signs and symptoms, and initial emergency care for an accelerated junctional rhythm.
6. Describe the ECG characteristics, possible causes, signs and symptoms, and initial emergency care for junctional tachycardia.

KEY TERMS

accelerated junctional rhythm: Dysrhythmia originating in the atrioventricular (AV) bundle with a rate between 61 and 100 beats per minute (beats/min).

junctional bradycardia: A rhythm that begins in the AV bundle with a rate of less than 40 beats/min.

junctional escape rhythm: A rhythm that begins in the AV bundle; characterized by a very regular ventricular rate of 40 to 60 beats/min.

junctional tachycardia: A rhythm that begins in the AV bundle with a ventricular rate of more than 100 beats/min.

retrograde: Moving backward; moving in the opposite direction to that which is considered normal.

INTRODUCTION

The atrioventricular (AV) node is a group of specialized cells located in the lower part of the right atrium above the base of the tricuspid valve (Fig. 5.1). The AV node's main job is to delay an electrical impulse, allowing the atria to contract and complete filling of the ventricles with blood before the next ventricular contraction.

After passing through the AV node, the electrical impulse enters the bundle of His. The bundle of His, also called the common bundle or the AV bundle, is located in the upper part of the interventricular septum. It connects the AV node with the right and left bundle branches. The bundle of His has pacemaker cells capable of discharging at a rhythmic rate of 40 to 60 beats/min. The AV node and the nonbranching portion of the bundle of His are called the AV junction (Fig. 5.2).

The bundle of His conducts the electrical impulse to the bundle branches.

Remember that the sinoatrial (SA) node is usually the heart's pacemaker. The AV junction may assume responsibility for pacing the heart if:

- The SA node fails to discharge (e.g., sinus arrest).
- An SA node impulse is generated but blocked as it exits the SA node (e.g., SA block).
- The rate of discharge of the SA node is slower than that of the AV junction (e.g., sinus bradycardia or the slower phase of a sinus arrhythmia).
- An impulse from the SA node is generated and is conducted through the atria but is not conducted to the ventricles (e.g., an AV block).

Rhythms that begin in the AV junction used to be called nodal rhythms until electrophysiologic studies proved the

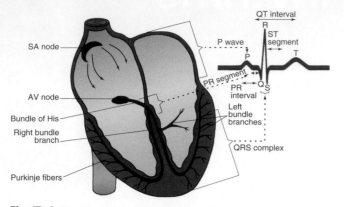

Fig. 5.1 The atrioventricular *(AV)* node is located in the lower portion of the right atrium. The bundle of His is located in the upper part of the interventricular septum. *SA,* Sinoatrial. (From Ignatavicius, D. D., Workman, M. L., & Rebar, C. R. (2021). *Medical-surgical nursing: concepts for interprofessional collaborative care* (10th ed.). St. Louis: Elsevier.)

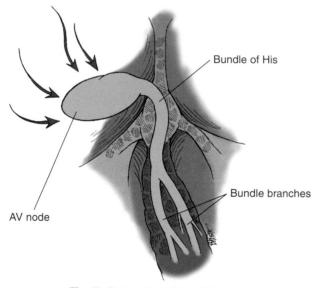

Fig. 5.2 The atrioventricular *(AV)* junction.

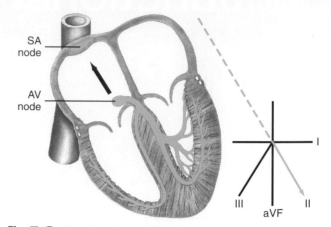

Fig. 5.3 If the atrioventricular *(AV)* junction paces the heart, the electrical impulse must travel in a backward (retrograde) direction to activate the atria. If a P wave is seen, it will be inverted in leads II, III, and aVF because the impulse is traveling away from the positive electrode. *SA,* Sinoatrial. (From Grauer, K. (1998). *A practical guide to ECG interpretation* (2nd ed.). St. Louis: Mosby.)

distorts the end of the QRS complex, and an inverted P wave will appear *after* the QRS. The QRS duration associated with a rhythm that begins in the AV junction measures 0.11 second or less if conduction through the bundle branches, Purkinje fibers, and ventricles is normal.

⟳ ECG Pearl

P waves are usually positive (i.e., upright) in lead I. Inverted P waves may be seen in some, all, or none of the chest leads.

PREMATURE JUNCTIONAL COMPLEXES

How Do I Recognize Them?

ECG characteristics of PJCs include the following:

Rhythm:	Irregular because of the premature beats
Rate:	Usually within normal range but depends on underlying rhythm
P waves:	May occur before, during, or after the QRS; if visible, the P wave is inverted in leads II, III, and aVF
PR interval:	If a P wave occurs before the QRS, the PR interval will usually be 0.12 second or less; if no P wave occurs before the QRS, there will be no PR interval
QRS duration:	0.11 second or less unless abnormally conducted

A PJC occurs when an irritable site (i.e., focus) within the AV junction fires before the next SA node impulse is ready to fire, interrupting the underlying rhythm. Because the impulse is conducted through the ventricles in the usual

AV node does not contain pacemaker cells. The cells nearest the bundle of His are actually responsible for secondary pacing function. Rhythms originating from the AV junction are now called junctional dysrhythmias.

If the AV junction paces the heart, the electrical impulse must travel backward (retrograde) to activate the atria. If a P wave is seen, it will be inverted in leads II, III, and aVF because the impulse is traveling away from the positive electrode (Fig. 5.3). If the atria depolarize before the ventricles, an inverted P wave will be seen *before* the QRS complex, and the PR interval will usually measure 0.12 second or less (Fig. 5.4). The PR interval is shorter than usual because an impulse that begins in the AV junction does not have to travel as far to stimulate the ventricles. If the atria and ventricles depolarize at the same time, a P wave will not be visible because it will be hidden in the QRS complex. When the atria are depolarized after the ventricles, the P wave typically

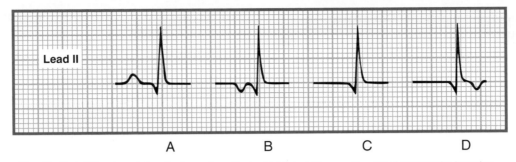

Fig. 5.4 A, With a sinus rhythm, the P wave is positive (upright) in lead II because the wave of depolarization is moving toward the positive electrode. The P wave associated with a junctional beat (in lead II) may be inverted (retrograde) and appear before the QRS (B), be hidden by the QRS (C), or appear after the QRS (D). (From Grauer, K. (1998). *A practical guide to ECG interpretation* (2nd ed.). St. Louis: Mosby.)

manner, the QRS complex will usually measure 0.11 second or less. PJCs are sometimes called premature junctional extrasystoles. A noncompensatory (incomplete) pause often follows a PJC. This pause represents the delay during which the SA node resets its rhythm for the next beat. PJCs may occur in patterns—couplets, bigeminy, trigeminy, and quadrigeminy.

ECG Pearl

You can usually tell the difference between a PAC and a PJC by the P wave. A PAC typically has an upright P wave before the QRS complex in leads II, III, and aVF. A P wave may or may not be present with a PJC. If a P wave is present, it is inverted (retrograde) and may precede or follow the QRS. PJCs can be misdiagnosed when the P wave of a PAC is buried in the preceding T wave.

Junctional complexes may come early or late (i.e., before or after the next expected beat of the underlying rhythm). If the complex is *early*, it is called a *premature junctional complex*. If the complex is *late*, it is called a *junctional escape beat*. To determine if a complex is early or late, we need to see at least two beats in a row of the underlying rhythm to establish its regularity.

Let's look at Fig. 5.5. Looking at the overall rhythm, it appears to be irregular. Because the rhythm is irregular, we

estimate the rate using the 6-second method of rate calculation at 140 beats/min. All QRS complexes appear to be narrow, so we assume that all impulses started from above the ventricles. Using a pen or pencil, mark an "S" for SA node above each normal-looking P wave. Mark a "J" for junctional above those P waves that are inverted or absent. When you are finished, you should have a "J" marked over the P waves in beats 2, 5, 8, and 11. The rest of the P waves should be marked with an "S." Now take your calipers or a piece of paper and mark the third and fourth complexes in Fig. 5.5. We already determined that these complexes came from the SA node. These beats reflect the underlying rhythm. We now know that the underlying rhythm is a sinus tachycardia at about 140 beats/min. Now move your calipers or paper to the right. If beat 5 occurred on time (i.e., when the next sinus beat was expected), it would line up with your calipers or paper. The fifth complex is early; it occurred *before* the next expected sinus beat; therefore, this complex is a PJC. The other beats that have an inverted P wave before the QRS are also PJCs.

A PJC is not an entire rhythm; rather, it is a single beat. When identifying a rhythm, be sure to specify the underlying rhythm and the origin of the ectopic beat(s). In this rhythm strip, we found that the underlying rhythm was a sinus tachycardia at about 140 beats/min. All of the ectopic beats were early and came from the AV junction; therefore, we interpret this rhythm strip as sinus tachycardia at 140 beats/min with frequent PJCs.

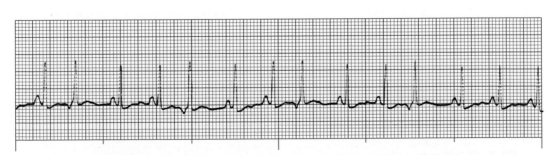

Fig. 5.5 Sinus tachycardia at 140 beats/min with frequent premature junctional complexes.

Box **5.1**	Premature Junctional Complexes— Causes

- Acute coronary syndromes
- Digitalis toxicity
- Electrolyte imbalance
- Heart failure
- Hypoxia
- Mental and physical fatigue
- Rheumatic heart disease
- Stimulants (e.g., caffeine, tobacco, cocaine)
- Sympathomimetics (e.g., epinephrine)
- Valvular heart disease

What Causes Them?

PJCs are less common than either PACs or PVCs. Causes of PJCs are shown in Box 5.1.

What Do I Do About Them?

PJCs do not generally require treatment because most individuals who have PJCs are asymptomatic. However, PJCs may lead to symptoms of palpitations or the feeling of skipped beats. Lightheadedness, dizziness, and other signs of decreased cardiac output can occur if PJCs are frequent. If PJCs occur because of ingestion of stimulants or digitalis toxicity, these substances should be withheld.

ECG Pearl

Keep in mind that inverted P waves are normal in lead V₁. To determine if a beat or rhythm came from the AV junction using this lead, look for a short PR interval. Use lead II, III, or aVF to confirm your findings.

JUNCTIONAL ESCAPE BEATS OR RHYTHM

How Do I Recognize It?

A junctional escape beat begins in the AV junction and appears *late* (i.e., after the next expected beat of the underlying

rhythm). The ECG characteristics of junctional escape beats include the following:

Rhythm:	Irregular because of *late* beats
Rate:	Usually within normal range but depends on underlying rhythm
P waves:	May occur before, during, or after the QRS; if visible, the P wave is inverted in leads II, III, and aVF
PR interval:	If a P wave occurs before the QRS, the PR interval will usually be 0.12 second or less; if no P wave occurs before the QRS, there will be no PR interval
QRS duration:	0.11 second or less unless abnormally conducted

Junctional escape beats frequently occur during episodes of sinus arrest or follow pauses of nonconducted PACs. Look at Fig. 5.6. Looking at the rhythm strip, you can see that the rhythm is irregular. There are three normal-looking beats on the left and two more on the far right. In the center of the strip is an odd-looking beat that appears in the middle of a long pause between beats 3 and 5. Looking more closely at beats 1, 2, 3, 5, and 6, you can see an upright P wave before each QRS complex. These beats came from the SA node. Based on this information, we know that the underlying rhythm is sinus in origin. Using your calipers or a piece of paper, mark the first and second complexes. When you move the calipers or paper to the right, you can see that beat 4 came *late*—that is, after the next expected sinus beat.

Now let's try to figure out where beat 4 came from and why. If you put your finger over beat 4, can you explain what happened? The long pause between beats 3 and 5 is an episode of sinus arrest. Remember that if the SA node fails to initiate an impulse, an escape pacemaker site (i.e., the AV junction or ventricles) should assume responsibility for pacing the heart. Look closely at beat 4. The QRS complex is narrow, and there is no P wave before the QRS complex. The narrow QRS complex and absence of a positive P wave before the QRS complex tell us the beat came from the AV junction. Because the beat is late, it is a junctional escape beat. If beat 4 had been *early*, we would call it a PJC. What happened here? The SA node fired in beats 1, 2, and 3. When the sinus did not fire again when it

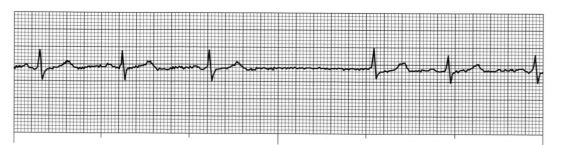

Fig. 5.6 Sinus rhythm at 60 beats/min with an episode of sinus arrest and a junctional escape beat. (From Aehlert, B. (2004). *ECG study cards.* St. Louis: Mosby.)

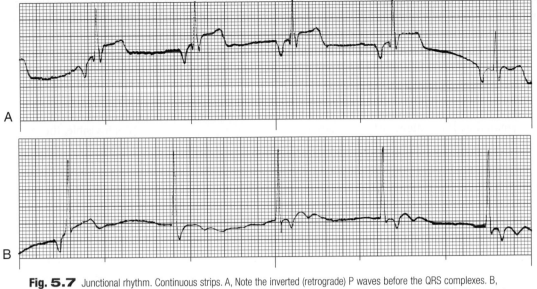

Fig. 5.7 Junctional rhythm. Continuous strips. A, Note the inverted (retrograde) P waves before the QRS complexes. B, Note the change in the location of the P waves. In the first beat, the retrograde P wave is seen before the QRS. In the second beat, no P wave is seen. In the remaining beats, the P wave is seen after the QRS complexes. (From Aehlert, B. (2004). *ECG study cards*. St. Louis: Mosby.)

should have, the AV junction kicked in and fired. Thus, a junctional escape beat is *protective*—preventing cardiac standstill. Two sinus beats follow this beat. Complete identification of the events in this rhythm strip would be as follows: Sinus rhythm at 60 beats/min with an episode of sinus arrest and a junctional escape beat.

ECG Pearl

Junctional escape beats and rhythms occur when the SA node fails to pace the heart or AV conduction fails.

A junctional rhythm is several sequential junctional escape beats. The terms *junctional rhythm* and *junctional escape rhythm* are used interchangeably. Remember that the intrinsic rate of the AV junction is 40 to 60 beats/min. Because a junctional rhythm starts from above the ventricles, the QRS complex is usually narrow, and its rhythm is very regular. The ECG characteristics of a junctional rhythm include the following:

Rhythm:	Very regular
Rate:	40 to 60 beats/min
P waves:	May occur before, during, or after the QRS; if visible, the P wave is inverted in leads II, III, and aVF
PR interval:	If a P wave occurs before the QRS, the PR interval will usually be 0.12 second or less; if no P wave occurs before the QRS, there will be no PR interval
QRS duration:	0.11 second or less unless abnormally conducted

If the AV junction paces the heart at a rate slower than 40 beats/min, the resulting rhythm is called **junctional bradycardia**. This terminology may seem confusing because the AV junction's normal pacing rate of 40 to 60 beats/min *is* bradycardic. However, the term *junctional bradycardia* refers to a rate slower than expected for the AV junction. A junctional rhythm is shown in Fig. 5.7.

What Causes It?

Junctional escape beats frequently occur during episodes of sinus arrest or after pauses of nonconducted PACs. Junctional escape beats may also be observed in healthy individuals during sinus bradycardia. Causes of a junctional rhythm appear in Box 5.2.

What Do I Do About It?

Patients may be asymptomatic with a junctional escape rhythm, or they may experience signs and symptoms

Box **5.2**   **Junctional Rhythm—Causes**
• Acute coronary syndromes (notably inferior wall myocardial infarction [MI])
• Effects of medications (e.g., amiodarone, beta-blockers, calcium blockers, digitalis)
• Hypokalemia
• Immediately after cardiac surgery
• Increased parasympathetic tone
• Obstructive sleep apnea
• Rheumatic heart disease
• SA node disease
• Valvular disease

associated with the slow heart rate and decreased cardiac output. Signs and symptoms may include lightheadedness, weakness, chest pain or pressure, syncope, altered mental status, effort intolerance, and hypotension. If the patient is experiencing symptoms, try to determine their frequency, timing, duration, severity, longevity, circumstances, triggers, and alleviating factors. Be sure to ask about any prescribed and over-the-counter medications (including herbal supplements) that the patient may be taking because these agents can cause or worsen a bradycardia.

Treatment depends on the cause of the dysrhythmia, the patient's presenting signs and symptoms, and the frequency and severity of those symptoms. Patients who experience frequent symptoms may be asked to undergo continuous ambulatory ECG monitoring to determine if a dysrhythmia is a precipitating cause. Laboratory tests (e.g., electrolytes, thyroid function) may be ordered to help identify the cause of the dysrhythmia.

If a junctional rhythm results from the effects of a medication that slows the sinus rate, the medication should be withheld to allow the SA node to resume its pacing function. When a patient experiences serious signs and symptoms related to a slow heart rate, treatment should include applying a pulse oximeter, administering supplemental oxygen (if indicated), establishing intravenous (IV) access, and obtaining a 12-lead ECG. Atropine, given IV, is the first medication given for symptomatic bradycardia (Kusumoto et al., 2018). Reassess the patient's response and continue monitoring. Implantation of a permanent pacemaker may be necessary if the patient is symptomatic and the junctional rhythm is the result of sinus node dysfunction.

ACCELERATED JUNCTIONAL RHYTHM

How Do I Recognize It?

If the AV junction speeds up and fires at 61 to 100 beats/min, the resulting rhythm is called an **accelerated junctional rhythm**. This rhythm is caused by altered automaticity of the bundle of His. The only ECG difference between a junctional rhythm and an accelerated junctional rhythm is the increase in the ventricular rate. An example of an accelerated junctional rhythm is shown in Fig. 5.8. The ECG characteristics of this rhythm include the following:

Rhythm:	Very regular
Rate:	61 to 100 beats/min
P waves:	May occur before, during, or after the QRS; if visible, the P wave is inverted in leads II, III, and aVF
PR interval:	If a P wave occurs before the QRS, the PR interval will usually be 0.12 second or less; if no P wave occurs before the QRS, there will be no PR interval
QRS duration:	0.11 second or less unless abnormally conducted

What Causes It?

An accelerated junctional rhythm is associated with altered automaticity or triggered activity (Page et al., 2016). Causes of this dysrhythmia include acute MI, cardiac surgery, chronic obstructive pulmonary disease, digitalis toxicity, hypokalemia, and rheumatic fever. It may also be observed transiently after ablation for AV nodal reentrant tachycardia.

What Do I Do About It?

The patient is usually asymptomatic because the ventricular rate is 61 to 100 beats/min; however, the patient should be monitored closely. If the patient is symptomatic, treatment is focused on addressing the underlying cause of the dysrhythmia. For example, if the rhythm is caused by digitalis toxicity, this medication should be withheld.

JUNCTIONAL TACHYCARDIA

How Do I Recognize It?

Junctional tachycardia is an ectopic rhythm that begins in the pacemaker cells found in the bundle of His. A junctional

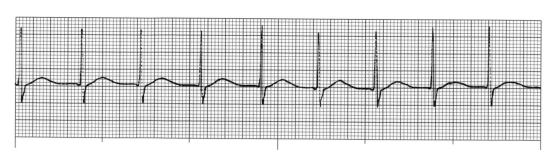

Fig. 5.8 Accelerated junctional rhythm at 93 beats/min.

tachycardia exists when three or more sequential PJCs occur at a rate of more than 100 beats/min. ECG characteristics of junctional tachycardia include the following:

Rhythm:	Ventricular rhythm usually regular, but may be irregular
Rate:	101 to 220 beats/min
P waves:	May occur before, during, or after the QRS; if visible, the P wave is inverted in leads II, III, and aVF
PR interval:	If a P wave occurs before the QRS, the PR interval will usually be 0.12 second or less; if no P wave occurs before the QRS, there will be no PR interval
QRS duration:	0.11 second or less unless abnormally conducted

Junctional tachycardias are usually regular but may be irregular with variable conduction to the atria (Page et al., 2016). *Nonparoxysmal* (i.e., gradual onset) *junctional tachycardia* is a benign dysrhythmia that is usually associated with a gradual increase in rate (i.e., a warm-up pattern) to more than 100 beats/min; it rarely exceeds 120 beats/min (Zimetbaum, 2020). *Paroxysmal junctional tachycardia*, which is also known as *focal* or *automatic junctional tachycardia*, is an uncommon dysrhythmia that starts and ends suddenly and is often precipitated by a PJC. The ventricular rate for paroxysmal junctional tachycardia is generally faster, at a rate of 140 beats/min or more. When the ventricular rate is faster than 150 beats/min, it is challenging to distinguish junctional tachycardia from other supraventricular tachycardias. An example of junctional tachycardia is shown in Fig. 5.9.

What Causes It?

Junctional tachycardia is caused by a disorder of impulse formation (i.e., automaticity) (Miller et al., 2019). It is uncommon in adults but may occur because of an acute coronary syndrome, digitalis toxicity, heart failure, or theophylline administration. Junctional tachycardia is more often seen in infants after cardiac surgery for congenital heart disease (Page et al., 2016).

What Do I Do About It?

Patients experiencing a junctional tachycardia may be asymptomatic. With sustained ventricular rates of 150 beats/min or more, the patient may complain of fatigue, palpitations, or chest discomfort or may experience syncope. Because of the fast ventricular rate, the ventricles may be unable to fill completely, resulting in decreased cardiac output. The more rapid the rate, the greater the incidence of symptoms because of increased myocardial oxygen demand. Junctional tachycardia associated with an acute coronary syndrome may do the following:
- Cause heart failure, hypotension, or cardiogenic shock
- Extend the size of an MI
- Increase myocardial ischemia
- Increase the frequency and severity of chest pain
- Predispose the patient to ventricular dysrhythmias

Treatment depends on the severity of the patient's signs and symptoms, and expert consultation is advised. If the patient tolerates the rhythm, observation is often all that is needed. If the patient is symptomatic because of the rapid rate, initial treatment should include applying a pulse oximeter, administering supplemental oxygen (if indicated), establishing IV access, and obtaining a 12-lead ECG. Because it is often difficult to distinguish junctional tachycardia from other narrow-QRS tachycardias, vagal maneuvers and, if necessary, IV adenosine may be ordered to help determine the origin of the rhythm. If the rhythm is the result of digitalis toxicity, the medication should be withheld. If the rhythm is the result of theophylline administration, the infusion should be slowed or stopped. A beta-blocker (e.g., propranolol) or calcium blocker (e.g., diltiazem, verapamil) may be ordered (if no contraindications exist) to slow conduction through the AV node and thereby slow the ventricular rate. Synchronized cardioversion is not indicated for junctional tachycardia because it typically recurs within seconds after the shock, and a release of endogenous catecholamines following the shock can worsen the dysrhythmia (Miller et al., 2019). A summary of junctional rhythm characteristics appears in Table 5.1.

ECG Pearl

Patients who do not tolerate treatment with antiarrhythmic medications or who have recurring episodes of junctional tachycardia may be referred for radiofrequency ablation.

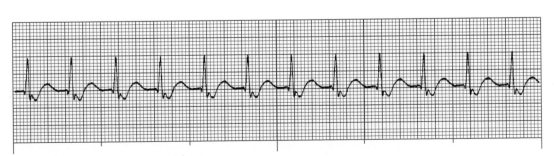

Fig. 5.9 Junctional tachycardia at 115 beats/min.

TABLE 5.1 Junctional Rhythms: Summary of Characteristics

Dysrhythmia	Rhythm	Rate (beats/min)	P waves (lead II)	PR interval	QRS duration
PJCs	Irregular because of *premature* beats	Usually within normal range but depends on underlying rhythm	May occur before, during, or after the QRS; if visible, P wave is inverted	If a P wave occurs before the QRS, the PR interval will usually be 0.12 sec or less; if no P wave occurs before the QRS, there will be no PR interval	0.11 sec or less unless abnormally conducted
Junctional escape beat	Irregular because of *late* beats	Usually within normal range but depends on the underlying rhythm	May occur before, during, or after the QRS; if visible, P wave is inverted	0.12 to 0.20 sec and constant from beat to beat	0.11 sec or less unless abnormally conducted
Junctional escape rhythm	Regular	40 to 60	May occur before, during, or after the QRS; if visible, P wave is inverted	0.12 to 0.20 sec and constant from beat to beat	0.11 sec or less unless abnormally conducted
Accelerated junctional rhythm	Regular	61 to 100	May occur before, during, or after the QRS; if visible, P wave is inverted	0.12 to 0.20 sec and constant from beat to beat	0.11 sec or less unless abnormally conducted
Junctional tachycardia	Ventricular rhythm usually regular	101 to 220	May occur before, during, or after the QRS; if visible, P wave is inverted	When present, 0.12 to 0.20 sec and constant from beat to beat	0.11 sec or less unless abnormally conducted

PJC, Premature junctional complex.

REFERENCES

Kusumoto, F. M., Schoenfeld, M. H., Barrett, C., Edgerton, J. R., Ellenbogen, K. A., Gold, M. R., ... Varosy, P. D. (2018). 2018 ACC/AHA/HRS guideline on the evaluation and management of patients with bradycardia and cardiac conduction delay. *Circulation, 140*(8), e382–e482.

Miller, J. M., Tomaselli, G. F., & Zipes, D. P. (2019). Therapy for cardiac arrhythmias. In D. P. Zipes, P. Libby, R. O. Bonow, D. L. Mann, G. F. Tomaselli, & E. Braunwald (Eds.), *Braunwald's heart disease: A textbook of cardiovascular medicine* (11th ed.). Philadelphia, PA: Elsevier.

Page, R. L., Joglar, J. A., Caldwell, M. A., Calkins, H., Conti, J. B., Deal, B. J., ... Al-Khatib, S. M. (2016). 2015 ACC/AHA/HRS guideline for the management of adult patients with supraventricular tachycardia. *Circulation, 133*(14), e506–e574.

Zimetbaum, P. (2020). Supraventricular cardiac arrhythmias. In L. Goldman, & A. I. Schafer (Eds.), *Goldman-Cecil medicine* (26th ed.) (pp. 331–343). Philadelphia, PA: Elsevier.

STOP & REVIEW

Identify one or more choices that best complete the statement or answer the question.

1. Select the correct statements about PJCs.
   a. A noncompensatory (incomplete) pause often follows a PJC.
   b. Unlike premature atrial complexes, PJCs do not occur in patterns.
   c. If seen, the P wave of a PJC is negative and may appear before or after the QRS complex.
   d. A PJC begins within the AV junction and appears earlier than the next expected beat of the underlying rhythm.

2. An accelerated junctional rhythm is identified by a regular ventricular response occurring at a rate of
   a. 20 to 40 beats/min.
   b. 40 to 60 beats/min.
   c. 61 to 100 beats/min.
   d. 101 to 180 beats/min.

3. The term *junctional bradycardia* is used to describe a rhythm that is junctional in origin with
   a. an atrial rate of 40 to 60 beats/min.
   b. an atrial rate slower than 60 beats/min.
   c. a ventricular rate of 40 to 60 beats/min.
   d. a ventricular rate slower than 40 beats/min.

4. When viewing a junctional rhythm in lead II, where is the P wave location on the ECG if ventricular depolarization precedes atrial depolarization?
   a. Before the QRS complex
   b. During the QRS complex
   c. After the QRS complex

5. In rhythms originating from the AV junction, the QRS duration is typically _____ or less unless an intraventricular conduction delay exists.
   a. 0.04 second
   b. 0.11 second
   c. 0.14 second
   d. 0.20 second

6. Select the correct statements regarding junctional dysrhythmias.
   a. The intrinsic rate of the AV junction is 40 to 60 beats/min.
   b. Junctional dysrhythmias may be seen in acute coronary syndromes.
   c. An accelerated junctional rhythm is a potentially life-threatening dysrhythmia.
   d. The ventricular rhythm associated with junctional dysrhythmias is usually very regular.

7. The primary waveform used to differentiate PJCs from PACs is the
   a. P wave.
   b. Q wave.
   c. R wave.
   d. T wave.

Questions 8—10 Pertain to the Following Scenario

A 63-year-old man is complaining of dizziness that began about 45 minutes ago while cleaning his garage. Because the patient's oxygen saturation level on room air was 88%, supplemental oxygen is being administered. The cardiac monitor has been applied, revealing the rhythm in Fig. 5.10. A coworker is attempting to establish intravenous access.

8. Which of the following statements are true about this patient's cardiac rhythm?
   a. The atrial rhythm is regular.
   b. The QRS complex is narrow.
   c. ST segment elevation is present.
   d. The ventricular rhythm is regular.
   e. There are more P waves than QRS complexes.

9. The rhythm shown on the cardiac monitor is
   a. sinus bradycardia.
   b. junctional bradycardia.
   c. junctional escape rhythm.
   d. accelerated junctional rhythm.

10. The patient's blood pressure is 82/50 mm Hg, ventilations 16. He states his normal blood pressure is about 130/80 mm Hg. The patient denies chest discomfort and states that he takes no prescription medications. His skin is cool, pink, and moist, and his breath sounds are clear. Intravenous access has been successfully established. Based on the information provided, which of the following statements is true regarding this patient situation?
   a. Because the patient is symptomatic with this rhythm, a vagal maneuver should be attempted.
   b. The patient is symptomatic with this rhythm. Obtain a 12-lead ECG and then administer atropine IV.
   c. Therapeutic interventions are not indicated because there is no evidence of ST-segment elevation on the cardiac monitor.
   d. Although the patient is complaining of dizziness, this symptom does not warrant any further intervention other than cardiac monitoring at this time.

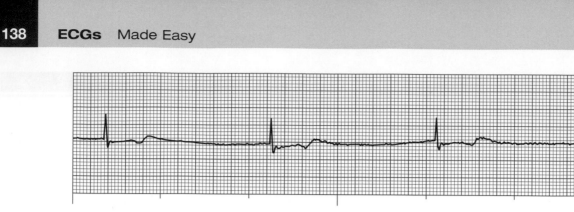

Fig. 5.10 (From Aehlert, B. (2004). *ECG study cards.* St. Louis: Mosby.)

Junctional Rhythms—Practice Rhythm Strips

Use the five steps of rhythm interpretation to interpret each of the following rhythm strips. All rhythms were recorded in lead II unless otherwise noted.

11. Identify the rhythm.

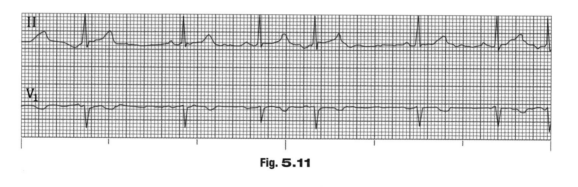

Fig. 5.11

Rhythm: _____ Rate: _____ P waves: _____
PR interval: _____ QRS duration: _____ QT interval: _____
Interpretation: _____

12. Identify the rhythm (lead III).

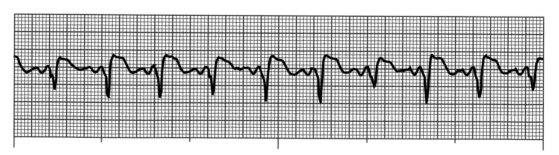

Fig. 5.12 (From Aehlert, B. (2004). *ECG study cards.* St. Louis: Mosby.)

Rhythm: _____ Rate: _____ P waves: _____
PR interval: _____ QRS duration: _____ QT interval: _____
Interpretation: _____

13. This rhythm strip is from a 74-year-old woman with chest pain. She rates her pain 9/10.

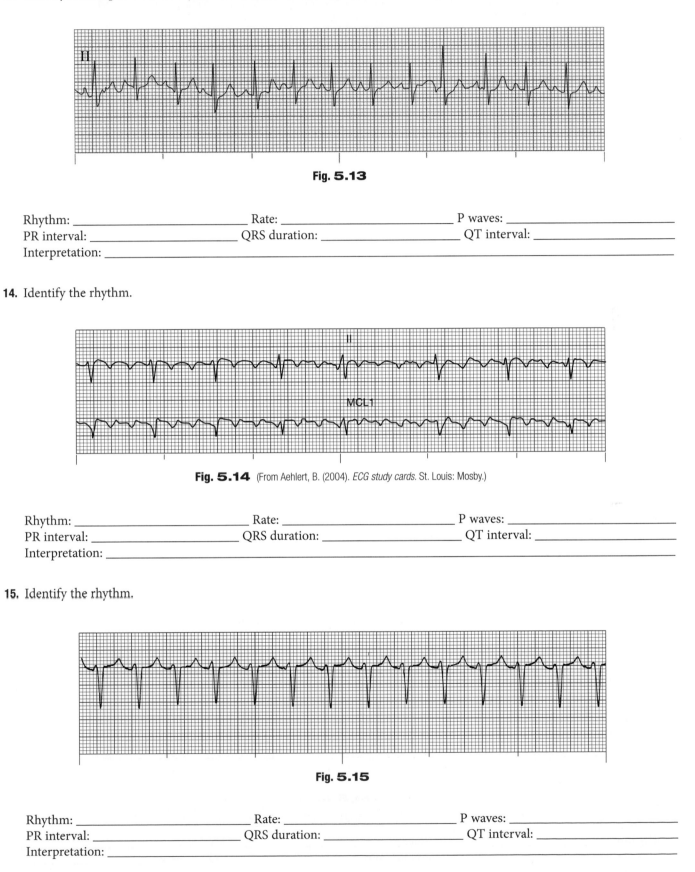

Fig. 5.13

Rhythm: _____ Rate: _____ P waves: _____

PR interval: _____ QRS duration: _____ QT interval: _____

Interpretation: _____

14. Identify the rhythm.

Fig. 5.14 (From Aehlert, B. (2004). *ECG study cards.* St. Louis: Mosby.)

Rhythm: _____ Rate: _____ P waves: _____

PR interval: _____ QRS duration: _____ QT interval: _____

Interpretation: _____

15. Identify the rhythm.

Fig. 5.15

Rhythm: _____ Rate: _____ P waves: _____

PR interval: _____ QRS duration: _____ QT interval: _____

Interpretation: _____

16. Identify the rhythm.

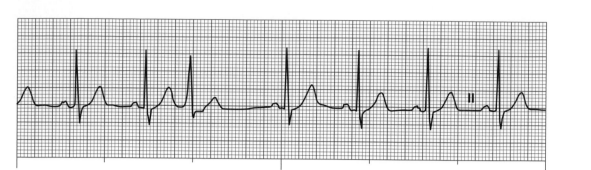

Fig. 5.16 (From Aehlert, B. (2004). *ECG study cards.* St. Louis: Mosby.)

Rhythm: _____ Rate: _____ P waves: _____
PR interval: _____ QRS duration: _____ QT interval: _____
Interpretation: _____

17. This rhythm strip is from an 80-year-old woman who states, "The room is spinning."

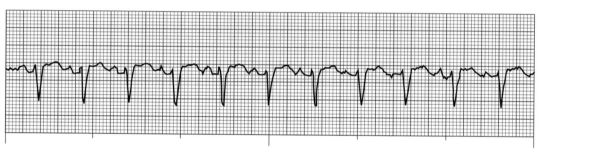

Fig. 5.17 (From Aehlert, B. (2004). *ECG study cards.* St. Louis: Mosby.)

Rhythm: _____ Rate: _____ P waves: _____
PR interval: _____ QRS duration: _____ QT interval: _____
Interpretation: _____

18. This rhythm strip is from an 88-year-old woman who experienced a syncopal episode. Her medical history includes a myocardial infarction 9 years ago, a stroke 5 years ago, hypertension, and diabetes.

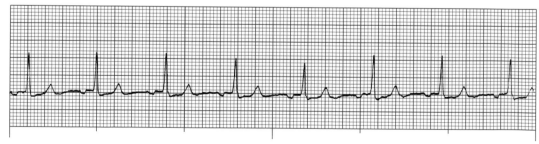

Fig. 5.18

Rhythm: _____ Rate: _____ P waves: _____
PR interval: _____ QRS duration: _____ QT interval: _____
Interpretation: _____

19. This rhythm strip is from a 72-year-old man presenting with left-sided weakness. He has a history of a brain tumor.

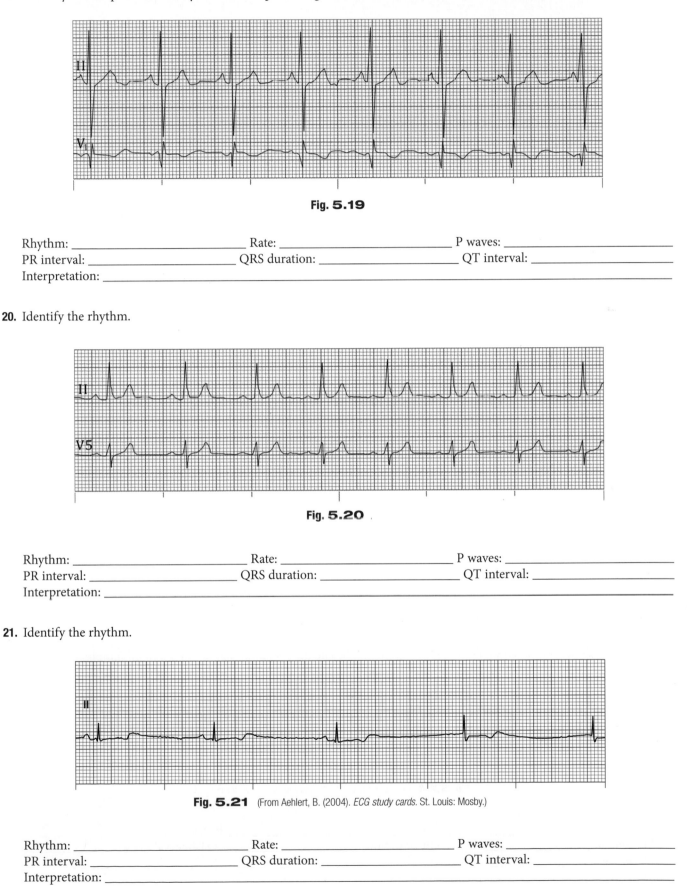

Fig. 5.19

Rhythm: _____ Rate: _____ P waves: _____
PR interval: _____ QRS duration: _____ QT interval: _____
Interpretation: _____

20. Identify the rhythm.

Fig. 5.20

Rhythm: _____ Rate: _____ P waves: _____
PR interval: _____ QRS duration: _____ QT interval: _____
Interpretation: _____

21. Identify the rhythm.

Fig. 5.21   (From Aehlert, B. (2004). *ECG study cards.* St. Louis: Mosby.)

Rhythm: _____ Rate: _____ P waves: _____
PR interval: _____ QRS duration: _____ QT interval: _____
Interpretation: _____

22. Identify the rhythm.

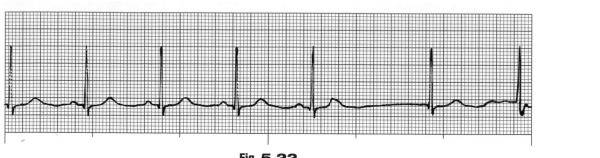

Fig. 5.22

Rhythm: _____ Rate: _____ P waves: _____
PR interval: _____ QRS duration: _____ QT interval: _____
Interpretation: _____

23. Identify the rhythm.

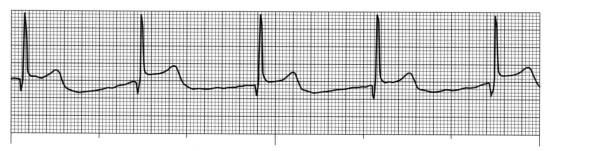

Fig. 5.23 (From Aehlert, B. (2004). *ECG study cards.* St. Louis: Mosby.)

Rhythm: _____ Rate: _____ P waves: _____
PR interval: _____ QRS duration: _____ QT interval: _____
Interpretation: _____

24. This rhythm strip is from a 43-year-old woman who was complaining of palpitations. The patient had a history of supraventricular tachycardia and stated that she could not tolerate adenosine.

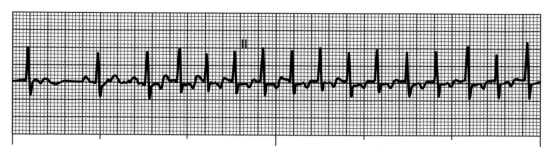

Fig. 5.24 (From Aehlert, B. (2004). *ECG study cards.* St. Louis: Mosby.)

Rhythm: _____ Rate: _____ P waves: _____
PR interval: _____ QRS duration: _____ QT interval: _____
Interpretation: _____

25. This rhythm strip is from a 43-year-old man after a seizure.

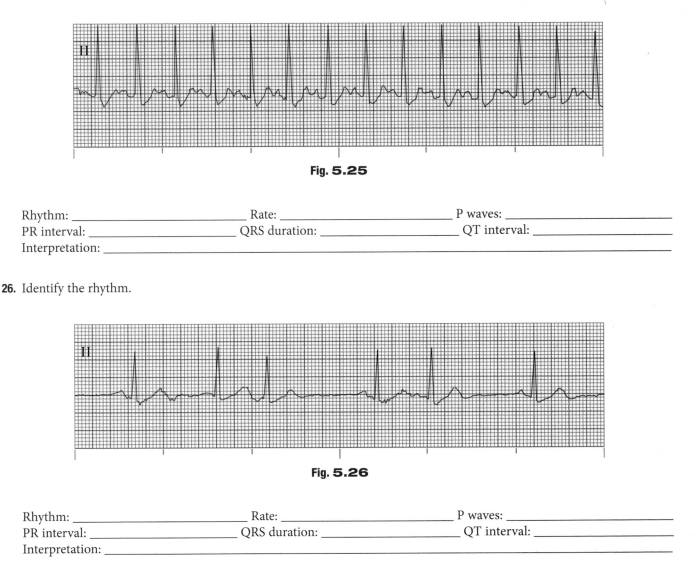

Fig. 5.25

Rhythm: _____ Rate: _____ P waves: _____
PR interval: _____ QRS duration: _____ QT interval: _____
Interpretation: _____

26. Identify the rhythm.

Fig. 5.26

Rhythm: _____ Rate: _____ P waves: _____
PR interval: _____ QRS duration: _____ QT interval: _____
Interpretation: _____

27. This rhythm strip is from a 96-year-old man experiencing chest pain and palpitations.

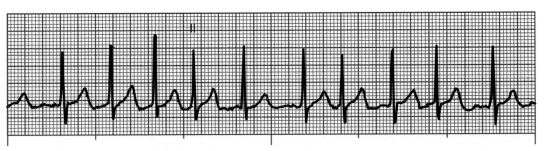

Fig. 5.27   (From Aehlert, B. (2004). *ECG study cards.* St. Louis: Mosby.)

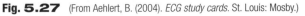

Rhythm: _____ Rate: _____ P waves: _____
PR interval: _____ QRS duration: _____ QT interval: _____
Interpretation: _____

28. This rhythm strip is from a 79-year-old man complaining of palpitations. His initial blood pressure was 112/84 mm Hg. His second blood pressure, 8 minutes after the first, was 78/P mm Hg.

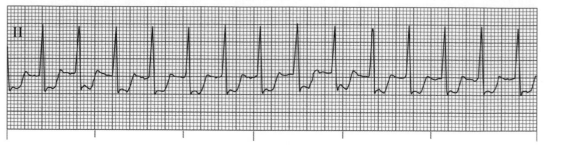

Fig. 5.28

Rhythm: _____ Rate: _____ P waves: _____
PR interval: _____ QRS duration: _____ QT interval: _____
Interpretation: _____

29. Identify the rhythm.

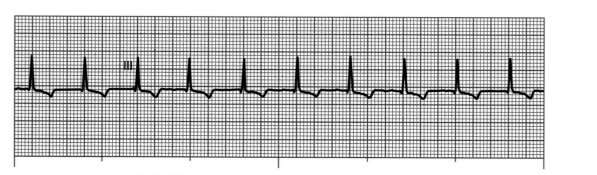

Fig. 5.29 (From Aehlert, B. (2004). *ECG study cards.* St. Louis: Mosby.)

Rhythm: _____ Rate: _____ P waves: _____
PR interval: _____ QRS duration: _____ QT interval: _____
Interpretation: _____

30. Identify the rhythm.

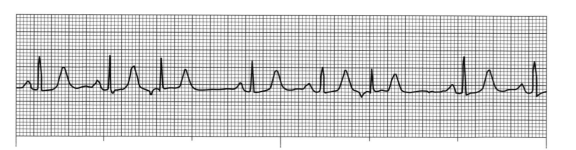

Fig. 5.30 (From Aehlert, B. (2004). *ECG study cards.* St. Louis: Mosby.)

Rhythm: _____ Rate: _____ P waves: _____
PR interval: _____ QRS duration: _____ QT interval: _____
Interpretation: _____

31. Identify the rhythm.

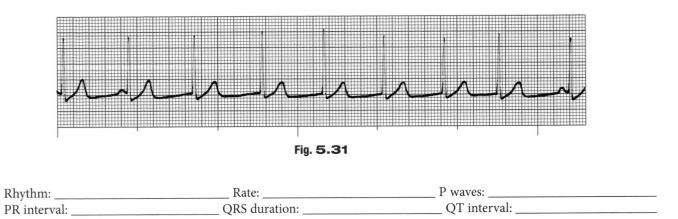

Fig. 5.31

Rhythm: _____ Rate: _____ P waves: _____
PR interval: _____ QRS duration: _____ QT interval: _____
Interpretation: _____

32. This rhythm strip (lead I) is from a 51-year-old man found unresponsive. He has a history of esophageal varices and gastrointestinal bleeding.

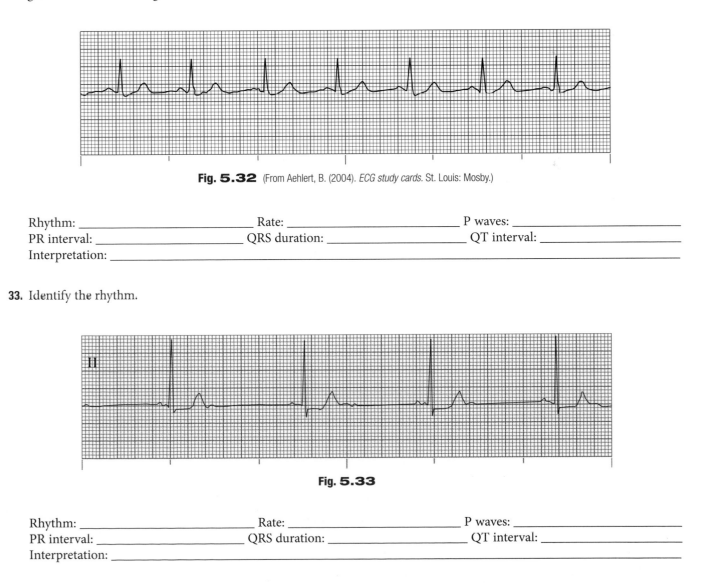

Fig. 5.32 (From Aehlert, B. (2004). *ECG study cards.* St. Louis: Mosby.)

Rhythm: _____ Rate: _____ P waves: _____
PR interval: _____ QRS duration: _____ QT interval: _____
Interpretation: _____

33. Identify the rhythm.

II

Fig. 5.33

Rhythm: _____ Rate: _____ P waves: _____
PR interval: _____ QRS duration: _____ QT interval: _____
Interpretation: _____

34. This rhythm strip is from a 75-year-old man complaining of chest pain that has been present for 20 minutes. He rates his pain 8/10.

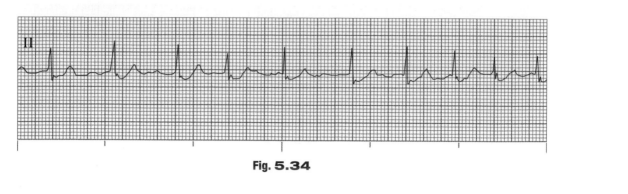

Fig. 5.34

Rhythm: _____ Rate: _____ P waves: _____
PR interval: _____ QRS duration: _____ QT interval: _____
Interpretation: _____

35. This rhythm strip is from a 76-year-old woman complaining of weakness.

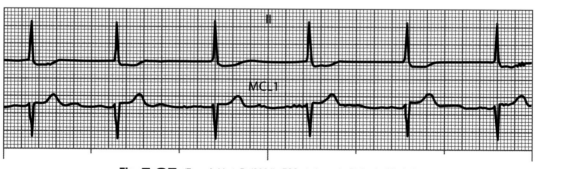

Fig. 5.35 (From Aehlert, B. (2004). *ECG study cards*. St. Louis: Mosby.)

Rhythm: _____ Rate: _____ P waves: _____
PR interval: _____ QRS duration: _____ QT interval: _____
Interpretation: _____

STOP & REVIEW ANSWERS

1. **A, C, D.** A PJC occurs when an irritable site within the AV junction fires before the next SA node impulse is ready to fire, interrupting the underlying rhythm. PJCs may occur as single beats or in patterns (e.g., couplets, bigeminy, trigeminy, quadrigeminy). A noncompensatory (incomplete) pause often follows a PJC. This pause represents the delay during which the SA node resets its rhythm for the next beat. When the P wave of a PJC is seen, it is negative and may appear before or after the QRS complex.

2. **C.** An accelerated junctional rhythm is a dysrhythmia originating in the AV bundle with a ventricular rate between 61 and 100 beats/min.

3. **D.** If the AV junction paces the heart at a rate slower than 40 beats/min, the resulting rhythm is called junctional bradycardia. This wording may seem confusing because the AV junction's normal pacing rate (40 to 60 beats/min) *is* bradycardic. However, the term *junctional bradycardia* refers to a rate slower than normal for the AV junction.

4. **C.** If the AV junction paces the heart, the electrical impulse must travel in a backward (retrograde) direction to activate the atria. If a P wave is seen, it will be inverted in leads II, III, and aVF because the impulse is traveling away from the positive electrode. If the atria depolarize before the ventricles, an inverted P wave will be seen *before* the QRS complex, and the PR interval will usually measure 0.12 second or less. The PR interval is shorter than usual because an impulse that begins in the AV junction does not have to travel as far to stimulate the ventricles. If the atria and ventricles depolarize at the same time, a P wave will not be visible because it will be hidden in the QRS complex. When the atria are depolarized after the ventricles, the P wave typically distorts the end of the QRS complex, and an inverted P wave will appear *after* the QRS.

5. **B.** The QRS duration associated with a rhythm that begins in the AV junction measures 0.11 second or less if conduction through the bundle branches, Purkinje fibers, and ventricles is normal.

6. **A, B, D.** The patient with an accelerated junctional rhythm is usually asymptomatic because the ventricular rate is 61 to 100 beats/min, which is the same rate as a sinus rhythm.

7. **A.** You can usually tell the difference between a PAC and a PJC by the P wave. A PAC typically has an upright P wave before the QRS complex in leads II, III, and aVF. A P wave may or may not be present with a PJC. If a P wave is present, it is inverted (retrograde) and may precede or follow the QRS. PJCs can be misdiagnosed when the P wave of a PAC is buried in the preceding T wave.

8. **B, D.** In this rhythm strip, the atrial rate and rhythm cannot be determined because P waves are not visible. The ventricular rhythm is regular and the QRS is narrow, measuring 0.08 second.

9. **B.** The cardiac monitor shows junctional bradycardia at 32 beats/min with ST-segment depression and inverted T waves.

10. **B.** Although there is no evidence of ST-segment elevation on the cardiac monitor, this patient is symptomatic with his slow heart rate, evidenced by his dizziness and hypotension. Treatment of symptomatic bradycardia should include applying a pulse oximeter, administering supplemental oxygen (if indicated), and establishing IV access, which has already been done. Next, obtain a 12-lead ECG and then administer atropine IV. Reassess the patient's response to your interventions and continue monitoring. Because vagal maneuvers are used to attempt to slow the heart rate of some *tachycardias*, and this patient is *bradycardic*, vagal maneuvers are contraindicated in this situation.

Practice Rhythm Strip Answers

Note: The rate and interval measurements provided here were obtained using electronic calipers.

26. Fig. 5.11
    Rhythm: Irregular
    Rate: 70 beats/min
    P waves: Positive; one precedes each QRS; P waves of beats 1, 4, and 7 are early and inverted
    PR interval: 0.16 second (sinus beats)
    QRS duration: 0.06 second
    QT interval: 0.36 second
    Interpretation: Sinus rhythm at 70 beats/min with PJCs (junctional trigeminy)

27. Fig. 5.12
    Rhythm: Regular
    Rate: 100 beats/min
    P waves: One inverted P wave precedes each QRS
    PR interval: 0.14 second
    QRS duration: 0.10 second
    QT interval: 0.28 second (approximate, T-wave end is not clearly visible with all beats)
    Interpretation: Accelerated junctional rhythm at 100 beats/min with ST-segment elevation (STE)

28. Fig. 5.13
Rhythm: Irregular
Rate: 130 beats/min
P waves: Positive; one precedes each QRS but the shape and amplitude of some differ; P wave of beat 10 is early and hidden in the T wave of the preceding beat
PR interval: 0.14 second
QRS duration: 0.07 second
QT interval: 0.28 second
Interpretation: Sinus tachycardia at 130 beats/min with a PAC

29. Fig. 5.14
Rhythm: Irregular
Rate: 80 beats/min
P waves: Flutter waves present
PR interval: None
QRS duration: 0.09 second
QT interval: Unable to determine
Interpretation: Atrial flutter at 80 beats/min

30. Fig. 5.15
Rhythm: Regular
Rate: 136 beats/min
P waves: None visible; hidden in T waves
PR interval: Unable to determine
QRS duration: 0.11 second
QT interval: 0.33 second
Interpretation: Narrow-QRS tachycardia, probably junctional tachycardia, at 136 beats/min

31. Fig. 5.16
Rhythm: Irregular
Rate: 70 beats/min
P waves: Sinus P waves are positive before each QRS and some are notched; P wave of beat 3 is early, inverted, and appears after the QRS
PR interval: 0.16 second
QRS duration: 0.09 second
QT interval: 0.36 second
Interpretation: Sinus rhythm at 70 beats/min with a PJC (beat 3 is the PJC)

32. Fig. 5.17
Rhythm: Regular
Rate: 115 beats/min
P waves: Positive before each QRS, but some differ in shape
PR interval: 0.16 second
QRS duration: 0.11 second
QT interval: 0.32 second
Interpretation: Sinus tachycardia at 115 beats/min with STE

33. Fig. 5.18
Rhythm: Regular
Rate: 75 beats/min
P waves: Inverted before each QRS
PR interval: 0.16 second
QRS duration: 0.06 second
QT interval: 0.32 second
Interpretation: Accelerated junctional rhythm at 75 beats/min; artifact is present

34. Fig. 5.19
Rhythm: Regular
Rate: 75 beats/min
P waves: Positive; one precedes each QRS
PR interval: 0.12 second
QRS duration: 0.09 second
QT interval: 0.35 second
Interpretation: Sinus rhythm at 75 beats/min

35. Fig. 5.20
Rhythm: Irregular
Rate: 80 beats/min
P waves: Positive; one precedes each QRS
PR interval 0.18 second
QRS duration: 0.07 second
QT interval: 0.30 second
Interpretation: Sinus arrhythmia at 80 beats/min

36. Fig. 5.21
Rhythm: Irregular
Rate: 33 beats/min (sinus beats); 32 beats/min (junctional beats)
P waves: Sinus P waves positive before QRS; none visible for junctional beats
PR interval: 0.16 second (sinus beats)
QRS duration: 0.07 second
QT interval: 0.37 second
Interpretation: Sinus bradycardia at 33 beats/min to junctional bradycardia at 32 beats/min; artifact is present

37. Fig. 5.22
Rhythm: Irregular
Rate: 70 beats/min
P waves: Sinus P waves are positive before each QRS; an early P wave appears after beat 5 and distorts the T wave; beat 6 has no P wave
PR interval: 0.16 second
QRS duration: 0.08 second
QT interval: 0.38 second
Interpretation: Sinus rhythm at 70 beats/min with a nonconducted PAC (note distortion of the T wave of the beat preceding the pause) and a junctional escape beat

38. Fig. 5.23
Rhythm: Regular
Rate: 45 beats/min
P waves: None visible
PR interval: None
QRS duration: 0.08 second
QT interval: 0.49 second (prolonged)
Interpretation: Junctional rhythm at 45 beats/min with STE and a prolonged QT interval

39. Fig. 5.24
Rhythm: Irregular; regular during the tachycardia
Rate: 160 beats/min; 188 beats/min during the tachycardia
P waves: Inverted after QRS in beat 1; sinus P wave in beats 2 and 3; cannot differentiate with certainty between inverted P waves and inverted T waves in beats associated with the tachycardia
PR interval: 0.16 second (sinus beats)
QRS duration: 0.08 second
QT interval: 0.24 second if the inverted waveforms during the tachycardia are T waves
Interpretation: Junctional beat, two sinus beats, changing to a narrow QRS tachycardia that is probably junctional tachycardia at 188 beats/min; ST-segment depression

40. Fig. 5.25
Rhythm: Regular
Rate: 136 beats/min
P waves: Positive; one precedes each QRS; some are notched, some are pointed, others are smooth and rounded
PR interval: 0.15 second
QRS duration: 0.08 second
QT interval: 0.25 second
Interpretation: Sinus tachycardia at 136 beats/min with ST-segment depression

41. Fig. 5.26
Rhythm: Irregular
Rate: 60 beats/min
P waves: Positive before sinus beats, early and inverted before the QRS in beat 3, early and upright in beat 5
PR interval: 0.18 second (sinus beats)
QRS duration: 0.06 second
QT interval: 0.43 second
Interpretation: Sinus rhythm at 60 beats/min with a PJC (beat 3), a PAC (beat 5), and ST-segment depression; artifact is present

42. Fig. 5.27
Rhythm: Irregular
Rate: 100 beats/min
P waves: Fibrillatory waves present
PR interval: None
QRS duration: 0.09 second
QT interval: 0.32 second
Interpretation: Atrial fibrillation at 100 beats/min

43. Fig. 5.28
Rhythm: Regular
Rate: 143 beats/min
P waves: None visible before each QRS; cannot differentiate with certainty between inverted P waves and inverted T waves after each QRS
PR interval: None
QRS duration: 0.07 second
QT interval: 0.21 second if the inverted waveforms after each QRS are T waves
Interpretation: Narrow-QRS tachycardia, probably junctional tachycardia, at 143 beats/min with ST-segment depression; artifact is present

44. Fig. 5.29
Rhythm: Regular
Rate: 97 beats/min
P waves: None visible
PR interval: None
QRS duration: 0.08 second
QT interval: 0.31 second
Interpretation: Accelerated junctional rhythm at 97 beats/min; inverted T waves

45. Fig. 5.30
Rhythm: Irregular
Rate: 80 beats/min
P waves: Positive before sinus beats; early inverted P waves appear in beats 3 and 6
PR interval: 0.17 second (sinus beats)
QRS duration: 0.06 second (sinus beats)
QT interval: 0.35 second (sinus beats)
Interpretation: Sinus rhythm at 80 beats/min with PJCs (beats 3 and 6)

46. Fig. 5.31
Rhythm: Irregular
Rate: 77 beats/min (junctional beats)
P waves: Positive for sinus beats; not visible for junctional beats
PR interval: 0.12 second (sinus beats)
QRS duration: 0.06 second
QT interval: 0.33 second
Interpretation: Sinus rhythm changing to an accelerated junctional rhythm at 77 beats/min, back to a sinus rhythm

47. Fig. 5.32
Rhythm: Regular
Rate: 74 beats/min
P waves: Positive; one precedes each QRS
PR interval: 0.14 second
QRS duration: 0.07 second
QT interval: 0.37 second
Interpretation: Sinus rhythm at 74 beats/min; artifact is present

48. Fig. 5.33
Rhythm: Irregular
Rate: 40 beats/min
P waves: Low amplitude but positive; one precedes each QRS; some are notched
PR interval: 0.13 to 0.16 second
QRS duration: 0.06 to 0.08 second
QT interval: 0.41 second
Interpretation: Sinus bradyarrhythmia at 40 beats/min with ST-segment depression; U waves are present

49. Fig. 5.34
Rhythm: Irregular
Rate: 100 beats/min
P waves: Fibrillatory waves present
PR interval: None
QRS duration: 0.06 second
QT interval: 0.30 second
Interpretation: Atrial fibrillation at 100 beats/min with ST-segment depression

50. Fig. 5.35
Rhythm: Irregular
Rate: 60 beats/min
P waves: None visible
PR interval: None
QRS duration: 0.06 second
QT interval: 0.36 second
Interpretation: Junctional rhythm at 60 beats/min; STE in MCL_1

Ventricular Rhythms 6

LEARNING OBJECTIVES

After reading this chapter, you should be able to:

1. Describe the electrocardiogram (ECG) characteristics, possible causes, signs and symptoms, and initial emergency care for premature ventricular complexes (PVCs).
2. Explain the terms *bigeminy, trigeminy, quadrigeminy*, and *run* as used to describe premature complexes.
3. Explain the difference between PVCs and ventricular escape beats.
4. Describe the ECG characteristics of ventricular escape beats.
5. Describe the ECG characteristics, possible causes, signs and symptoms, and initial emergency care for an idioventricular rhythm (IVR).
6. Explain the term *pulseless electrical activity* (PEA).
7. Describe the ECG characteristics, possible causes, signs and symptoms, and initial emergency care for an accelerated idioventricular rhythm (AIVR).
8. Explain the terms *sustained and nonsustained ventricular tachycardia* (VT), monomorphic VT, and polymorphic VT (PMVT).
9. Describe the ECG characteristics, possible causes, signs and symptoms, and initial emergency care for monomorphic VT.
10. Describe the ECG characteristics, possible causes, signs and symptoms, and initial emergency care for PMVT.
11. Describe the ECG characteristics, possible causes, signs and symptoms, and initial emergency care for ventricular fibrillation (VF).
12. State the purpose and indications for defibrillation.
13. Describe the ECG characteristics, possible causes, signs and symptoms, and initial emergency care for asystole.

KEY TERMS

accelerated idioventricular rhythm (AIVR): Dysrhythmia originating in the ventricles with a rate between 41 and 100 beats per minute (beats/min).

asystole: A total absence of ventricular electrical activity.

atrioventricular (AV) dissociation: Any dysrhythmia in which the atria and ventricles beat independently (e.g., VT, complete AV block).

automated external defibrillator (AED): A machine with a sophisticated computer system that analyzes a patient's heart rhythm using an algorithm to distinguish shockable rhythms from nonshockable rhythms and providing visual and auditory instructions to the rescuer to deliver an electrical shock, if a shock is indicated.

defibrillation: Delivery of an electrical current across the heart muscle over a very brief period to terminate an abnormal heart rhythm; also called unsynchronized countershock or asynchronous countershock

because the delivery of current has no relationship to the cardiac cycle.

fusion beat: Beat that occurs because of simultaneous activation of one cardiac chamber by two sites (foci); in pacing, the ECG waveform that results when an intrinsic depolarization and a pacing stimulus coincide and both contribute to depolarization of that cardiac chamber.

interpolated PVC: PVC that occurs between two normally conducted QRS complexes and that does not disturb the next ventricular depolarization or sinoatrial (SA) node activity.

torsades de pointes (TdP): Type of PMVT associated with a prolonged QT interval; the QRS changes in shape, amplitude, and width and appears to twist around the isoelectric line, resembling a spindle.

ventricular tachycardia (VT): Dysrhythmia originating in the ventricles with a ventricular rate greater than 100 beats/min.

INTRODUCTION

The ventricles may assume responsibility for pacing the heart if the sinoatrial (SA) node fails to discharge, an impulse from the SA node is generated but blocked as it exits the SA node, the rate of discharge of the SA node is slower than that of the ventricles, or an irritable site in either ventricle produces an early beat or rapid rhythm. If the ventricles function as the heart's pacemaker, they typically generate impulses at a rate of 20 to 40 beats per minute (beats/min) (Fig. 6.1).

The shape of the QRS complex is influenced by the site of origin of the electrical impulse. Typically, an electrical impulse that begins in the SA node, atria, or atrioventricular (AV) junction results in depolarization of the right and left ventricles at about the same time. The resulting QRS complex is usually narrow, measuring 0.11 second or less in duration.

If an area of either ventricle becomes ischemic or injured, it can become irritable. This irritability affects how impulses are conducted. Ventricular beats and rhythms can start in any part of the ventricles and may occur because of reentry, altered automaticity, or triggered activity (Garan, 2020). When an ectopic site within a ventricle assumes responsibility for pacing the heart, the electrical impulse bypasses the normal intraventricular conduction pathway, which results in stimulation of the ventricles at slightly different times. As a result, ventricular beats and rhythms usually have QRS complexes that are abnormally shaped and longer than normal (e.g., greater than 0.11 second). If the atria are depolarized after the ventricles, retrograde P waves may be seen.

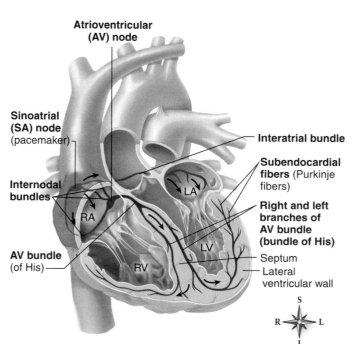

Fig. 6.1 The ventricles are the heart's least efficient pacemaker. (From Patton, K., & Thibodeau, G. (2020). *Structure & function of the body* (16th ed.). St. Louis: Elsevier.)

Because ventricular depolarization is abnormal, ventricular repolarization is also abnormal and results in ST segment and T wave changes. The T waves are usually in a direction opposite that of the QRS complex; if the major QRS deflection is negative, the ST segment is usually elevated, and the T wave is positive (i.e., upright). If the major QRS deflection is positive, the ST segment is usually depressed, and the T wave is usually negative (i.e., inverted). P waves are usually not seen with ventricular dysrhythmias; however, if they are visible, they have no consistent relationship to the QRS complex (i.e., **AV dissociation**).

⏺ ECG Pearl _____

When a ventricular rhythm is present, the appearance of ST segments and T waves in the opposite direction of the last portion of the QRS complex can complicate matters when looking for ECG signs of myocardial injury and infarction. For example, when the QRS complexes of a ventricular rhythm are negative, the ST segment is usually elevated. The resulting ST-segment elevation may result from abnormal repolarization and not because of any infarction-related causes. Assess the patient's clinical presentation and the results of other diagnostic studies in addition to your ECG findings.

PREMATURE VENTRICULAR COMPLEXES

How Do I Recognize Them?

A PVC, also called a premature ventricular extrasystole, ventricular premature beat, or premature ventricular depolarization, arises from an irritable site (i.e., focus) within either ventricle. By definition, a PVC is *premature*, occurring earlier than the next expected beat of the underlying rhythm. The general ECG characteristics of PVCs include the following:

Rhythm:	Irregular because of the early beats; if the PVC is an interpolated PVC, the rhythm will be regular
Rate:	Usually within normal range, but depends on the underlying rhythm
P waves:	Usually absent or, with retrograde conduction to the atria, may appear after the QRS (usually upright in the ST segment or T wave)
PR interval:	None with the PVC because the ectopic beat originates in the ventricles
QRS duration:	Usually 0.12 second or greater; T wave is usually in the opposite direction of the QRS complex

The shape of the QRS of a PVC depends on the location of the irritable focus within the ventricles (Fig. 6.2). The width of the QRS of a PVC is typically 0.12 second or greater because the PVC causes the ventricles to fire prematurely and in an abnormal manner (Fig. 6.3). The T wave usually points in a direction opposite that of the QRS complex.

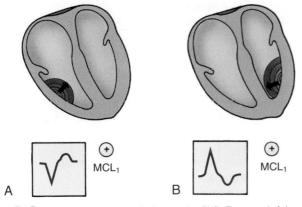

Fig. 6.2 A, Right premature ventricular complex (PVC). The spread of depolarization is from right to left, away from the positive electrode in lead V$_1$ (*MCL$_1$*), resulting in a wide, negative QRS complex. B, Left ventricular PVC. The spread of depolarization is from left to right, toward the positive electrode in lead V$_1$ (MCL$_1$). The QRS complex is wide and upright. (From Urden, L. D., Stacy, K. M., & Lough, M. E. (2022). *Critical care nursing: Diagnosis and management* (9th ed.). St. Louis: Elsevier.)

A compensatory pause often follows a PVC and occurs because the SA node is usually not affected by the PVC (Fig. 6.4). The SA node discharges at its regular rate and rhythm, including the period during and after the PVC. It is important to note that the presence of a full compensatory pause does not reliably differentiate ventricular ectopy from atrial ectopy; this is because atrial ectopy may produce a similar compensatory pattern if it does not reset the SA node (Crawford & Spence, 1995). In addition, when backward (i.e., retrograde) conduction occurs and a PVC is conducted to the atria, as in slow sinus rates, the PVC can reset the SA node, thereby resulting in a noncompensatory pause (Berger et al., 2016; Crawford & Spence, 1995).

A **fusion beat** is a result of an electrical impulse from a supraventricular site (e.g., SA node) discharging at the same time as an ectopic site in the ventricles (Fig. 6.5). Because fusion beats result from both supraventricular and ventricular depolarization, these beats do not resemble normally conducted beats, nor do they resemble true ventricular beats.

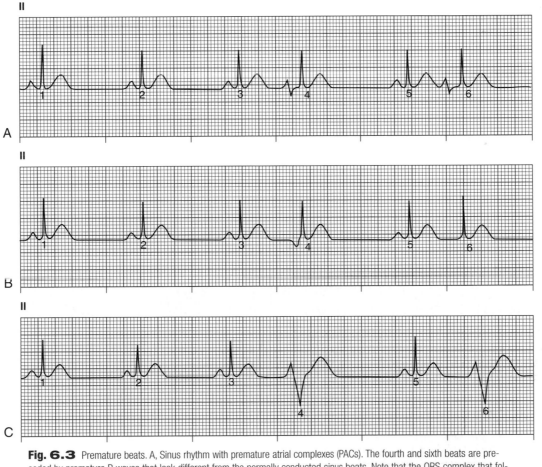

Fig. 6.3 Premature beats. A, Sinus rhythm with premature atrial complexes (PACs). The fourth and sixth beats are preceded by premature P waves that look different from the normally conducted sinus beats. Note that the QRS complex that follows each of these PACs is narrow and identical in appearance to that of the sinus-conducted beats. B, Sinus rhythm with premature junctional complexes (PJCs). The fourth and sixth beats are PJCs. Beat No. 4 is preceded by an inverted P wave with a short PR interval. There is no identifiable atrial activity associated with beat No. 6. C, Sinus rhythm with premature ventricular complexes (PVCs). The fourth and sixth beats are very different in appearance from the normally conducted sinus beats. Beats 4 and 6 are PVCs. P waves do not precede them. (From Grauer, K. (1998). *A practical guide to ECG interpretation* (2nd ed.). St. Louis: Mosby.)

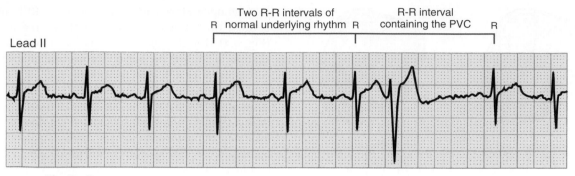

Fig. 6.4 A full compensatory pause often follows a premature ventricular complex (*PVC*). A compensatory pause is present if the period between the complex before and after a premature beat is the same as two normal R-R intervals. (From Paul, S., & Hebra, J. D. (1998). *The nurse's guide to cardiac rhythm interpretation: Implications for patient care.* Philadelphia: Saunders.)

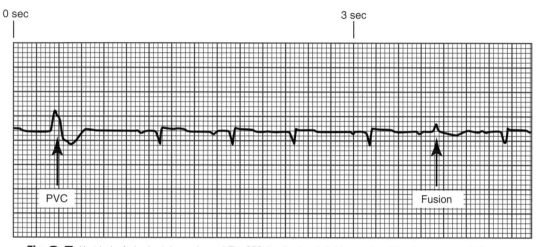

Fig. 6.5 Ventricular fusion beat *(second arrow)*. The QRS duration is only 0.08 second, and the shape represents the normal QRS and the previous premature ventricular complex (*PVC*). (From Urden, L. D., Stacy, K. M., & Lough, M. E. (2022). *Critical care nursing: Diagnosis and management* (9th ed.). St. Louis: Elsevier.)

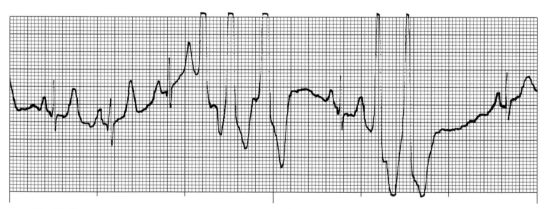

Fig. 6.6 Sinus rhythm with a run of ventricular tachycardia and one episode of ventricular couplets. (From Aehlert, B. (2004). *ECG study cards.* St. Louis: Mosby.)

PATTERNS OF PREMATURE VENTRICULAR COMPLEXES

PVCs may occur alone or in groups (i.e., patterns). Frequent PVCs are defined as the presence of at least 1 PVC on a 12-lead ECG or more than 30 PVCs per hour (Al-Khatib et al., 2018). PVCs that infrequently occur with no identifiable pattern are called isolated PVCs.

Two consecutive PVCs are called a pair or couplet (Fig. 6.6). Couplets are also referred to as "two PVCs in a row" or "back-to-back PVCs." The appearance of couplets indicates the ventricular ectopic site is very irritable. Three or more sequential PVCs are termed a run, a salvo, or burst, and three or more PVCs that occur in a row at a rate of more than 100 beats/min is considered a run of VT.

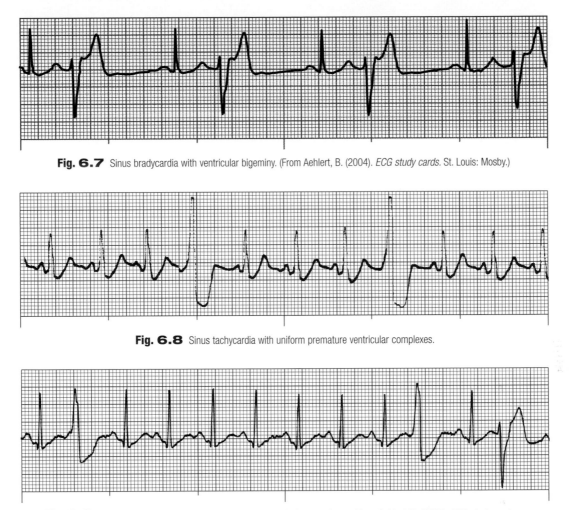

Fig. 6.7 Sinus bradycardia with ventricular bigeminy. (From Aehlert, B. (2004). *ECG study cards.* St. Louis: Mosby.)

Fig. 6.8 Sinus tachycardia with uniform premature ventricular complexes.

Fig. 6.9 Sinus tachycardia with multiform premature ventricular complexes. (From Aehlert, B. (2004). *ECG study cards.* St. Louis: Mosby.)

Ventricular bigeminy describes a rhythm in which every other beat is a PVC (Fig. 6.7); with ventricular trigeminy, every third beat is a PVC; and with ventricular quadrigeminy, every fourth beat is a PVC.

TYPES OF PREMATURE VENTRICULAR COMPLEXES

Uniform and Multiform Premature Ventricular Complexes

PVCs that look alike in the same lead and begin from the same anatomic site (i.e., focus) are called uniform PVCs (Fig. 6.8). PVCs that look different from one another in the same lead are called multiform PVCs (Fig. 6.9). The terms *unifocal* and *multifocal* are sometimes used to describe PVCs that are similar or different in appearance. Uniform PVCs are unifocal; that is, they arise from the same anatomic site within the ventricles. Multiform PVCs often, but do not always, arise from different anatomic sites; therefore, multiform PVCs are not necessarily multifocal (Goldberger et al., 2018). Multiform PVCs are generally considered more serious than uniform PVCs because they suggest a greater area of irritable myocardial tissue.

A PVC can occur with any supraventricular dysrhythmia. When identifying the rhythm, first describe the patient's underlying rhythm and then describe the ectopic beats present (i.e., "Sinus tachycardia with uniform PVCs at 110 beats/min" or "Sinus tachycardia with multiform PVCs at 120 beats/min").

Interpolated Premature Ventricular Complexes

When a PVC occurs between two normally conducted QRS complexes without interfering with the normal cardiac cycle, it is called an **interpolated PVC** (Fig. 6.10). An interpolated PVC does not have a full compensatory pause; instead, it is squeezed between two normally conducted QRS complexes (i.e., the R-R intervals between sinus beats remain the same) and does not disturb the next ventricular depolarization or SA node activity. An interpolated PVC usually occurs when the PVC is very early or when the patient's underlying heart rate is relatively slow.

R-on-T Premature Ventricular Complexes

An R-on-T PVC occurs when the R wave of a PVC falls on the T wave of the preceding beat (Fig. 6.11). Because ventricular repolarization is not yet complete during the last half of the T wave (i.e., the relative refractory period), it is possible that a PVC that occurs during this period will precipitate VT or VF. R-on-T phenomenon refers to the start of a ventricular tachydysrhythmia because of an improperly timed electrical impulse on the T wave (Spotts, 2017).

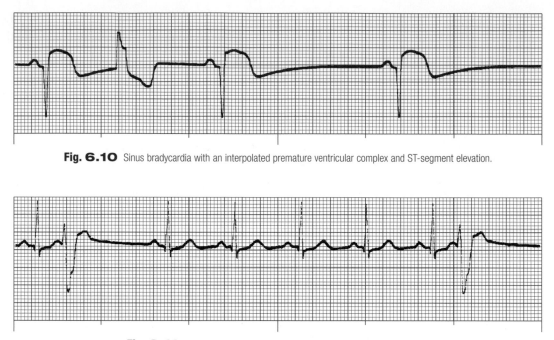

Fig. 6.10 Sinus bradycardia with an interpolated premature ventricular complex and ST-segment elevation.

Fig. 6.11 Sinus rhythm with two R-on-T premature ventricular complexes.

What Causes Them?

PVCs are common, occurring in about 50% of all people with and without heart disease (Al-Khatib et al., 2018). They can occur at rest, or they can be associated with exercise. PVCs can occur for no apparent cause, and the frequency with which they occur increases with age. Frequent PVCs are associated with increased cardiovascular risk and increased mortality (Al-Khatib et al., 2018). The frequency of PVCs progressively increases during the first several weeks after a myocardial infarction (MI) and decreases at about 6 months (Miller et al., 2019). Common causes of PVCs include the following:

- Acid–base imbalance
- Acute coronary syndromes
- Digitalis toxicity
- Electrolyte imbalance (e.g., potassium, magnesium)
- Emotional stress, anxiety
- Exercise
- Heart failure
- Hypoxia
- Medications (e.g., sympathomimetics)
- Normal variant
- Stimulants (e.g., caffeine, tobacco)
- Structural heart disease (e.g., ischemic heart disease, cardiomyopathy, valvular heart disease, adult congenital heart disease)
- Ventricular aneurysm

What Do I Do About Them?

The signs and symptoms associated with PVCs vary, and their effect on cardiac output generally depends on their frequency. Some patients experiencing PVCs are asymptomatic; others may experience palpitations, lightheadedness,

fatigue, or a pounding sensation in their neck or chest. Symptoms are particularly likely when they occur in patterns (e.g., bigeminy, trigeminy).

Treatment of PVCs depends on the cause, the patient's signs and symptoms, and the clinical situation. Most patients experiencing PVCs do not require treatment with antiarrhythmic medications; rather, treatment of PVCs focuses on searching for and treating potentially reversible causes. For example, reassure the patient who complains of palpitations while searching for possible triggers for their PVCs (e.g., excessive caffeine ingestion, nicotine use, emotional stress). Ambulatory monitoring can help identify the type and frequency of ventricular ectopy. Beta-blockers, calcium blockers, and some antiarrhythmics may be prescribed to reduce symptoms of palpitations (Al-Khatib et al., 2018). In the setting of an acute coronary syndrome, treatment is directed at ensuring adequate oxygenation; relieving pain; and rapidly identifying and correcting hypoxia, heart failure, and electrolyte or acid–base abnormalities.

ECG Pearl

When PVCs cause serious symptoms, antiarrhythmic medications (e.g., amiodarone, procainamide, lidocaine) are sometimes used to reduce the frequency with which they occur or to eliminate them. However, antiarrhythmics can cause a proarrhythmic effect, which means that they have the potential to cause serious adverse effects, more serious dysrhythmias, or both than those that they were intended to treat. For example, the treatment of occasional PVCs, which are not critical, may initiate a life-threatening sustained ventricular tachydysrhythmia.

VENTRICULAR ESCAPE BEATS OR RHYTHM

How Do I Recognize It?

Remember that premature beats are *early*, and escape beats are *late*. We need to see at least two sinus beats in a row to establish the regularity of the underlying rhythm and to determine if a complex is early or late.

Although ventricular escape beats share some physical characteristics with PVCs (e.g., wide QRS complexes, T waves deflected in a direction opposite the QRS), they differ in some critical areas. A PVC appears *early*, before the next expected beat of the underlying rhythm. PVCs often reflect ventricular irritability. A ventricular escape beat occurs after a pause in which a supraventricular pacemaker failed to fire; thus, the escape beat is *late*, appearing after the next expected normal beat. A ventricular escape beat is a *protective* mechanism, safeguarding the heart from more extreme slowing or even **asystole**. Because it is protective, you do not want to administer any medication that would wipe out the escape beat.

The ECG characteristics of ventricular escape beats include the following:

Rhythm:	Irregular because of *late* beats; the ventricular escape beat occurs *after* the next expected beat of the underlying rhythm
Rate:	Usually within normal range, but depends on the underlying rhythm
P waves:	Usually absent or, with retrograde conduction to the atria, may appear after the QRS (usually upright in the ST segment or T wave)
PR interval:	None with the ventricular escape beat because the ectopic beat originates in the ventricles
QRS duration:	0.12 second or greater; the T wave is frequently in the opposite direction of the QRS complex

Let's take a look at Fig. 6.12. One of the first things you notice is that the rhythm is irregular at a rate of about 60 beats/min, and there is a QRS complex that differs from the others. Although this beat looks interesting, let's use our systematic approach to examine the rhythm strip. There are upright P waves

before beats 1, 2, 3, 5, and 6. Now we know that the underlying rhythm is sinus in origin. Next, let's examine the wide-QRS beat more closely and see what happened here. Look to the left of the wide-QRS beat and see if anything looks amiss. When you look closely at the T wave of beat 3, it has an extra protrusion or hump. Now take a moment to plot P waves across the strip. You will find that this extra hump is an early P wave that was not conducted. This waveform is a nonconducted premature atrial complex (PAC). When plotting the P waves, notice that the wide-QRS complex occurred *late*—after the next expected sinus beat. This late complex is an escape beat. Because the QRS associated with it is *wide*, it is a *ventricular* escape beat. A *junctional* escape beat is also late, but it usually has a *narrow* QRS. Notice that the T wave of this beat is deflected in a direction opposite its QRS complex. When you look at the PR intervals and ST segment, you will find that the PR interval is longer than expected, measuring about 0.24 second. For now, we will simply say that it is prolonged. We will explore the reasons for this and give it a name in the next chapter. ST-segment depression is also present. Our interpretation of this rhythm strip would be something like this: "Sinus rhythm with a prolonged PR interval, nonconducted PAC, ventricular escape beat, and ST-segment depression at 60 beats/min." My goodness! That was one complicated rhythm strip!

An IVR, also called a ventricular escape rhythm, exists when three or more ventricular escape beats occur in a row at a rate of 20 to 40 beats/min. The QRS complexes seen in IVR are wide because the impulses begin in the ventricles, bypassing the normal conduction pathway. Characteristics of IVR include the following:

Rhythm:	Ventricular rhythm is essentially regular
Rate:	Ventricular rate 20 to 40 beats/min
P waves:	Usually absent or, with retrograde conduction to the atria, may appear after the QRS (usually upright in the ST segment or T wave)
PR interval:	None
QRS duration:	0.12 second or greater; the T wave is frequently in the opposite direction of the QRS complex

When the ventricular rate slows to less than 20 beats/min, some practitioners refer to the rhythm as an agonal rhythm or dying heart. An example of IVR is shown in Fig. 6.13.

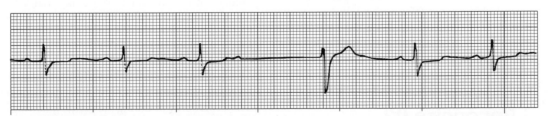

Fig. 6.12 Sinus rhythm with a prolonged PR interval, nonconducted premature atrial complex, ventricular escape beat, and ST-segment depression. (From Chou, T., & Ramaiah, L. S. (1996). *Electrocardiography in clinical practice: Adult and pediatric* (4th ed.). Philadelphia: Saunders.)

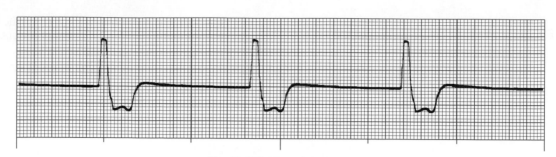

Fig. 6.13 Idioventricular rhythm.

What Causes It?

A ventricular escape rhythm may occur if the SA node and the AV junction fail to initiate an electrical impulse; if the SA node or AV junction discharge at a rate less than that of the intrinsic rate of the Purkinje fibers; or if the impulses generated by a supraventricular pacemaker site are blocked. A ventricular escape rhythm may also result from an acute coronary syndrome, digitalis toxicity, or metabolic imbalances.

What Do I Do About It?

Because the ventricular rate associated with IVR is slow (i.e., 20 to 40 beats/min) with a loss of atrial kick, the patient may experience serious signs and symptoms because of decreased cardiac output. If the patient has a pulse and is symptomatic because of the slow rate, apply a pulse oximeter and administer supplemental oxygen if indicated. Establish intravenous (IV) access and obtain a 12-lead ECG. Atropine may be ordered to treat the symptomatic bradycardia. If atropine is administered, reassess the patient's response and continue monitoring. Transcutaneous pacing (TCP) or a dopamine or epinephrine IV infusion may be ordered if atropine is ineffective. Ventricular antiarrhythmic medications should be avoided when managing patients with this rhythm. These drugs may abolish ventricular activity, possibly causing asystole in a patient with a ventricular escape rhythm.

If the patient is not breathing and has no pulse despite the appearance of organized electrical activity on the cardiac monitor, PEA exists. Therapeutic interventions for PEA include performing cardiopulmonary resuscitation (CPR), giving oxygen, starting an IV, administering epinephrine, possibly placing an advanced airway, and aggressively searching for the underlying cause (Box 6.1).

ACCELERATED IDIOVENTRICULAR RHYTHM

How Do I Recognize It?

An **accelerated idioventricular rhythm (AIVR)** exists when three or more ventricular beats occur in a row at a rate of

Box 6.1	Reversible Causes of Cardiac Emergencies

The Hs and Ts is a memory aid that can be used to recall the potentially reversible causes of cardiac emergencies, including cardiac arrest:

Hs and Ts

Hypovolemia	**T**amponade, cardiac
Hypoxia	**T**ension pneumothorax
Hypothermia	**T**hrombosis: lungs (massive pulmonary embolism)
Hypo-/hyperkalemia	**T**hrombosis: heart (acute coronary syndromes)
Hydrogen ion (acidosis)	**T**ablets or toxins: drug overdose

41 to 100 beats/min (Fig. 6.14). ECG characteristics of AIVR include the following:

Rhythm:	Ventricular rhythm is essentially regular
Rate:	41 to 100 (41 to 120 per some cardiologists) beats/min
P waves:	Usually absent or, with retrograde conduction to the atria, may appear after the QRS (usually upright in the ST segment or T wave)
PR interval:	None
QRS duration:	0.12 second or greater; the T wave is frequently in the opposite direction of the QRS complex

AIVR is usually considered a benign escape rhythm. It appears when the sinus rate slows and disappears when the sinus rate speeds up. Episodes of AIVR usually last a few seconds to 1 minute. Because AIVR usually begins and ends gradually, it is also called nonparoxysmal VT. Fusion beats are often seen at the onset and end of the rhythm.

What Causes It?

AIVR is often seen during the early hours of an acute MI, after successful reperfusion therapy, after interventional coronary artery procedures, or during the period following cardiac arrest. AIVR has also been observed in patients with the following:

- Acute myocarditis
- Cardiomyopathies

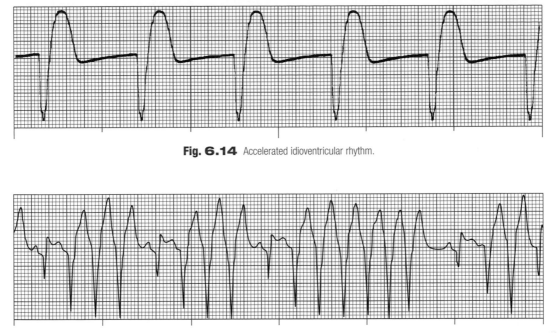

Fig. 6.14 Accelerated idioventricular rhythm.

Fig. 6.15 Nonsustained ventricular tachycardia. (From Crawford, M. V., & Spence, M. I. (1994). *Commonsense approach to coronary care* (Rev. ed. 6). St. Louis: Mosby.)

- Cocaine toxicity
- Digitalis toxicity
- Electrolyte imbalances
- Hypertensive heart disease
- Subarachnoid hemorrhage

What Do I Do About It?

AIVR generally requires no treatment because the rhythm is protective and often transient, spontaneously resolving on its own; however, possible dizziness, lightheadedness, or other signs of hemodynamic compromise may occur because of the loss of atrial kick. When treatment is indicated, apply a pulse oximeter and administer supplemental oxygen if indicated. Establish IV access and obtain a 12-lead ECG. IV atropine may be ordered to stimulate the SA node and improve AV conduction (Gildea & Levis, 2018). If atropine is given, reassess the patient's response and continue monitoring.

VENTRICULAR TACHYCARDIA

Ventricular tachycardia (VT) exists when three or more sequential PVCs occur at a rate of more than 100 beats/min. VT may occur with or without pulses, and the patient may be stable or unstable with this rhythm.

How Do I Recognize It?

VT may occur as a short run that lasts less than 30 seconds and spontaneously ends (i.e., nonsustained VT) (Fig. 6.15). Episodes of nonsustained VT may be recorded in up to 3% of apparently healthy individuals with no identifiable heart disease (Garan, 2020). The frequency with which nonsustained VT occurs increases with age and the presence and severity of underlying heart disease (Garan, 2020). In patients with heart disease, nonsustained VT is often a predictor of high risk for sustained VT or VF (Martin & Wharton, 2001).

Sustained VT persists for more than 30 seconds or requires termination because of resulting hemodynamic compromise in less than 30 seconds (Al-Khatib et al., 2018) (Fig. 6.16). The rapid heart rate associated with sustained VT can cause a marked decrease in ventricular function and cardiac output, particularly in patients with underlying heart disease, resulting in acute heart failure, syncope, hypotension, or circulatory collapse within several seconds to minutes after the onset of VT (Garan, 2020).

MONOMORPHIC VENTRICULAR TACHYCARDIA

Similar to PVCs, VT may originate from an ectopic focus in either ventricle. When the QRS complexes of VT are of the same shape and amplitude, the rhythm is called monomorphic VT (Fig. 6.17). Monomorphic VT with a ventricular rate of 150 to 300 beats/min is called ventricular flutter by some experts (Olgin et al., 2019). The ECG characteristics of monomorphic VT include the following:

Rhythm:	Ventricular rhythm is essentially regular
Rate:	101 to 250 (121 to 250 per some cardiologists) beats/min
P waves:	Usually not seen; if present, they have no set relationship with the QRS complexes that appear between them at a rate different from that of the VT

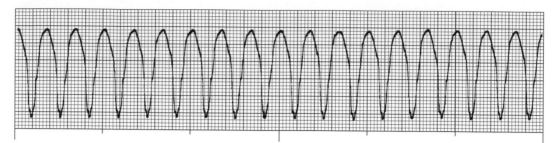

Fig. 6.16 If this rhythm lasts longer than 30 seconds or requires termination because of resulting hemodynamic compromise in less than 30 seconds, it is called sustained ventricular tachycardia.

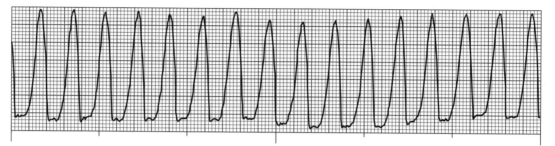

Fig. 6.17 Monomorphic ventricular tachycardia. (From Aehlert, B. (2004). *ECG study cards.* St. Louis: Mosby.)

PR interval: None
QRS duration: 0.12 second or greater; often difficult to differentiate between the QRS and T wave

What Causes It?

Mechanisms of VT include disorders of impulse formation, such as altered automaticity or triggered activity, or disorders of conduction, such as reentry. Sustained monomorphic VT is often associated with chronic heart disease. Other possible causes of VT include the following:

- Acid–base imbalance
- Acute coronary syndromes
- Cocaine or methamphetamine abuse
- Electrolyte imbalance (e.g., potassium, calcium, magnesium)
- Structural heart disease (e.g., ischemic heart disease, cardiomyopathy, valvular heart disease, adult congenital heart disease)
- Trauma (e.g., myocardial contusion, invasive cardiac procedures)
- Tricyclic antidepressant overdose

What Do I Do About It?

Signs and symptoms associated with VT vary. Because episodes of nonsustained VT come and go, they typically don't cause symptoms; however, a beta-blocker may be prescribed if episodes are frequent and accompanied by symptoms such as palpitations or syncope. Because nonsustained VT is associated with an increased risk of death and other cardiovascular adverse outcomes, including stroke (Al-Khatib et al., 2018), patients should receive follow-up and ongoing management by a cardiologist. Ambulatory monitoring or use of an implanted cardiac monitor may be ordered to diagnose the dysrhythmia,

ascertain its frequency, establish if it is the cause of the patient's symptoms, and assess the patient's response to treatment.

During sustained VT, the severity of the patient's symptoms is related to several factors, including how rapid the ventricular rate is, how long the tachycardia has been present, current medications, the presence and extent of underlying heart disease, and the presence and severity of peripheral vascular disease (Olgin et al., 2019). The patient may experience palpitations, dizziness, chest discomfort, shortness of breath, or lightheadedness. Syncope, near-syncope, or a seizure may occur because of an abrupt onset of VT.

⊙ ECG Pearl

Signs and symptoms of hemodynamic instability related to VT may include an acute altered mental status, acute heart failure, chest pain or discomfort, hypotension, pulmonary congestion, shock, or shortness of breath.

Monomorphic VT can degenerate into PMVT or VF, particularly when the ventricular rate is very fast or myocardial ischemia is present. Treatment is based on the patient's signs and symptoms and the type of VT. In all cases, a search for the cause of the VT is essential. For example, VT that results from hypokalemia may be terminated with potassium replacement. When possible, obtain a 12-lead ECG before attempting pharmacologic or electrical conversion of the dysrhythmia; doing so enables proper rhythm interpretation, diagnosis, and treatment (De Ponti et al., 2017).

If the rhythm is monomorphic VT (and the tachycardia causes the patient's symptoms):

- CPR and defibrillation are used to treat the pulseless patient with VT.

- Stable but symptomatic patients are treated with oxygen (if indicated), IV access, and ventricular antiarrhythmics (e.g., procainamide, amiodarone, sotalol) to suppress the rhythm. Procainamide should be avoided if the patient has a prolonged QT interval or signs of heart failure. Sotalol should also be avoided if the patient has a prolonged QT interval. Echocardiography is typically performed to assess cardiac structure and function in patients with structural heart disease.
- Unstable patients (usually a sustained heart rate of 150 beats/min or more) are treated with oxygen, IV access, and sedation (if the patient is awake and time permits), followed by synchronized cardioversion.

After the acute event is resolved, the patient will require a thorough evaluation to identify the underlying cause, reduce the likelihood of recurrence of symptomatic sustained VT, and prevent sudden cardiac death. Interventions may include genetic testing, invasive cardiac imaging (e.g., cardiac catheterization, computed tomography angiography), electrophysiologic testing with possible catheter ablation, antiarrhythmic medications, or insertion of an implantable cardioverter-defibrillator.

ECG Pearl

A supraventricular tachycardia (SVT) with an intraventricular conduction delay may be difficult to distinguish from VT. Keep in mind that VT is considered a potentially life-threatening dysrhythmia. If you are unsure whether a regular, wide-QRS tachycardia is VT or SVT with an intraventricular conduction delay, treat the rhythm as VT until proven otherwise. Obtaining a 12-lead ECG may help differentiate VT from SVT, but do not delay treatment if the patient is symptomatic.

POLYMORPHIC VENTRICULAR TACHYCARDIA

With PMVT, the QRS complexes vary in shape and amplitude from beat to beat and appear to twist from upright to negative or negative to upright and back, resembling a spindle (Fig. 6.18). The twisting may not always be seen,

especially if the episode is nonsustained or if only a limited number of leads are available (Al-Khatib et al., 2018). PMVT is a dysrhythmia of intermediate severity between monomorphic VT and VF (Fig. 6.19). It may be challenging to distinguish PMVT from VF when the rate of PMVT is very fast (Garan, 2020). The ECG characteristics of PMVT include the following:

Rhythm:	Ventricular rhythm may be regular or irregular
Rate:	Ventricular rate 150 to 300 beats/min; typically 200 to 250 beats/min
P waves:	None
PR interval:	None
QRS duration:	0.12 second or more; there is a gradual alteration in the amplitude and direction of the QRS complexes; a typical cycle consists of 5 to 20 QRS complexes

What Causes It?

Several types of PMVT and their possible causes have been identified. Most PMVTs are associated with a normal QT interval (Jebberi et al., 2019) and are simply referred to as normal-QT PMVT. PMVT that occurs in the presence of a long QT interval (typically 0.45 second or more and often 0.50 second or more) is called **torsades de pointes (TdP)**. A long QT interval may be congenital, acquired (typically precipitated by antiarrhythmic drugs that lengthen the QT interval or hypokalemia, which are often associated with bradycardia), or idiopathic (neither familial nor with an identifiable acquired cause). PMVT can occur in the presence of an abnormally short QT interval (typically less than 0.32 second). This type of PMVT is called short-QT PMVT. PMVT that occurs in the setting of an acute MI is associated with increased mortality (Virani et al., 2021).

What Do I Do About It?

The signs and symptoms associated with PMVT are usually related to the decreased cardiac output that occurs because of the fast ventricular rate. Signs of shock are often present. The patient may experience a syncopal episode or seizures.

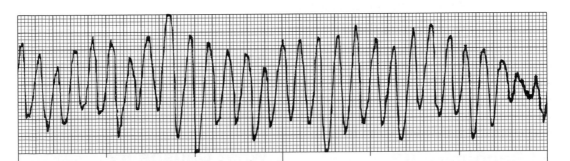

Fig. 6.18 Polymorphic ventricular tachycardia. This rhythm strip is from a 77-year-old man 3 days after MI. His chief complaint at the onset of this episode was chest pain. He had a past medical history of a previous MI and an abdominal aortic aneurysm repair. The patient was given a ventricular antiarrhythmic and defibrillated several times without success. Laboratory work revealed a serum potassium (K^+) level of 2.0. Intravenous K^+ was administered, and the patient converted to a sinus rhythm with the next defibrillation.

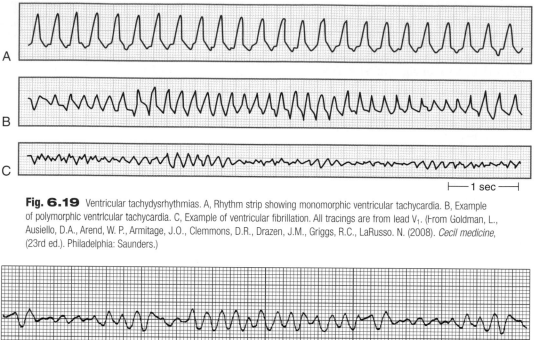

Fig. 6.19 Ventricular tachydysrhythmias. A, Rhythm strip showing monomorphic ventricular tachycardia. B, Example of polymorphic ventricular tachycardia. C, Example of ventricular fibrillation. All tracings are from lead V₁. (From Goldman, L., Ausiello, D.A., Arend, W. P., Armitage, J.O., Clemmons, D.R., Drazen, J.M., Griggs, R.C., LaRusso. N. (2008). *Cecil medicine*, (23rd ed.). Philadelphia: Saunders.)

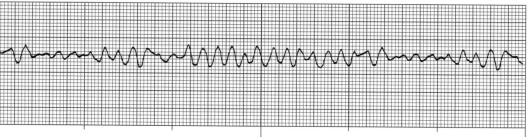

Fig. 6.20 Ventricular fibrillation (VF) with waves that are 3 mm high or more is called coarse VF.

The rhythm may occasionally terminate spontaneously and recur after several seconds or minutes, or it may deteriorate to VF and cause cardiac arrest. The patient with sustained PMVT is rarely hemodynamically stable.

It is best to consult a cardiologist when treating a patient with PMVT because of the diverse mechanisms of PMVT, as there may or may not be clues as to its specific cause at the time of the patient's presentation. Treatment options vary and can be contradictory. For example, a medication that may be appropriate for treating a patient with TdP may be contraindicated when treating a patient with another form of PMVT. In general, if the patient is symptomatic because of the tachycardia, treat ischemia (if it is present), correct electrolyte abnormalities, and discontinue any medications that the patient may be taking that prolong the QT interval. If the patient is stable, the use of IV amiodarone (if the QT interval is normal), magnesium, or beta-blockers may be effective, depending on the cause of the PMVT. Defibrillate if the patient is unstable or has no pulse.

VENTRICULAR FIBRILLATION

How Do I Recognize It?

VF is a chaotic rhythm that begins in the ventricles. In VF, there is no organized ventricular depolarization. The ventricular muscle quivers, and as a result, there is no effective myocardial contraction and no pulse. The resulting rhythm looks chaotic with deflections that vary in shape and amplitude. No normal-looking waveforms are visible. VF with waves that are 3 mm or more high is called coarse VF (Fig. 6.20). As VF continues, myocardial energy stores become depleted, and the amplitude of the fibrillating waves decreases. VF with low amplitude waves (i.e., less than 3 mm) is called fine VF (Fig. 6.21). In general, coarse VF is more likely to respond to defibrillation than fine VF. If untreated, VF will eventually degenerate to asystole. The ECG characteristics of VF include the following:

Rhythm:	Rapid and chaotic with no pattern or regularity
Rate:	Cannot be determined because there are no discernible waves or complexes to measure
P waves:	None
PR interval:	None
QRS duration:	None

Fig. 6.22 illustrates a comparison of ventricular dysrhythmias.

What Causes It?

Factors that increase the susceptibility of the myocardium to fibrillate include the following:
- Acute coronary syndromes
- Dysrhythmias

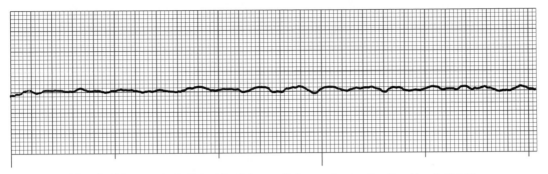

Fig. 6.21 Ventricular fibrillation (VF) with low-amplitude waves (i.e., less than 3 mm) is called fine VF.

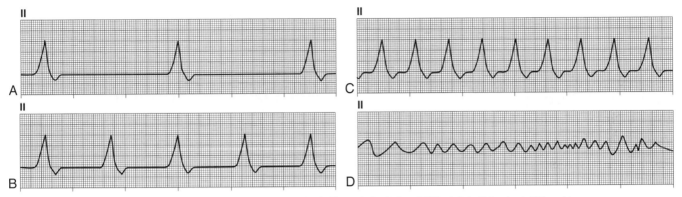

Fig. 6.22 Comparison of ventricular dysrhythmias. A, Idioventricular rhythm at 38 beats/min. B, Accelerated idioventric-ular rhythm at 75 beats/min. C, Monomorphic ventricular tachycardia at 150 beats/min. D, Coarse ventricular fibrillation. (From Grauer, K. (1998). *A practical guide to ECG interpretation* (2nd ed.). St. Louis: Mosby.)

- Electrolyte imbalance
- Environmental factors (e.g., electrocution)
- Hypertrophy
- Increased sympathetic nervous system activity
- Proarrhythmic effect of antiarrhythmics and other medi-cations
- Severe heart failure
- Structural heart disease (e.g., ischemic heart disease, car-diomyopathy, valvular heart disease, adult congenital heart disease)
- Vagal stimulation

🕐 ECG Pearl _____

Of patients hospitalized with acute MI, 5% to 10% have VF or sustained VT before they arrive at the hospital, and another 5% will have VF or sustained VT after hospital arrival, most within 48 hours of admission (Al-Khatib et al., 2018).

What Do I Do About It?

The patient in VF is unresponsive, apneic, and pulseless. The priorities of care in cardiac arrest resulting from pulseless VT or VF are high-quality CPR and defibrillation. Use the Hs and Ts to recall possible reversible causes of pulseless VT or VF. Administer medications and perform additional in-terventions per current resuscitation guidelines.

🕐 ECG Pearl _____

Because artifact can mimic VF, *always* check the patient's pulse before beginning treatment.

DEFIBRILLATION

Defibrillation is the delivery of an electrical current across the heart muscle over a very brief period to terminate an abnormal heart rhythm. Defibrillation is also called unsyn-chronized countershock or asynchronous countershock because current delivery has no relationship to the cardiac cycle. The shock attempts to deliver a uniform electrical cur-rent of sufficient intensity to depolarize myocardial cells (including fibrillating cells) at the same time. By briefly stun-ning the heart, an opportunity is provided for the heart's natural pacemakers to resume normal activity. When the cells repolarize, the pacemaker with the highest degree of automaticity should assume pacing responsibility.

Manual defibrillation refers to the placement of adhesive pads on a patient's chest, the interpretation of the patient's cardiac rhythm by a trained health care professional, and the health care professional's decision to deliver a shock, if indicated. Automated external defibrillation refers to the placement of pads on a patient's chest and the interpretation of the patient's cardiac rhythm by an **automated external defibrillator (AED)**. The AED has a sophisticated computer system that analyzes a patient's heart rhythm using an algorithm to distinguish shockable rhythms from nonshockable rhythms and providing visual and auditory instructions to the rescuer to deliver an electrical shock, if a shock is indicated. Defibrillation is indicated in the treatment of pulseless monomorphic VT, sustained PMVT, and VF.

ECG Pearl

Cardiac arrest rhythms include asystole, PEA, VF, and pulseless VT. VF and pulseless VT are *shockable* rhythms, which means that delivering a shock to the heart with a defibrillator may result in the termination of the rhythm. Asystole and PEA are *nonshockable* rhythms.

ASYSTOLE (CARDIAC STANDSTILL)

How Do I Recognize It?

Asystole, also called cardiac standstill, is a total absence of atrial and ventricular electrical activity (Fig. 6.23). There is no atrial or ventricular rate or rhythm, no pulse, and no

cardiac output. If atrial electrical activity is present, the rhythm is called P wave asystole or ventricular standstill (Fig. 6.24). The ECG characteristics of asystole include the following:

Rhythm:	Ventricular not discernible; atrial may be discernible
Rate:	Ventricular not discernible, but atrial activity may be observed (i.e., P-wave asystole)
P waves:	Usually none
PR interval:	None
QRS duration:	Absent

What Causes It?

Use the Hs and Ts to recall possible reversible causes of asystole. Ventricular asystole may occur temporarily after the termination of a tachycardia with medications, defibrillation, or synchronized cardioversion (Fig. 6.25).

What Do I Do About It?

When asystole is observed on a cardiac monitor, quickly confirm that the patient is unresponsive and has no pulse, and then begin high-quality CPR. Additional care includes

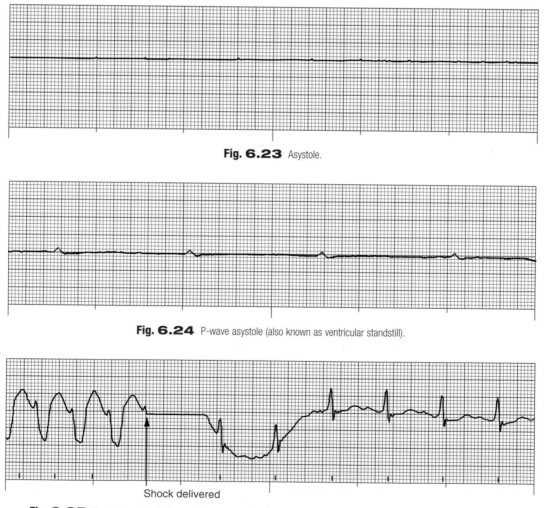

Fig. 6.23 Asystole.

Fig. 6.24 P-wave asystole (also known as ventricular standstill).

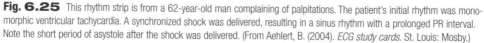

Shock delivered

Fig. 6.25 This rhythm strip is from a 62-year-old man complaining of palpitations. The patient's initial rhythm was monomorphic ventricular tachycardia. A synchronized shock was delivered, resulting in a sinus rhythm with a prolonged PR interval. Note the short period of asystole after the shock was delivered. (From Aehlert, B. (2004). *ECG study cards.* St. Louis: Mosby.)

TABLE 6.1 Ventricular Rhythms: Summary of Characteristics

Dysrhythmia	Rhythm	Rate (beats/min)	P Waves (Lead II)	PR Interval	QRS Duration
PVCs	Irregular because of *early* beats	Usually within normal range but depends on underlying rhythm	Usually absent or, with retrograde conduction to the atria, may appear after the QRS (usually upright in the ST segment or T wave)	None with the PVC because the ectopic beat originates in the ventricles	Usually 0.12 sec or greater
Ventricular escape beat	Irregular because of *late* beats	Usually within normal range but depends on the underlying rhythm	Usually absent or, with retrograde conduction to the atria, may appear after the QRS	None because the ectopic beat originates in the ventricles	0.12 sec or greater
Idioventricular rhythm	Ventricular rhythm essentially regular	20 to 40	Usually absent or, with retrograde conduction to the atria, may appear after the QRS	None	0.12 sec or greater
Accelerated idioventricular rhythm	Ventricular rhythm essentially regular	41 to 100; 41 to 120 per some experts	Usually absent or, with retrograde conduction to the atria, may appear after the QRS	None	0.12 sec or greater
Monomorphic VT	Ventricular rhythm essentially regular	101 to 250; 121 to 250 per some experts	Usually not seen	None	0.12 sec or greater
Polymorphic VT	Ventricular rhythm may be regular or irregular	150 to 300 beats/min	None	None	0.12 sec or greater
Ventricular fibrillation	Rapid, chaotic with no pattern or regularity	Not discernible	None	None	Not discernible
Asystole	Ventricular not discernible; atrial may be discernible	Ventricular not discernible, but atrial activity may be observed	Usually none	None	Absent

PVC, Premature ventricular complex; *VT*, ventricular tachycardia.

establishing vascular access, considering possible reversible causes of the arrest, administering medications (i.e., epinephrine), and performing additional interventions per current resuscitation guidelines. Defibrillation is not indicated in the treatment of asystole. A summary of ventricular rhythm characteristics appears in Table 6.1.

REFERENCES

Al-Khatib, S. M., Stevenson, W. G., Ackerman, M. J., Bryant, W. J., Callans, D. J., Curtis, A. B., ... Page, R. L. (2018). 2017 AHA/ACC/HRS guideline for management of patients with ventricular arrhythmias and the prevention of sudden cardiac death. *J Am Coll Cardiol, 72*(14), e91–e220.

Berger, M. G., Rubenstein, J. C., & Roth, J. A. (2016). Cardiac arrhythmias. In I. J. Benjamin, R. C. Griggs, E. J. Wing, & J. G. Fitz (Eds.), *Andreoli & Carpenter's Cecil essentials of medicine* (9th ed., pp. 110–135). Philadelphia, PA: Saunders.

Crawford, M. V., & Spence, M. I. (1995). Electrical complications in coronary artery disease: Arrhythmias. In *Common sense approach to coronary care* (6th ed., p. 220). St. Louis, MO: Mosby.

De Ponti, R., Bagliani, G., Padeletti, L., & Natale, A. (2017). General approach to a wide QRS complex. *Card Electrophysiol Clin, 9*(3), 461–485.

Garan, H. (2020). Ventricular arrhythmias. In L. Goldman, & A. I. Schafer (Eds.), *Goldman-Cecil medicine* (26th ed., pp. 343–350). Philadelphia, PA: Elsevier.

Gildea, T. H., & Levis, J. T. (2018). ECG diagnosis: Accelerated idioventricular rhythm. *Perm J, 22*(2), 87–88.

Goldberger, A. L., Goldberger, Z. D., & Shvilkin, A. (2018). Ventricular arrhythmias. In *Goldberger's clinical electrocardiography* (9th ed., pp. 156–171). Philadelphia, PA: Elsevier.

Jebberi, Z., Marazzato, J., De Ponti, R., Bagliani, G., Leonelli, F. M., & Boveda, S. (2019). Polymorphic wide QRS complex tachycardia: Differential diagnosis. *Card Electrophysiol Clin, 11*(2), 333–344.

Martin, D., & Wharton, J. M. (2001). Sustained monomorphic ventricular tachycardia. In P. J. Podrid, & P. R. Kowey (Eds.), *Cardiac arrhythmia: Mechanisms, diagnosis, and management* (2nd ed., pp. 573–601). Philadelphia, PA: Lippincott Williams & Wilkins.

Miller, J. M., Tomaselli, G. F., & Zipes, D. P. (2019). Diagnosis of cardiac arrhythmias. In D. P. Zipes, P. Libby, R. O. Bonow, D. L. Mann, G. F. Tomaselli, & E. Braunwald (Eds.), *Braunwald's heart disease: A textbook of cardiovascular medicine* (11th ed., pp. 648–669). Philadelphia, PA: Elsevier.

Olgin, J., Tomaselli, G. F., & Zipes, D. P. (2019). Ventricular arrhythmias. In D. P. Zipes, P. Libby, R. O. Bonow, D. L. Mann, G. F. Tomaselli, & E. Braunwald (Eds.), *Braunwald's heart disease—A textbook of cardiovascular medicine* (11th ed., pp. 753–771). Philadelphia, PA: Elsevier.

Spotts, V. (2017). Temporary transcutaneous (external) pacing. In D. L. Wiegand (Ed.), *AACN procedure manual for critical care* (7th ed., pp. 399–406). St. Louis, MO: Elsevier.

Virani, S. S., Alonso, A., Aparicio, H. J., Benjamin, E. J., Bittencourt, M. S., Callaway, C. W., … Tsao, C. W. (2021). Heart disease and stroke statistics—2021 update: A report from the American Heart Association. *Circulation, 143*(8), e254–e743.

STOP & REVIEW

Identify one or more choices that best complete the statement or answer the question.

1. Identify the ECG characteristics of an IVR.
   a. Essentially regular ventricular rhythm
   b. Ventricular rate is 40 to 60 beats/min
   c. QRS complexes measure 0.12 second or greater
   d. P waves may occur before, during, or after the QRS
   e. Gradual alteration in the amplitude and direction of the QRS

2. A 74-year-old man experienced a syncopal episode at the grocery store. His blood pressure is 74/50 mm Hg, heart rate is 30 beats/min, and ventilatory rate is 18 breaths/min. Breath sounds are clear, his oxygen saturation on room air is 97%, and his blood glucose is normal. The cardiac monitor reveals a ventricular escape rhythm. Based on the information provided, which of the following are possible therapeutic interventions to consider?
   a. Prepare for TCP.
   b. Establish IV access.
   c. Obtain a 12-lead ECG.
   d. Administer atropine IV.
   e. Administer amiodarone IV.

3. How would you differentiate a junctional escape rhythm at 40 beats/min from an idioventricular rhythm at the same rate?
   a. It is impossible to differentiate a junctional escape rhythm from an idioventricular rhythm.
   b. The junctional escape rhythm will have a narrow QRS complex; the idioventricular rhythm will have a wide QRS complex.
   c. The rate (i.e., 40 beats/min) would indicate a junctional escape rhythm, not an idioventricular rhythm.
   d. The junctional escape rhythm will have a wide QRS complex; an idioventricular rhythm will have a narrow QRS complex.

4. The term for three or more PVCs occurring in a row at a rate of more than 100/min is
   a. ventricular trigeminy.
   b. ventricular fibrillation.
   c. a run of ventricular tachycardia.
   d. a run of ventricular escape beats.

5. Which of the following are the priorities of care in cardiac arrest resulting from pulseless VT or VF?
   a. Performing defibrillation
   b. Performing high-quality CPR
   c. Inserting an advanced airway
   d. Giving resuscitation medications

6. Select the shockable cardiac arrest rhythms from the choices below.
   a. VF
   b. PEA
   c. Asystole
   d. Pulseless VT

7. The primary difference between a PVC and a ventricular escape beat is
   a. a PVC is early and an escape beat is late.
   b. a PVC has a narrow QRS and a ventricular escape beat has a wide QRS.
   c. the ventricular rate associated with escape beats is faster than that of PVCs.
   d. the ventricular rhythm with a PVC is irregular, but it is regular with an escape beat._

8. Which of the following statements are true about asystole?
   a. Begin TCP as soon as the equipment is available.
   b. Defibrillation is the treatment of choice for this rhythm.
   c. Use the Hs and Ts when considering possible reversible causes of the rhythm.
   d. If a flat line is present but atrial activity is seen, the rhythm is called P wave asystole or ventricular standstill.

9. An 83-year old woman with a history of ischemic heart disease presents with a sudden onset of sustained monomorphic VT. Which of the following should be anticipated when caring for this patient?
   a. Stroke
   b. Syncope
   c. Heart failure
   d. Hypotension
   e. Circulatory collapse

10. Antiarrhythmics can cause a ____ effect, which means that they have the potential to cause serious adverse effects, more serious dysrhythmias, or both, than those that they were intended to treat.
    a. probiotic
    b. proactive
    c. polymorphic
    d. proarrhythmic

11. Which of the following is a type of PVC that occurs between two normally conducted QRS complexes and does not disturb the next ventricular depolarization or SA node activity?
    a. A fusion beat
    b. A uniform PVC
    c. An escape beat
    d. An interpolated PVC

12. The ECG characteristics of monomorphic VT include
    a. a PR interval of 0.12 to 0.20 second.
    b. a ventricular rate of 101 to 250 beats/min.
    c. a ventricular rhythm that is essentially regular.
    d. a QRS that is 0.12 second or greater in duration.

Ventricular Rhythms—*Practice Rhythm Strips*

Use the five steps of rhythm interpretation to interpret each of the following rhythm strips. All rhythms were recorded in lead II unless otherwise noted.

13. Identify the rhythm.

Rhythm: _____ Rate: _____ P waves: _____

PR interval: _____ QRS duration: _____ QT interval: _____

Interpretation: _____

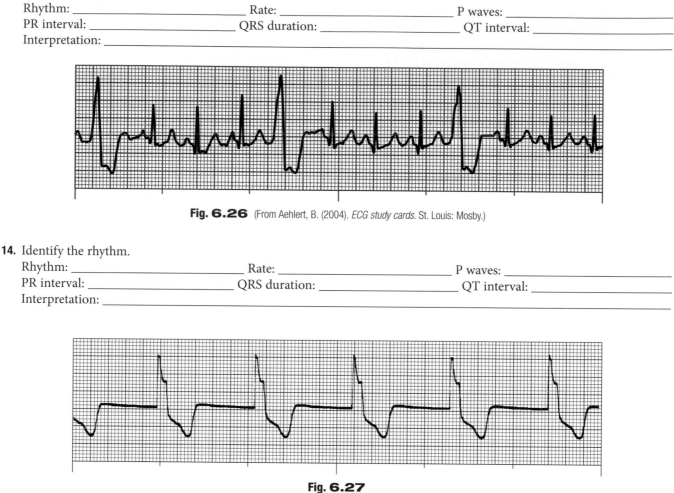

Fig. 6.26 (From Aehlert, B. (2004). *ECG study cards.* St. Louis: Mosby.)

14. Identify the rhythm.

Rhythm: _____ Rate: _____ P waves: _____

PR interval: _____ QRS duration: _____ QT interval: _____

Interpretation: _____

Fig. 6.27

15. This rhythm strip is from a 63-year-old man who collapsed on the kitchen floor. He is unresponsive, apneic, and pulseless. His past medical history includes a coronary artery bypass graft 8 years ago and pacemaker implantation 5 years ago.

Rhythm: _____ Rate: _____ P waves: _____

PR interval: _____ QRS duration: _____ QT interval: _____

Interpretation _____

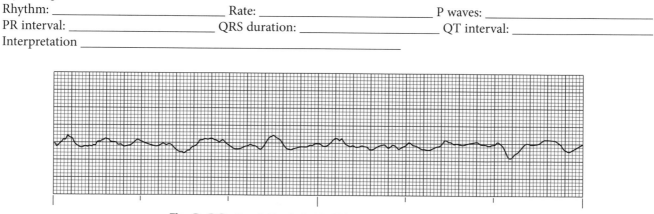

Fig. 6.28 (From Aehlert, B. (2004). *ECG study cards.* St. Louis: Mosby.)

16. This rhythm strip is from a 1-month-old infant after a 3-minute seizure.

Rhythm: _____ Rate: _____ P waves: _____

PR interval: _____ QRS duration: _____ QT interval: _____

Interpretation: _____

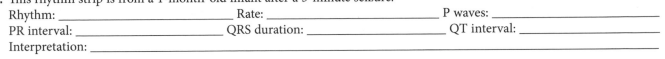
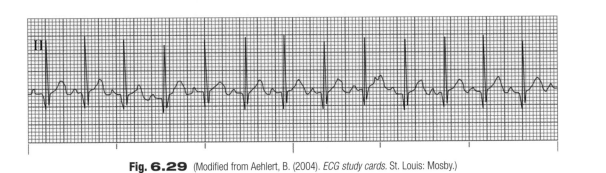

Fig. 6.29 (Modified from Aehlert, B. (2004). *ECG study cards*. St. Louis: Mosby.)

17. Identify the rhythm.

Rhythm: _____ Rate: _____ P waves: _____

PR interval: _____ QRS duration: _____ QT interval: _____

Interpretation: _____

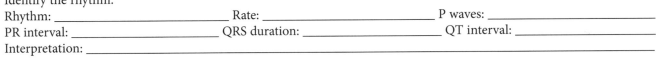
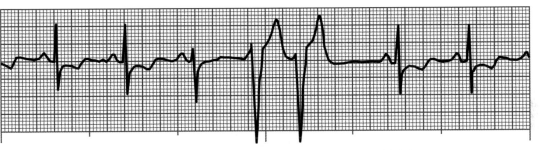
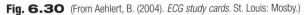

Fig. 6.30 (From Aehlert, B. (2004). *ECG study cards*. St. Louis: Mosby.)

18. Identify the rhythm.

Rhythm: _____ Rate: _____ P waves: _____

PR interval: _____ QRS duration: _____ QT interval: _____

Interpretation: _____

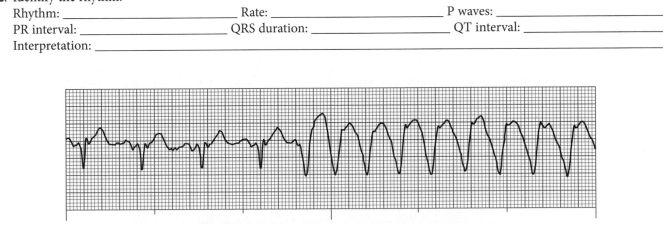

Fig. 6.31 (From Aehlert, B. (2004). *ECG study cards*. St. Louis: Mosby.)

19. Identify the rhythm.

Rhythm: _____ Rate: _____ P waves: _____

PR interval: _____ QRS duration: _____ QT interval: _____

Interpretation: _____

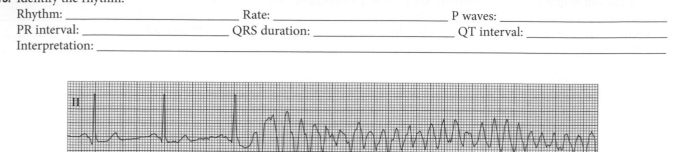

Fig. 6.32

20. Identify the rhythm.

Rhythm: _____ Rate: _____ P waves: _____

PR interval: _____ QRS duration: _____ QT interval: _____

Interpretation: _____

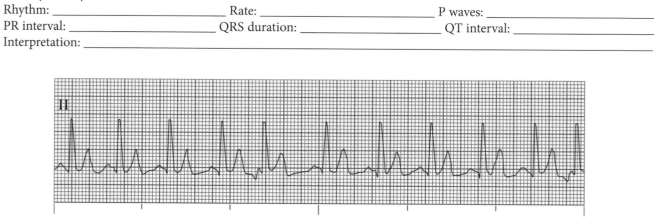

Fig. 6.33 (Modified from Aehlert, B. (2004). *ECG study cards*. St. Louis: Mosby.)

21. This rhythm strip is from a 73-year-old woman complaining of chest pain.

Rhythm: _____ Rate: _____ P waves: _____

PR interval: _____ QRS duration: _____ QT interval: _____

Interpretation: _____

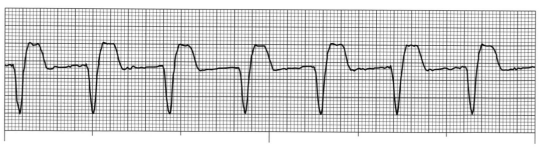

Fig. 6.34 (From Aehlert, B. (2004). *ECG study cards*. St. Louis: Mosby.)

22. This rhythm strip is from a 25-year-old man with an altered mental status because of alcohol.

Rhythm: _____ Rate: _____ P waves: _____

PR interval: _____ QRS duration: _____ QT interval: _____

Interpretation: _____

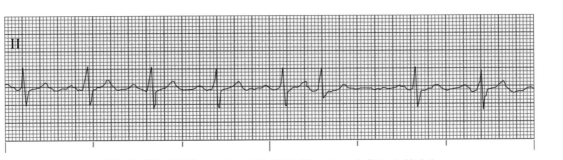

Fig. 6.35 (Modified from Aehlert, B. (2004). *ECG study cards.* St. Louis: Mosby.)

23. Identify the rhythm.

Rhythm: _____ Rate: _____ P waves: _____

PR interval: _____ QRS duration: _____ QT interval: _____

Interpretation: _____

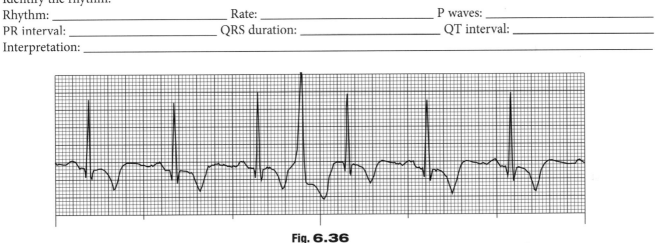

Fig. 6.36

24. Identify the rhythm.

Rhythm: _____ Rate: _____ P waves: _____

PR interval: _____ QRS duration: _____ QT interval: _____

Interpretation: _____

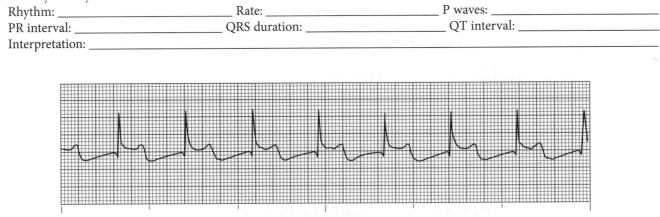

Fig. 6.37

25. Identify the rhythm.

Rhythm: _____ Rate: _____ P waves: _____
PR interval: _____ QRS duration: _____ QT interval: _____
Interpretation: _____

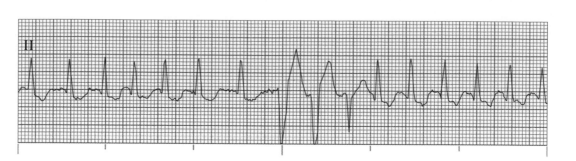

Fig. 6.38 (Modified from Aehlert, B. (2004). *ECG study cards.* St. Louis: Mosby.)

26. Identify the rhythm.

Rhythm: _____ Rate: _____ P waves: _____
PR interval: _____ QRS duration: _____ QT interval: _____
Interpretation: _____

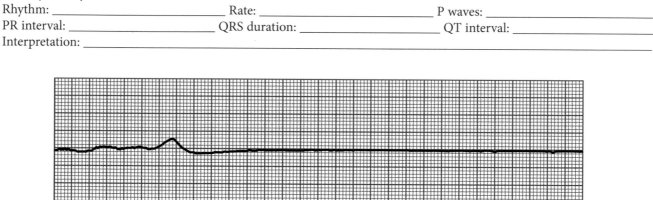

Fig. 6.39 (From Aehlert, B. (2004). *ECG study cards.* St. Louis: Mosby.)

27. This rhythm strip is from a 47-year-old man with an altered mental status. His blood pressure is 118/86 mm Hg, and his blood sugar is 37 mg/dL.

Rhythm: _____ Rate: _____ P waves: _____
PR interval: _____ QRS duration: _____ QT interval: _____
Interpretation: _____

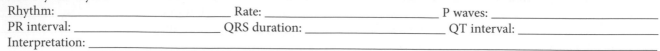

Fig. 6.40 (Modified from Aehlert, B. (2004). *ECG study cards.* St. Louis: Mosby.)

28. This rhythm strip is from a 69-year-old man who is complaining of substernal chest pain. He rates his discomfort
as 9/10.

Rhythm: _____   Rate: _____   P waves: _____

PR interval: _____   QRS duration: _____   QT interval: _____

Interpretation: _____

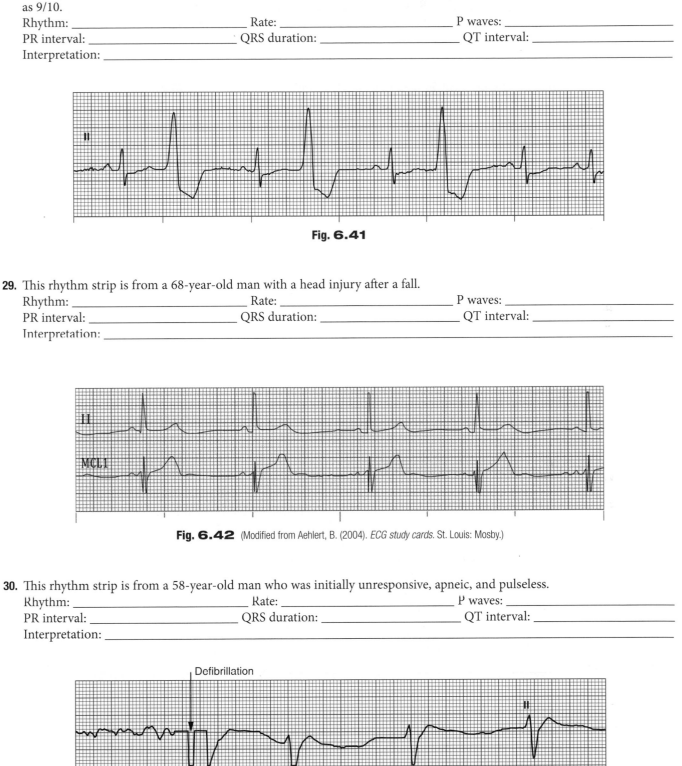

Fig. 6.41

29. This rhythm strip is from a 68-year-old man with a head injury after a fall.

Rhythm: _____   Rate: _____   P waves: _____

PR interval: _____   QRS duration: _____   QT interval: _____

Interpretation: _____

Fig. 6.42   (Modified from Aehlert, B. (2004). *ECG study cards.* St. Louis: Mosby.)

30. This rhythm strip is from a 58-year-old man who was initially unresponsive, apneic, and pulseless.

Rhythm: _____   Rate: _____   P waves: _____

PR interval: _____   QRS duration: _____   QT interval: _____

Interpretation: _____

Fig. 6.43   (From Aehlert, B. (2004). *ECG study cards.* St. Louis: Mosby.)

31. Identify the rhythm.
Rhythm: _____ Rate: _____ P waves: _____
PR interval: _____ QRS duration: _____ QT interval: _____
Interpretation: _____

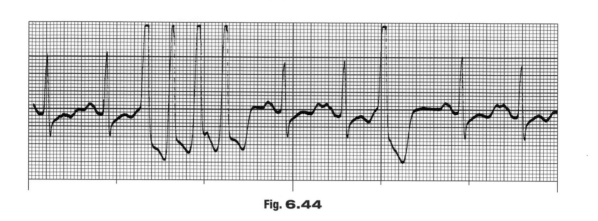

Fig. 6.44

32. This rhythm strip is from a 61-year-old woman who is complaining of shortness of breath.
Rhythm: _____ Rate: _____ P waves: _____
PR interval: _____ QRS duration: _____ QT interval: _____
Interpretation: _____

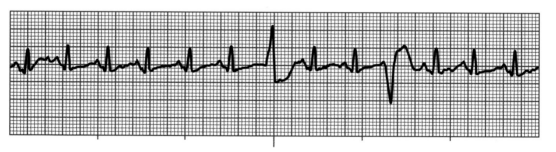

Fig. 6.45 (From Aehlert, B. (2004). *ECG study cards.* St. Louis: Mosby.)

33. Identify the rhythm.
Rhythm: _____ Rate: _____ P waves: _____
PR interval: _____ QRS duration: _____ QT interval: _____
Interpretation: _____

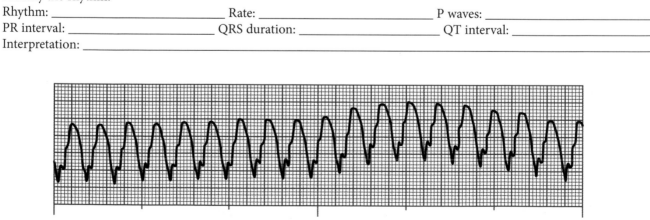

Fig. 6.46 (From Aehlert, B. (2004). *ECG study cards.* St. Louis: Mosby.)

34. Identify the rhythm.

Rhythm: _____ Rate: _____ P waves: _____

PR interval: _____ QRS duration: _____ QT interval: _____

Interpretation: _____

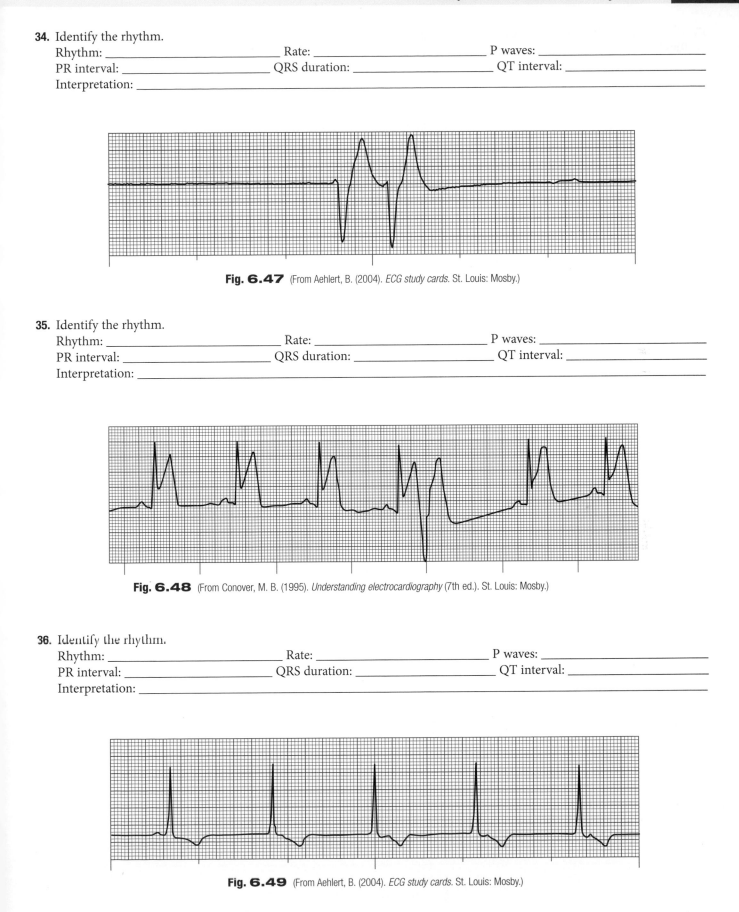

Fig. 6.47 (From Aehlert, B. (2004). *ECG study cards.* St. Louis: Mosby.)

35. Identify the rhythm.

Rhythm: _____ Rate: _____ P waves: _____

PR interval: _____ QRS duration: _____ QT interval: _____

Interpretation: _____

Fig. 6.48 (From Conover, M. B. (1995). *Understanding electrocardiography* (7th ed.). St. Louis: Mosby.)

36. Identify the rhythm.

Rhythm: _____ Rate: _____ P waves: _____

PR interval: _____ QRS duration: _____ QT interval: _____

Interpretation: _____

Fig. 6.49 (From Aehlert, B. (2004). *ECG study cards.* St. Louis: Mosby.)

37. This rhythm strip is from a 90-year-old unresponsive woman who has a history of heart failure.

Rhythm: _____ Rate: _____ P waves: _____

PR interval: _____ QRS duration: _____ QT interval: _____

Interpretation: _____

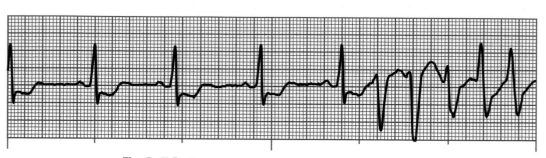

Fig. 6.50 (From Aehlert, B. (2004). *ECG study cards.* St. Louis: Mosby.)

STOP & REVIEW ANSWERS

1. **A, C.** The ECG characteristics of an idioventricular rhythm include an essentially regular ventricular rhythm with QRS complexes measuring 0.12 second or greater; P waves are usually absent or, with retrograde conduction to the atria, may appear after the QRS (usually upright in the ST segment or T wave); and a ventricular rate 20 to 40 beats/min.

2. **A, B, C, D.** Establish IV access and obtain a 12-lead ECG. Atropine may be ordered to treat the symptomatic bradycardia. TCP or a dopamine or epinephrine IV infusion may be ordered if atropine is ineffective. Ventricular antiarrhythmic medications (e.g., amiodarone, lidocaine, procainamide) should be avoided when managing patients with this rhythm. These drugs may abolish ventricular activity, possibly causing asystole.

3. **B.** A junctional escape rhythm has a narrow QRS complex and an intrinsic rate of 40 to 60 beats/min. An idioventricular rhythm has a wide QRS complex and an intrinsic rate of 20 to 40 beats/min.

4. **C.** Three or more sequential PVCs are termed a run or burst, and three or more PVCs that occur in a row at a rate of more than 100 beats/min are considered a run of VT.

5. **A, B.** The priorities of care in cardiac arrest resulting from pulseless VT or VF are high-quality CPR and defibrillation. Other interventions, such as administering medications and inserting and advanced airway, are less important.

6. **A, D.** VF and pulseless VT are shockable rhythms, which means that delivering a shock to the heart with a defibrillator may result in the termination of the rhythm. Asystole and PEA are nonshockable rhythms.

7. **A.** A PVC occurs *before* and a ventricular escape beat occurs *after* the next expected beat of the underlying rhythm.

8. **C, D.** Defibrillation is performed to briefly stun the heart with electrical current of sufficient intensity to allow the heart's natural pacemakers to resume normal activity. With asystole, there is no electrical activity to reset. Similarly, TCP is not indicated. Instead, focus your efforts on performing high-quality CPR, establishing IV access, giving epinephrine, and using the Hs and Ts to identify possible reversible causes of the event. Asystole is also called cardiac standstill because there is a total absence of atrial and ventricular electrical activity. If a flat line is present and atrial activity is seen (i.e., P waves are present), the rhythm is called P wave asystole or ventricular standstill.

9. **B, C, D, E.** The rapid heart rate associated with sustained VT can cause a marked decrease in ventricular function and cardiac output, particularly in patients with underlying heart disease, resulting in acute heart failure, syncope, hypotension, or circulatory collapse within several seconds to minutes after the onset of VT.

10. **D.** Antiarrhythmics can cause a proarrhythmic effect, which means that they have the potential to cause serious adverse effects, more serious dysrhythmias, or both, than those that they were intended to treat.

11. **D.** An interpolated PVC occurs between two normally conducted QRS complexes and does not disturb the next ventricular depolarization or SA node activity.

12. **B, C, D.** ECG characteristics of monomorphic VT include a ventricular rhythm that is essentially regular, a ventricular rate of 101 to 250 beats/min, and a QRS that is 0.12 second or greater in duration. There is no PR interval associated with VT because the rhythm originates below the AV node.

Practice Rhythm Strip Answers

Note: The rate and interval measurements provided here were obtained using electronic calipers.

13. Fig. 6.26
    Rhythm: Irregular
    Rate: 120 beats/min
    P waves: Positive, one precedes each QRS (sinus beats)
    PR interval: 0.13 second (sinus beats)
    QRS duration: 0.08 second (sinus beats)
    QT interval: 0.32 second (sinus beats)
    Interpretation: Sinus tachycardia at 120 beats/min with ventricular quadrigeminy; baseline artifact is present

14. Fig. 6.27
    Rhythm: Regular
    Rate: 55 beats/min
    P waves: None visible
    PR interval: None
    QRS duration: 0.12 second
    QT interval: 0.45 second (prolonged)
    Interpretation: AIVR at 55 beats/min with a prolonged QT interval

15. Fig. 6.28
    Rhythm: Irregular
    Rate: None
    P waves: None
    PR interval: None
    QRS duration: None
    QT interval: None
    Interpretation: Coarse VF

16. Fig. 6.29
    Rhythm: Regular
    Rate: 131 beats/min (within normal limits for age)
    P waves: Positive; one precedes each QRS; most are smooth and rounded; a few are pointed
    PR interval: 0.14 second
    QRS duration: 0.08 second
    QT interval: 0.24 second
    Interpretation: Sinus rhythm at 131 beats/min

17. Fig. 6.30
Rhythm: Irregular
Rate: 70 beats/min
P waves: Positive, one precedes each QRS before the sinus beats and the fusion beat
PR interval: 0.16 second (sinus beats)
QRS duration: 0.08 second (sinus beats)
QT interval: 0.34 second (sinus beats)
Interpretation: Sinus rhythm at 70 beats/min with a fusion beat, a pair of PVCs, ST-segment depression, and inverted T waves

18. Fig. 6.31
Rhythm: Irregular; two rhythms are present
Rate: 90 beats/min (sinus beats); 160 beats/min (VT) (because two rhythms are present, a rate for each should be documented)
P waves: Positive, one precedes each QRS before the sinus beats; none visible with VT
PR interval: 0.16 second (sinus beats)
QRS duration: 0.10 second (sinus beats); 0.14 second (VT)
QT interval: 0.33 second (sinus beats)
Interpretation: Sinus rhythm at 90 beats/min, a fusion beat, and then monomorphic VT at 160 beats/min; baseline artifact is present

19. Fig. 6.32
Rhythm: Irregular; two rhythms are present
Rate: 60 beats/min (sinus beats); 300 to 375 beats/min (PMVT)
P waves: Positive, one precedes each QRS before the sinus beats, one is notched; none visible with PMVT (because two rhythms are present, a rate for each should be documented)
PR interval: 0.16 second (sinus beats)
QRS duration: 0.09 second (sinus beats); 0.12 second (PMVT)
QT interval: 0.40 second (sinus beats)
Interpretation: Sinus rhythm at 60 beats/min to PMVT at 300 to 375 beats/min

20. Fig. 6.33
Rhythm: Irregular
Rate: 110 beats/min
P waves: Positive, one precedes each QRS before the sinus beats; early and inverted in beats 5 and 11
PR interval: 0.14 second
QRS duration: 0.09 second (sinus beats)
QT interval: 0.30 second (sinus beats)
Interpretation: Sinus tachycardia at 110 beats/min with two PJCs (beats 5 and 11)

21. Fig. 6.34
Rhythm: Regular
Rate: 68 beats/min
P waves: None visible
PR interval: None
QRS duration: 0.12 second

QT interval: 0.32 to 0.38 second (difficult to clearly identify end of T waves)
Interpretation: AIVR at 68 beats/min; artifact is present

22. Fig. 6.35
Rhythm: Irregular
Rate: 82 beats/min
P waves: Positive, one precedes each QRS before the sinus beats; early with beat 6, distorting the T wave of beat 5
PR interval: 0.19 second
QRS duration: 0.10 second
QT interval: 0.34 second
Interpretation: Sinus rhythm at 82 beats/min with a PAC (beat 5); artifact is present

23. Fig. 6.36
Rhythm: Irregular
Rate: 70 beats/min
P waves: Positive, one precedes each QRS before the sinus beats; none visible with beat 4
PR interval: 0.21 second
QRS duration: 0.11 second
QT interval: 0.40 second
Interpretation: Sinus rhythm at 70 beats/min with an interpolated PVC (beat 4) and inverted T waves; artifact is present

24. Fig. 6.37
Rhythm: Regular
Rate: 79 beats/min
P waves: None visible
PR interval: None
QRS duration: 0.08 second
QT interval: 0.32 second
Interpretation: Accelerated junctional rhythm at 79 beats/min with ST-segment elevation

25. Fig. 6.38
Rhythm: Irregular to regular
Rate: 143 to 167 beats/min (atrial beats); 150 beats/min with beats 11 through 16
P waves: None visible
PR interval: None
QRS duration: 0.08 second (atrial beats)
QT interval: 0.22 second
Interpretation: Atrial fibrillation (AFib) at 143 to 167 beats/min with two ventricular complexes and a fusion beat, changing to supraventricular tachycardia (SVT) at 150 beats/min; ST-segment depression and artifact present

26. Fig. 6.39
Rhythm: None
Rate: None
P waves: None
PR interval: None
QRS duration: None
QT interval: None
Interpretation: Asystole

27. Fig. 6.40.
Rhythm: Irregular
Rate: 70 beats/min
P waves: Positive, one precedes each QRS
PR interval: 0.16 second
QRS duration: 0.06 second
QT interval: 0.40 second
Interpretation: Sinus arrhythmia at 70 beats/min with ST-segment depression; artifact is present

28. Fig. 6.41
Rhythm: Irregular
Rate: 80 beats/min
P waves: Positive, one precedes each QRS with sinus beats; none with beats 2, 4, and 6
PR interval: 0.18 second (sinus beats)
QRS duration: 0.08 second (sinus beats)
QT interval: 0.38 second (sinus beats) (difficult to clearly identify end of T waves)
Interpretation: Sinus rhythm at 80 beats/min with uniform PVCs, artifact is present

29. Fig. 6.42
Rhythm: Regular
Rate: 48 beats/min
P waves: Positive, one precedes each QRS
PR interval: 0.15 second
QRS duration: 0.08 second
QT interval: 0.44 second
Interpretation: Sinus bradycardia at 48 beats/min; U waves are visible in lead MCL_1

30. Fig. 6.43
Rhythm: Irregular
Rate: None to 40 beats/min
P waves: None visible
PR interval: None
QRS duration: 0.16 second
QT interval: 0.36 second
Interpretation: Ventricular fibrillation, a shock (defibrillation), idioventricular rhythm at 40 beats/min

31. Fig. 6.44
Rhythm: Irregular
Rate: Sinus rate 88 beats/min; overall rate about 110 beats/min
P waves: Positive, one precedes each QRS with sinus beats; some are notched
PR interval: 0.20 second (sinus beats)
QRS duration: 0.08 second (sinus beats)
QT interval: 0.36 second (sinus beats)
Interpretation: Sinus rhythm at 88 beats/min with a run of VT and a PVC, ST-segment depression, and inverted T waves

32. Fig. 6.45
Rhythm: Irregular
Rate: 130 beats/min
P waves: Positive, one precedes each QRS with sinus beats; none visible with beats 7 and 10

PR interval: 0.12 second (sinus beats)
QRS duration: 0.06 second (sinus beats)
QT interval: Unable to determine because T waves are not visible
Interpretation: Sinus tachycardia at 130 beats/min with multiform PVCs (beats 7 and 10)

33. Fig. 6.46
Rhythm: Regular
Rate: 188 beats/min
P waves: None visible
PR interval: None
QRS duration: 0.14 to 0.18 second
QT interval: Unable to determine
Interpretation: Monomorphic VT at 188 beats/min

34. Fig. 6.47
Rhythm: Irregular
Rate: Two ventricular complexes to none
P waves: One visible on the far right of the strip; otherwise none
PR interval: None
QRS duration: 0.14 second to none
QT interval: 0.48 second to none
Interpretation: Agonal rhythm/asystole

35. Fig. 6.48
Rhythm: Irregular
Rate: 70 beats/min
P waves: Positive, one precedes each QRS with sinus beats; none visible with beat 5
PR interval: 0.20 second (sinus beats)
QRS duration: 0.09 second (sinus beats)
QT interval: 0.30 second (sinus beats)
Interpretation: Sinus rhythm at 70 beats/min with an R-on-T PVC (beat 5) and ST-segment elevation

36. Fig. 6.49
Rhythm: Regular
Rate: 52 beats/min
P waves: Positive before QRS in beat 1, none visible with remaining beats
PR interval: 0.14 second (sinus beat)
QRS duration: 0.07 second
QT interval: 0.44 second
Interpretation: Sinus beat to junctional rhythm at 52 beats/min; inverted T waves

37. Fig. 6.50
Rhythm: Irregular
Rate: 65 beats/min (sinus beats) to 167 to 214 beats/min (PMVT)
P waves: Positive, one precedes each QRS with sinus beats; none visible with PMVT
PR interval: 0.16 second (sinus beats)
QRS duration: 0.10 to 0.12 second (sinus beats)
QT interval: 0.32 second (sinus beats)
Interpretation: Sinus rhythm at 65 beats/min with ST-segment depression to PMVT at 167 to 214 beats/min

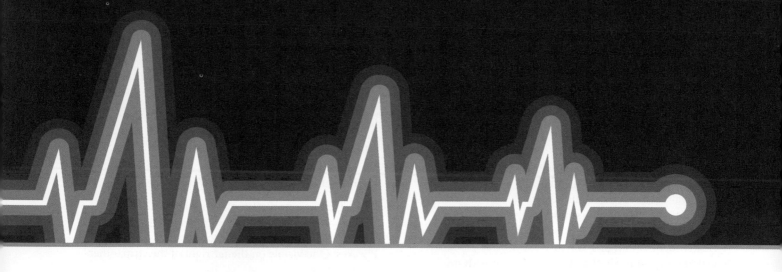

Atrioventricular Blocks

7

LEARNING OBJECTIVES

After reading this chapter, you should be able to:

1. Describe the electrocardiogram (ECG) characteristics, possible causes, signs and symptoms, and emergency management for first-degree atrioventricular (AV) block.
2. Describe the ECG characteristics, possible causes, signs and symptoms, and emergency management for second-degree AV block type I.
3. Describe the ECG characteristics, possible causes, signs and symptoms, and emergency management for second-degree AV block type II.
4. Describe 2:1 AV block and advanced second-degree AV block.
5. Describe the ECG characteristics, possible causes, signs and symptoms, and emergency management for third-degree AV block.

KEY TERM

atrioventricular (AV) block: A delay or interruption in impulse conduction from the atria to the ventricles that occurs because of a transient or permanent anatomic or functional impairment in the conduction system

INTRODUCTION

You have learned that the AV node and AV bundle have many essential functions (Fig. 7.1). First, a supraventricular impulse that enters the AV node is normally delayed, thereby allowing the atrial chambers to contract and empty blood into the ventricles before the next ventricular contraction begins. Second, a healthy AV node can filter some of the supraventricular impulses coming to it, thereby protecting the ventricles from excessively rapid rates. Third, the AV bundle has pacemaker cells with an intrinsic rate of 40 to 60 beats per minute (beats/min) and can function as an escape pacemaker if the sinoatrial (SA) node fails.

Depolarization and repolarization are slow in the AV node, making this area vulnerable to blocks in conduction. When impulse conduction from the atria to the ventricles is delayed or interrupted because of a transient or permanent anatomic or functional impairment in the conduction system, the resulting dysrhythmia is called an **AV block** (Issa et al., 2019).

When analyzing a rhythm strip, you can assess PR intervals to detect AV conduction disturbances. Remember that the PR interval is made up of the P wave and the PR segment. The normal PR interval measures 0.12 to 0.20 second.

AV block is classified into (1) first-degree AV block, (2) second-degree AV block, and (3) third-degree AV block (Fig. 7.2). With first-degree AV block, impulses from the SA node to the ventricles are *delayed*; they are not blocked. With second-degree AV blocks, there is an *intermittent* disturbance in the conduction of impulses between the atria and the ventricles. There is a *complete* block in the conduction of impulses between the atria and the ventricles with a third-degree AV block.

AV most often occurs in the absence of significant cardiac disease and is generally attributed to fibrosis of the conduction system that results from an unknown cause (Kerola et al., 2019). The evaluation of a patient with an AV block should include searching for possible reversible causes such as Lyme disease, myocardial ischemia, thyroid dysfunction, or the adverse effects of medications (Sidhu & Marine, 2020).

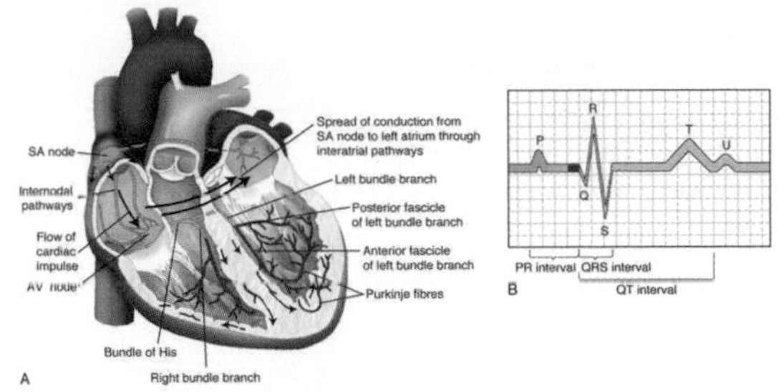

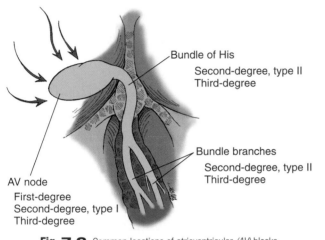

Fig. 7.1 Interruptions in impulse transmission between the atria and ventricles can be detected by assessing PR intervals. A, Conduction system of the heart. *AV,* Atrioventricular; *SA,* sinoatrial. B, The normal electrocardiogram pattern. (From Brown, D., Edwards, H., Buckley, T., & Aitken, R. L. (2017). *Lewis' medical-surgical nursing* (5th ed.). Australia: Elsevier.)

Fig. 7.2 Common locations of atrioventricular *(AV)* blocks.

First-degree AV block usually occurs because of a conduction delay within the AV node. Second- and third-degree AV blocks can occur at the level of the AV node, within the bundle of His, or below the bundle of His within the bundle branches. AV blocks located at the bundle of His or bundle branches are called infranodal or subnodal AV blocks.

AV blocks that occur at the level of the AV node have a tremendous advantage because there is usually a reliable junctional pacemaker available that can fire at 40 to 60 beats/min. However, when an AV block occurs below the AV junction, the only available pacemaker may be a slow ventricular one, firing at 20 to 40 beats/min. Not only are ventricular pacemakers slow, but they are also prone to long pauses, making them less than reliable. Therefore, AV blocks at the level of the AV node usually have a more effective and reliable escape pacemaker than do AV blocks at the bundle of His or below.

ECG Pearl

The clinical significance of an AV block depends on the following:
- The degree of the block
- The rate of the escape pacemaker (junctional versus ventricular)
- The patient's response to that ventricular rate

FIRST-DEGREE ATRIOVENTRICULAR BLOCK

With a first-degree AV block, all components of the cardiac cycle are usually within normal limits, except for the PR interval. The PR interval is abnormal because electrical impulses travel in their usual manner from the SA node through the atria but then encounter a delay in impulse conduction, usually at the level of the AV node (Fig. 7.3). Despite its name, the SA node impulse is not blocked during a first-degree AV block; instead, each sinus impulse is *delayed* for the same period before it is conducted to the ventricles. The terms *AV delay* and *delayed AV conduction* have been suggested as alternative names for first-degree AV block. Delayed AV conduction results in a PR interval that is longer than normal (i.e., more than 0.20 second in duration in adults) and constant before each QRS complex. Despite the prolonged PR interval, each P wave is followed by a QRS complex (i.e., there is a 1:1 relationship of P waves to QRS complexes). In adults, a severe first-degree AV block exists when the PR interval is longer than 0.30 second (Kusumoto et al., 2018).

When the QRS complex associated with a first-degree AV block is narrow, the conduction abnormality is usually within the AV node. When the QRS complex associated with a first-degree AV block is wide, the conduction abnormality may be located in the AV node, the bundle of His, or the bundle branches (Issa et al., 2019).

ECG Pearl

Not all AV blocks have a 1:1 relationship of P wave to QRS complex. When inspecting a rhythm strip, be sure to determine both atrial and ventricular regularity, identify P waves, assess the PR interval, and determine if the QRS complex is narrow or wide.

How Do I Recognize It?

ECG characteristics of first-degree AV block include the following:

Rhythm:	Regular
Rate:	Usually within normal range, but depends on underlying rhythm
P waves:	Normal in size and shape; one positive (upright) P wave before each QRS
PR interval:	Prolonged (i.e., more than 0.20 second) but constant
QRS duration:	Usually 0.11 second or less unless abnormally conducted

Let's look at the rhythm shown in Fig. 7.4. The ventricular rhythm is regular at a rate of 88 beats/min. A positive P wave precedes each QRS complex. The atrial rhythm is also regular at a rate of 88 beats/min. Based on these findings, we now know that the underlying rhythm is a sinus rhythm at 88 beats/min. The QRS duration is within normal limits; however, the PR interval measures 0.28 second, which is longer

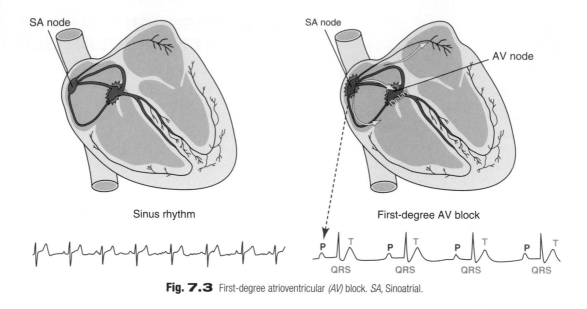

Fig. 7.3 First-degree atrioventricular *(AV)* block. *SA,* Sinoatrial.

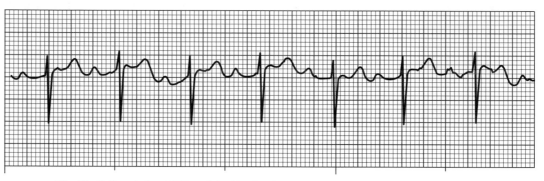

Fig. 7.4 Sinus rhythm at 88 beats/min with a first-degree atrioventricular block and ST-segment elevation.

than normal, and the interval is consistent before each QRS. The 1:1 relationship of P wave to QRS complex and a longer than normal PR interval fit the criteria for a first-degree AV block.

First-degree AV block is not a dysrhythmia itself; rather, it is a condition that describes the prolonged (but constant) PR interval that is seen on the rhythm strip. Our interpretation of the rhythm strip in Fig. 7.4 must include a description of the underlying rhythm, the ventricular rate, and then a description of anything that appears amiss. In this case, we will identify the rhythm as sinus rhythm at 88 beats/min with a first-degree AV block and ST-segment elevation (STE).

What Causes It?

First-degree AV block may be a normal finding in individuals with no history of cardiac disease, especially in athletes. In some people, mild prolongation of the PR interval may be a normal variant, especially with sinus bradycardia during rest or sleep. First-degree AV block may also occur because of the following:

- Acute myocardial infarction (MI)
- Acute myocarditis or endocarditis
- Cardiomyopathy
- Degenerative fibrosis and sclerosis of the conduction system
- Drug effect
- Hyperkalemia
- Ischemia or injury to the AV node or AV bundle
- Rheumatic heart disease
- Valvular heart disease

ECG Pearl

Examples of medications that can cause AV blocks include amiodarone, beta-blockers, digoxin, diltiazem, procainamide, and verapamil.

What Do I Do About It?

Patients with first-degree AV block are often asymptomatic; however, marked first-degree AV block can cause symptoms of fatigue or exertional intolerance (Kusumoto et al., 2018). First-degree AV block that occurs with acute MI should be monitored closely to detect progression to higher-degree AV block. If first-degree AV block accompanies symptomatic bradycardia, treat the bradycardia.

SECOND-DEGREE ATRIOVENTRICULAR BLOCKS

The term *second-degree AV block* is used when one or more, but not all, sinus impulses are blocked from reaching the ventricles. Because the SA node generates impulses normally, each P wave will occur at a regular interval across the rhythm strip (i.e., all P waves will plot through on time), although a QRS complex won't follow every P wave. This finding suggests that the atria are being depolarized normally, but not every impulse is being conducted to the ventricles (i.e., intermittent conduction). As a result, more P waves than QRS complexes are seen on the ECG.

Second-degree AV block is classified as type I or type II, depending on the behavior of the PR intervals associated with the dysrhythmia. The type I or type II designation is used to describe the *ECG pattern* of the PR intervals and should not be used to describe the anatomic site (i.e., location) of the AV block (Issa et al., 2019). At least two consecutively conducted PR intervals must be observed to determine their pattern.

SECOND-DEGREE ATRIOVENTRICULAR BLOCK TYPE I

Second-degree AV block type I is also known as type I block, Mobitz I, or Wenckebach (Fig. 7.5). Wenckebach phenomenon is a progressive lengthening of conduction time in any cardiac conduction tissue that eventually results in the dropping of a beat or a reversion to the initial conduction time. With type I AV block, atrial impulses arrive earlier and earlier during the relative refractory period of the AV node, resulting in longer and longer conduction delays and PR intervals, until an impulse arrives during the

absolute refractory period and fails to conduct (Issa et al., 2019). The nonconducted impulse appears on the ECG as a P wave with no QRS complex after it.

The following features are associated with classic Wenckebach phenomenon:

- Progressive prolongation of the PR intervals; the most significant increase in PR interval duration is noted in the second beat of a cycle
- Gradual shortening of R to R intervals
- A P wave not followed by a QRS complex
- A pause with an R to R interval less than the sum of two P to P intervals
- The first conducted atrial impulse after the pause shows a shorter or normal PR interval

All of the classic Wenckebach features are found in perhaps fewer than 50% of cases (Olgin & Zipes, 2019). For example, after a blocked impulse, the second conducted PR interval may fail to show the greatest increase in length; instead, the PR interval may shorten and then lengthen in the middle of a grouped beating pattern. Alternately, the duration of the PR intervals may show no apparent change in the middle or for a few beats just before the end of a group (Barold & Hayes, 2001).

When a second-degree AV block type I occurs with a narrow QRS complex, the conduction delay and site of the block are almost always within the AV node (Issa et al., 2019). When a second-degree AV block type I occurs with a wide QRS complex, the site of the block may be in the AV node, but it is more likely to lie within or below the His-Purkinje system.

How Do I Recognize It?

Second-degree AV block type I is characterized by a repeating pattern that consists of conducted P waves (i.e., each P wave is followed by a QRS) and then a P wave that is not conducted (i.e., the P wave is not followed by a QRS). In

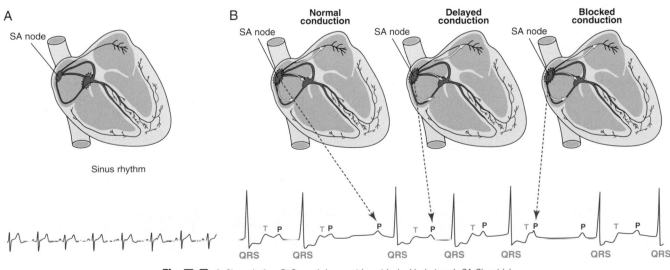

Fig. 7.5 A, Sinus rhythm. B, Second-degree atrioventricular block, type I. *SA,* Sinoatrial.

second-degree AV block type I, any P-to-QRS ratio may be seen. For example, an AV conduction ratio of 3:2 means that for every three P waves, two are followed by QRS complexes. Four conducted P waves to three QRS complexes results in 4:3 conduction, five conducted P waves to four QRS complexes results in 5:4 conduction, and so on. The P wave that is not conducted ends a *group* of beats. Because QRS complexes are periodically absent, the ventricular rhythm is irregular. The cycle then begins again. The repetition of this cyclic pattern is called *grouped beating*. It is important to note that this pattern of grouped beats occurs in fewer than 50% of patients with second-degree AV block type I (Olgin & Zipes, 2019). The ECG characteristics of second-degree AV block type I can be summarized as follows:

Rhythm:	Ventricular irregular; atrial regular (i.e., P waves plot through on time); grouped beating may be present
Rate:	Atrial rate is greater than the ventricular rate
P waves:	Normal in size and shape; some P waves are not followed by a QRS complex (i.e., more P waves than QRS complexes)
PR interval:	Lengthens with each cycle (although lengthening may be very slight) until a P wave appears without a QRS complex; the PR interval after a nonconducted P wave is shorter than the interval preceding the nonconducted beat
QRS duration:	Usually 0.11 second or less; complexes are periodically dropped

Let's look at the example of this type of AV block in Fig. 7.6. Label the QRS complexes on this rhythm strip 1 through 6. You can quickly see that the ventricular rhythm is irregular, with an overall rate of about 60 beats/min. Now look to the left of each QRS and label each P wave in the rhythm strip. Place your calipers or a piece of paper on two P waves and begin moving from the left side of the strip to the right to see if the P waves occur on time. You will find that there is an extra P wave after beat 3. The extra P wave occurs on time, but there is no QRS after it. The remainder of the P waves occur on time. The atrial rhythm is regular with a rate of about 68 beats/min.

Although we are discussing AV blocks in this chapter, how do you know that the extra P wave with no QRS after it isn't a nonconducted premature atrial complex (PAC)? Well, the difference is in the timing of the P waves. If you have not been plotting P waves when analyzing rhythm strips until now, it is *essential* that you do so when identifying AV blocks. There are more P waves than QRS complexes in second- and third-degree AV blocks, and the P waves occur *on time*. This happens because the problem in second- and third-degree AV blocks is not within the SA node. The problem occurs somewhere in the conduction system *below* the SA node. Therefore, the sinus fires regularly—as it is supposed to. The P wave that occurs after beat 3 is not a nonconducted PAC because all P waves are on time. By definition, the P wave of a nonconducted *premature* atrial complex is early.

The duration of the QRS complexes in Fig. 7.6 are within normal limits. Now, look closely at the PR intervals and determine if a pattern exists. To do this, we need to see at least two PQRST cycles in a row that do not contain extra waveforms. Beats 1, 2, and 3 allow us to do this because there is one P wave before each QRS. When you compare the PR intervals of these beats, the PR interval of beat 1 is short. The PR interval of beat 2 is longer than that of beat 1, and the PR interval of beat 3 is longer than that of the first two beats. The PR intervals of beats 1 through 3 can be described as *lengthening*. The blocked sinus impulse appears on the ECG as a P wave with no QRS after it (i.e., a dropped beat). The cycle begins again after the dropped beat. The PR interval of the first conducted beat *after* the blocked sinus impulse (i.e., beat 4) is shorter than the PR interval of the conducted beat *before* the blocked beat (i.e., beat 3). This finding is an important one in identifying second-degree AV block type I. We would interpret this rhythm strip as second-degree AV block type I at 60 beats/min.

What Causes It?

Remember that the right coronary artery (RCA) supplies the AV node in 90% of the population. The RCA also supplies the inferior wall of the left ventricle and the right ventricle in most individuals. Blockage of the RCA, resulting in an inferior MI or right ventricular infarction, can result in conduction delays such as first-degree AV block and second-degree AV block type I. Second-degree AV block type I can also occur in athletes and healthy individuals during sleep. Other possible causes of this dysrhythmia include aortic valve disease, atrial septal defect, medications (e.g., beta-blockers, calcium blockers, digoxin), mitral valve prolapse, and rheumatic heart disease.

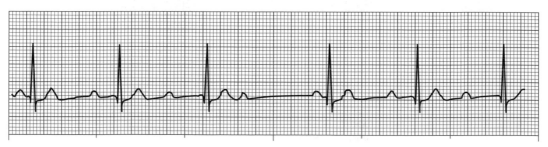

Fig. 7.6 Second-degree atrioventricular block type I at 60 beats/min.

What Do I Do About It?

The patient with type I AV block is usually asymptomatic because the ventricular rate often remains nearly normal, and cardiac output is not significantly affected. For some active, healthy individuals, type I AV block may occur during periods of exercise and result in symptoms such as dizziness and exertional intolerance (Kusumoto et al., 2018). Ambulatory monitoring may be ordered if the patient's initial physical examination and ECG do not reveal a clear cause for their symptoms. When type I AV block is associated with an acute inferior wall MI, this dysrhythmia is usually transient and resolves within 48 to 72 hours as the effects of parasympathetic stimulation disappear.

If the heart rate is slow and serious signs and symptoms occur because of the slow rate, apply a pulse oximeter, administer oxygen (if indicated), obtain the patient's vital signs, and establish intravenous (IV) access. Obtain a 12-lead ECG if doing so will not delay patient treatment. Atropine, administered intravenously, is the drug of choice. Reassess the patient's response and continue monitoring. When this rhythm occurs in conjunction with acute MI, observe the patient closely for increasing AV block.

⊘ ECG Pearl

If the patient with an AV block is symptomatic and the dysrhythmia results from medications, these agents should be withheld.

SECOND-DEGREE ATRIOVENTRICULAR BLOCK TYPE II

Second-degree AV block type II is also called type II block or Mobitz II AV block. The site of block in second-degree AV block type II is almost always below the AV node, occurring in the bundle of His about 30% of the time and within the bundle branches in the remainder (Issa et al., 2019). Although second-degree AV block type II is less common than type I, type II is more serious and is a cause for concern because it can progress to a third-degree AV block.

How Do I Recognize It?

As with second-degree AV block type I, there are more P waves than QRS complexes with second-degree AV block type II, and the P waves occur on time. The PR interval with type II block can be normal or prolonged, but it is constant for the conducted beats. Most important, the PR intervals before and after a blocked sinus impulse (i.e., P wave) are *constant*. The ECG characteristics of second-degree AV block type II include the following:

Rhythm:	Ventricular irregular; atrial regular (i.e., P waves plot through on time)
Rate:	Atrial rate is greater than the ventricular rate; ventricular rate is often slow
P waves:	Normal in size and shape; some P waves are not followed by a QRS complex (i.e., more P waves than QRS complexes)
PR interval:	Within normal limits or prolonged but constant for the conducted beats; the PR intervals before and after a blocked P wave are constant
QRS duration:	Within normal limits if the block occurs above or within the bundle of His; greater than 0.11 second if the block occurs below the bundle of His; complexes are periodically absent after P waves

Let's look at Fig. 7.7. You can see right away that the ventricular rhythm is irregular at an overall rate of about 70 beats/min. You can quickly see that there are more P waves than QRS complexes in this rhythm strip. Use your calipers or paper to plot the P waves and see whether they occur on time. Indeed, they occur regularly at a rate of about 94 beats/min, although a QRS complex doesn't follow every P wave. Each P wave occurs at a regular interval across the rhythm strip (i.e., all P waves plot through on time) because the SA node generates impulses in a normal manner. Impulses generated by the SA node are conducted to the ventricles until a sinus impulse is suddenly blocked—appearing on the ECG as a P wave with no QRS after it (i.e., a dropped beat); this results in an irregular ventricular rhythm. Looking at the QRS complexes in Fig. 7.7, you can see that they are slightly wider than normal, measuring about 0.12 second.

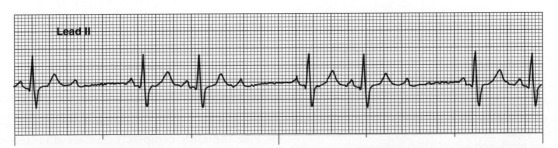

Fig. 7.7 Second-degree atrioventricular block type II at 70 beats/min. (From Aehlert, B. (2004). *ECG study cards*. St. Louis: Mosby.)

Now look closely at each of the PR intervals and compare them. Are they the same or different? In this rhythm strip, the PR intervals are the same, and then a P wave suddenly appears with no QRS after it. When the PR intervals measure the same, we say that they are *constant* or *fixed*. This finding is an important difference between second-degree AV block type I and second-degree AV block type II. In second-degree AV block type II, the PR interval may be within normal limits or prolonged, but it is constant for the conducted beats. Most important, the PR intervals before and after a blocked sinus impulse (i.e., P wave) are *constant*. Our interpretation of the rhythm in Fig. 7.7 is second-degree AV block type II at 70 beats/min.

What Causes It?

You will recall that the site of block in second-degree AV block type II is almost always below the AV node, occurring in the bundle branches about 70% of the time (Issa et al., 2019). Because a branch of the left coronary artery supplies the bundle branches and the anterior wall of the left ventricle, disease of the left coronary artery or an anterior MI is often associated with conduction defects within the bundle branches. Second-degree AV block type II may also occur because of acute myocarditis, aortic valve disease, cardiomyopathy, fibrosis of the conduction system, or rheumatic heart disease.

What Do I Do About It?

The patient's response to this rhythm is usually related to the ventricular rate. If the ventricular rate is within normal limits, the patient may be asymptomatic. More commonly, the ventricular rate is significantly slowed, and serious signs and symptoms result because of the slow rate and decreased cardiac output. The greater the number is of nonconducted beats, the greater the impact is on the cardiac output.

If the heart rate is slow and serious signs and symptoms occur because of the slow rate, treatment should include applying a pulse oximeter, administering oxygen (if indicated), obtaining the patient's vital signs, and establishing IV access. Obtain a 12-lead ECG and a cardiology consult. Temporary or permanent pacing may be necessary. Because second-degree AV block type II may abruptly progress to third-degree AV block, the patient should be closely monitored for increasing AV block.

⚙ ECG Pearl

Although atropine is the drug of choice for symptomatic narrow-QRS bradycardias, it is unlikely to be helpful with symptomatic wide-QRS bradycardias. Reports exist of occasional worsened AV conduction and/or hemodynamic compromise following atropine administration in such patients. For this reason, atropine should be used cautiously in patients with AV block and wide QRS complexes (Kusumoto et al., 2018).

2:1 ATRIOVENTRICULAR BLOCK

How Do I Recognize It?

Before we discuss 2:1 AV block, let's review a few crucial points regarding second-degree AV blocks. So far, you have learned how important it is to plot P waves to make sure that they occur on time. If there are more P waves than QRS complexes and the P waves occur on time, you know that you have some type of AV block. The ventricular rhythm is irregular with both second-degree AV block type I and type II. The QRS complex with a second-degree AV block type I is usually narrow; it is usually wide with a second-degree AV block type II, although exceptions exist with both types of second-degree blocks.

You have also learned that there are differences in the PR interval patterns with second-degree AV block type I and type II. These differences are vital in differentiating between type I and type II AV blocks. To compare PR intervals, we must see at least two PQRST cycles in a row. More importantly, we must look at the PR interval of the conducted beat *after* a dropped QRS complex and compare it with the PR interval of the last conducted beat *before* the dropped QRS. With this information, you can then begin to differentiate what type of second-degree AV block it is. For example, if the PR interval after a dropped QRS complex is shorter than the PR interval before the dropped complex, a pattern consistent with second-degree AV block type I is present. If the PR interval after a dropped QRS complex is the same as the PR interval before the dropped complex, a pattern consistent with second-degree AV block type II exists.

With second-degree AV block in the form of 2:1 AV block, there is one conducted P wave followed by a blocked P wave; thus, two P waves occur for every one QRS complex (i.e., 2:1 conduction) (Fig. 7.8). Because there are no two PQRST cycles in a row to compare PR intervals, the 2:1 AV block cannot be conclusively classified as type I or type II. To determine the type of block with certainty, it is necessary to continue close ECG monitoring of the patient until the conduction ratio of P waves to QRS complexes changes to 3:2, 4:3, and so on, which would enable PR interval comparison.

The ECG characteristics of 2:1 AV block can be summarized as follows:

Rhythm:	Ventricular regular; atrial regular (P waves plot through on time)
Rate:	Atrial rate is twice the ventricular rate
P waves:	Normal in size and shape; every other P wave is not followed by a QRS complex (i.e., more P waves than QRS complexes)
PR interval:	Constant
QRS duration:	May be narrow or wide; complexes are absent after every other P wave

If the QRS complex measures 0.11 second or less, the block is likely to be located within the AV node and a form of second-degree AV block type I (Fig. 7.9). A

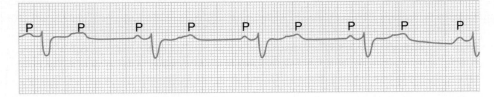

Fig. 7.8 2:1 atrioventricular block. (From Pappano, A. J., & Wier, W. G. (2019). *Cardiovascular physiology* (11th ed.). Philadelphia: Elsevier.)

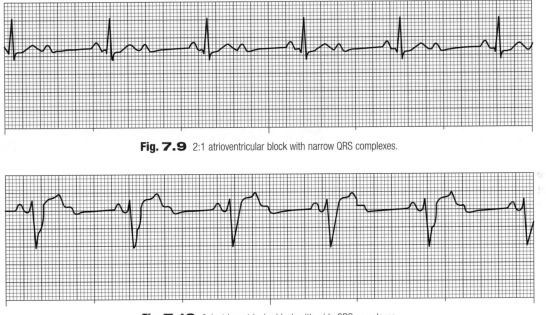

Fig. 7.9 2:1 atrioventricular block with narrow QRS complexes.

Fig. 7.10 2:1 atrioventricular block with wide QRS complexes.

2:1 AV block associated with a wide QRS complex (i.e., more than 0.11 second) is usually associated with a block below the AV node; thus, it is usually a type II block (Fig. 7.10). Patients with 2:1 AV block may experience symptoms of fatigue and dizziness, particularly if the dysrhythmia persists during exertion (Kusumoto et al., 2018). The causes and emergency management procedures for 2:1 AV block are those of type I or type II block previously described.

ADVANCED SECOND-DEGREE ATRIOVENTRICULAR BLOCK

The terms *advanced* or *high-grade second-degree AV block* may be used to describe three or more consecutive P waves at a normal rate that are not conducted. For example, with 3:1 AV block, every third P wave is conducted (i.e., followed by a QRS complex); with 4:1 AV block, every fourth P wave is conducted (Fig. 7.11). Advanced second-degree AV block is generally considered to originate within or below the bundle of His (Kusumoto et al., 2018).

Because of the frequency with which impulses from the SA node to the Purkinje fibers are blocked, the presence of advanced AV block is a cause for concern, and the development of third-degree AV block should be anticipated. Advanced AV block is considered a marker of worse outcomes in patients with ST-segment elevation myocardial infarction (STEMI) (Kosmidou et al., 2021).

ECG Pearl

A Quick Look at P Waves and Atrioventricular (AV) Blocks

AV Block	P Wave Conduction
First degree	All P waves conducted but delayed; slowed conduction
Second degree	Some P waves conducted, others blocked; intermittent conduction
Third degree	No P waves conducted; absent conduction

THIRD-DEGREE ATRIOVENTRICULAR BLOCK

Second-degree AV blocks are types of *incomplete* blocks because at least some of the impulses from the SA node are conducted to the ventricles (i.e., intermittent conduction). There is a *complete* block in impulse conduction between the atria and the ventricles with a third-degree AV block.

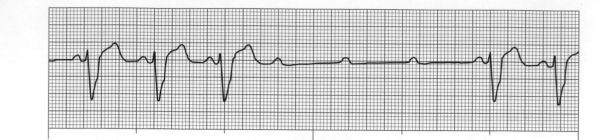

Fig. 7.11 An example of advanced second-degree atrioventricular block. (From Aehlert, B. (2004). *ECG study cards.* St. Louis: Mosby.)

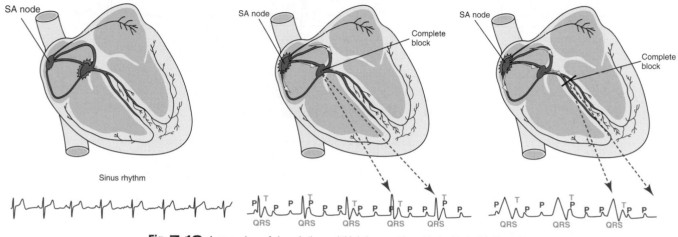

Fig. 7.12 A comparison of sinus rhythm and third-degree atrioventricular block. *SA,* Sinoatrial.

How Do I Recognize It?

With third-degree AV block, the block site may occur at the level of the AV node, the bundle of His, or distal to the bundle of His (Fig. 7.12). A secondary pacemaker (either junctional or ventricular) stimulates the ventricles; therefore, the QRS may be narrow or wide, depending on the location of the escape pacemaker and the condition of the intraventricular conduction system. ECG characteristics of third-degree AV block include the following:

Rhythm: Ventricular regular; atrial regular (P waves plot through); no relationship between the atrial and ventricular rhythms (i.e., AV dissociation is present)

Rate: Ventricular rate is determined by the origin of the escape pacemaker; atrial rate is greater than (and independent of) the ventricular rate

P waves: Normal in size and shape; some P waves are not followed by a QRS complex (i.e., more P waves than QRS complexes)

PR interval: None; the atria and the ventricles beat independently of each other, so there is no true PR interval

QRS duration: Narrow or wide, depending on the location of the escape pacemaker and the condition of the intraventricular conduction system

Fig. 7.13 shows an example of third-degree AV block with the P waves marked. Note the dissociation between the P waves and the QRS complexes. Now, let's look at the rhythm strip in Fig. 7.14. Determine the ventricular rhythm and then calculate the ventricular rate. You will find that the ventricular rhythm is regular and the ventricular rate is 29 beats/min. Next, locate the P waves. In locating P waves, it often helps to place your calipers, or to make marks on a piece of paper, on two clearly identifiable P waves and then move the calipers (or paper) left and right across the strip, marking the remaining P waves as you go. For example, it would be a good idea to mark P waves 2 and 3 first in this rhythm strip because they are readily seen; then move to the left, identifying P wave 1, and then move to the right, identifying P waves 4 through 7. P wave 4 is hidden in the T wave following the second QRS complex. When all of the P waves have been identified, determine their regularity and then determine their rate. You will find that the P waves occur regularly and that the atrial rate is 68 beats/ min. Because you have more P waves than QRS complexes and the P waves occur on time, you know that you have some type of AV block. To determine which one, you must look closely at the PR intervals. As you can see, there is no true PR interval because the atria and ventricles are beating independently of each other. The ECG characteristics discussed so far and the fact that there is no true PR interval fit the criteria for a third-degree AV block. The QRS is

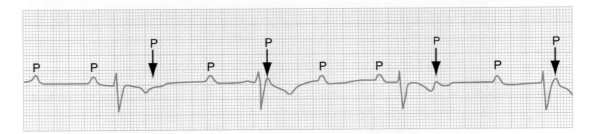

Fig. 7.13 Third-degree heart block; P waves are marked to show the dissociation between the P waves and the QRS complexes. (From Pappano, A. J., & Wier, W. G. (2019). *Cardiovascular physiology* (11th ed.). Philadelphia: Elsevier.)

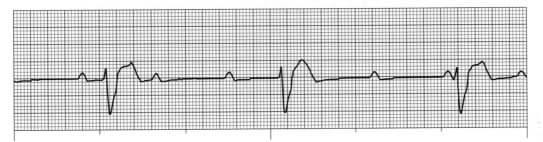

Fig. 7.14 Third-degree atrioventricular block at 29 beats/min with a wide QRS. (From Aehlert, B. (2004). *ECG study cards*. St. Louis: Mosby.)

wide, measuring 0.16 second, and the QT interval measures 0.36 to 0.38 second. Our interpretation of the dysrhythmia in Fig. 7.14 is third-degree AV block at 29 beats/min with a wide QRS.

What Causes It?

Causes of third-degree AV block include the following:
- Acute MI
- Acute myocarditis
- Congenital heart disease
- Drug effect
- Fibrosis of the conduction system
- Increased parasympathetic tone

Third-degree AV block associated with an inferior MI is thought to be the result of a block above the bundle of His. It often occurs after progression from first-degree AV block or second-degree AV block type I. The resulting rhythm is usually stable because the escape pacemaker is usually junctional (i.e., narrow QRS complexes) with a ventricular rate of more than 40 beats/min. Third-degree AV block that is associated with an anterior or an anteroseptal MI is often preceded by second-degree AV block type II or an intraventricular conduction delay (i.e., right or left bundle branch block) (Issa et al., 2019). The resulting rhythm is usually unstable because the escape pacemaker is usually ventricular (i.e., wide QRS complexes) with a ventricular rate of less than 40 beats/min. In the setting of an acute anterior MI, the development of third-degree AV block is associated with a higher risk of ventricular tachycardia and ventricular fibrillation, hypotension, pulmonary edema, and in-hospital mortality (Issa et al., 2019).

What Do I Do About It?

The patient's signs and symptoms will depend on the origin of the escape pacemaker (i.e., junctional versus ventricular) and the patient's response to a slower ventricular rate. Possible rate-related signs and symptoms include dizziness, lightheadedness, generalized weakness, seizures, and Adams-Stokes syndrome (which is also known as Stokes-Adams attacks). Adams-Stokes syndrome is sudden, recurring episodes of loss of consciousness caused by the transient interruption of cardiac output by incomplete or complete heart block; the ventricular rate is inadequate to maintain cerebral perfusion and results in a syncopal episode.

If the patient is symptomatic as a result of the slow rate, treatment should include applying a pulse oximeter and administering oxygen (if indicated), obtaining the patient's vital signs, establishing IV access, and obtaining a 12-lead ECG. IV administration of atropine may be tried. If the disruption in AV nodal conduction is caused by increased parasympathetic tone, the administration of atropine may be effective in reversing excess vagal tone and improving AV node conduction. Other interventions that may be used in the treatment of third-degree AV block include epinephrine or dopamine IV infusions or transcutaneous pacing. Frequent patient reassessment is essential. Most patients with third-degree AV block have an indication for permanent pacemaker placement.

Examples of most of the AV blocks discussed in this chapter appear in Fig. 7.15. A summary of AV block characteristics is given in Table 7.1.

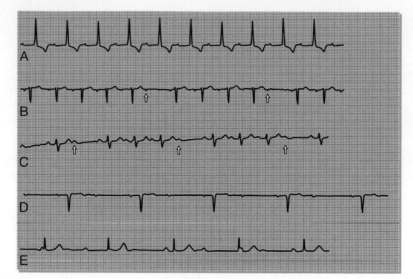

Fig. 7.15 Atrioventricular (AV) blocks. A, First-degree AV block; the PR interval is constant and more than 0.20 second. B, Second-degree AV block type I. The PR intervals after the nonconducted P waves *(arrows)* are shorter than the interval preceding the nonconducted beat. C, Second-degree AV block type II. Nonconducted P waves are seen *(arrows)*. The PR intervals before and after the nonconducted P waves are constant. D, 2:1 AV block during which every other P wave is conducted. E, Third-degree AV block with AV dissociation and a junctional escape rhythm. (From Andreoli, T. E., Griggs, R., Wing, W., & Fitz, J. G. (2016). *Andreoli and Carpenter's Cecil essentials of medicine* (9th ed.). Philadelphia: Saunders.)

TABLE **7.1**	Atrioventricular Blocks: Summary of Characteristics				
Dysrhythmia	Rhythm	Rate (beats/min)	P Waves (Lead II)	PRI	QRS Duration
First-degree block	Atrial regular, ventricular regular	Usually within normal range but depends on underlying rhythm	Normal; one P wave precedes each QRS	Greater than 0.20 sec and constant	Usually 0.11 sec or less unless abnormally conducted
Second-degree block type I	Atrial regular, ventricular irregular	Atrial rate greater than ventricular rate; both often within normal limits	Normal in size and shape; some P waves are not followed by a QRS complex (i.e., more Ps than QRSs)	Lengthening; the PRI after the nonconducted beat is shorter than the interval preceding the nonconducted beat	Usually 0.11 sec or less and is periodically dropped
Second-degree block type II	Atrial regular, ventricular irregular	Atrial rate greater than ventricular rate; ventricular rate often slow	Normal in size and shape; some P waves are not followed by a QRS complex (i.e., more Ps than QRSs)	Within normal limits or prolonged but constant for the conducted beats; the PRIs before and after a blocked sinus impulse (i.e., P wave) are constant	Within normal limits if the block occurs above or within the bundle of His; greater than 0.11 sec if the block occurs below the bundle of His
Second-degree 2:1 AV block	Atrial regular, ventricular regular	Atrial rate greater than ventricular rate	Normal in size and shape; every other P wave is not followed by a QRS complex (i.e., more Ps than QRSs)	Constant	Narrow or wide depending on the location of the escape pacemaker and condition of intraventricular conduction system
Third-degree block	Atrial regular, ventricular regular	Atrial rate greater than ventricular rate; ventricular rate determined by origin of escape rhythm	Normal in size and shape; some P waves are not followed by a QRS complex (i.e., more Ps than QRSs)	None; the atria and ventricles beat independently of each other, so there is no true PR interval	Narrow or wide depending on location of escape pacemaker and condition of intraventricular conduction system

AV, Atrioventricular; PRI, PR interval.

REFERENCES

Barold, S. S., & Hayes, D. L. (2001). Second-degree atrioventricular block: A reappraisal. *Mayo Clin Proc, 76*(1), 44–57.

Issa, Z. F., Miller, J. M., & Zipes, D. P. (2019). Atrioventricular conduction abnormalities. In Z. F. Issa, J. M. Miller, & D. P. Zipes (Eds.), *Clinical arrhythmology and electrophysiology: A companion to Braunwald's heart disease* (3rd ed., pp. 255–285). Philadelphia, PA: Elsevier.

Kerola, T., Eranti, A., Arol, A. L., Haukilahti, A., Holkeri, A., & Marcus, G. M. (2019). Risk factors associated with atrioventricular block. *JAMA Netw Open, 2*(5), e194176.

Kosmidou, I., Redfors, B., Dordi, R., Dizon, J. M., McAndrew, T., Mehran, R., ... Stone, G. W. (2021). Incidence, predictors, and outcomes of high-grade atrioventricular block in patients with ST-segment elevation myocardial infarction undergoing primary percutaneous coronary intervention (from the HORIZONS-AMI trial). *Am J Cardiol, 119*(9), 1295–1301.

Kusumoto, F. M., Schoenfeld, M. H., Barrett, C., Edgerton, J. R., Ellenbogen, K. A., Gold, M. R., ... Varosy, P. D. (2018). 2018 ACC/AHA/HRS guideline on the evaluation and management of patients with bradycardia and cardiac conduction delay. *Circulation, 140*(8), e382–e482.

Olgin, J. E., & Zipes, D. P. (2019). Bradyarrhythmias and atrioventricular block. In D. P. Zipes, P. Libby, R. O. Bonow, D. L. Mann, G. F. Tomaselli, & E. Braunwald (Eds.), *Braunwald's heart disease—A textbook of cardiovascular medicine* (11th ed., pp. 772–779). Philadelphia, PA: Elsevier.

Sidhu, S., & Marine, J. E. (2020). Evaluating and managing bradycardia. *Trends Cardiovasc Med, 30*(5), 265–272.

STOP & REVIEW

Multiple Response

Identify one or more choices that best complete the statement or answer the question.

1. Which of the following dysrhythmias may be a normal finding in individuals with no history of cardiac disease, especially in athletes?
   a. Atrial fibrillation
   b. First-degree AV block
   c. Third-degree AV block
   d. Ventricular tachycardia

2. Which of the following ECG components is used to detect AV conduction disturbances?
   a. P wave
   b. PR interval
   c. QT interval
   d. ST segment

3. The term *second-degree AV block type I* is synonymous with
   a. Mobitz I.
   b. Mobitz II.
   c. Wenckebach.
   d. AV dissociation.
   e. high-grade AV block.
   f. Wolff-Parkinson-White pattern.

4. Identify the ECG characteristics of 2:1 AV block.
   a. The ventricular rate is twice the atrial rate.
   b. Atrial and ventricular rhythms are regular.
   c. Every other P wave is not followed by a QRS complex.
   d. PR intervals progressively lengthen until a P wave appears without a QRS after it.

5. A key difference between second-degree type I and type II AV block is that with
   a. type I the P waves occur irregularly.
   b. type I the ventricular rhythm is regular.
   c. type II the QRS duration is consistently more than 0.12 second in duration.
   d. type II the PR intervals before and after a blocked P wave are constant.

6. With a third-degree AV block, the PR interval
   a. shortens.
   b. is absent.
   c. lengthens.
   d. remains constant.

7. Which of the following dysrhythmias is more commonly seen with an inferior wall myocardial infarction?
   a. Sinus arrhythmia
   b. Second-degree AV block type I
   c. Second-degree AV block type II
   d. Third-degree AV block with a wide-QRS

8. An ECG rhythm strip reveals an irregular ventricular rhythm at a rate of 46 to 54 beats/min, more P waves than QRS complexes with regular P-P intervals, PR intervals after nonconducted P waves are shorter than the interval preceding the nonconducted beats, and a QRS duration of 0.08 second. This rhythm is
   a. 2:1 AV block.
   b. third-degree AV block.
   c. second-degree AV block type I.
   d. second-degree AV block type II.

9. An ECG rhythm strip reveals an irregular ventricular rhythm at a rate of 28 to 40 beats/min, more P waves than QRS complexes, regular P-P intervals, a constant PR interval of 0.16 second, and a QRS duration of 0.14 second. This rhythm is
   a. 2:1 AV block.
   b. third-degree AV block.
   c. second-degree AV block type I.
   d. second-degree AV block type II.

10. A 67-year-old man presents with a blood pressure of 64/42 mm Hg, a heart rate of 38 beats/min, and an oxygen saturation on room air of 90%. The cardiac monitor reveals a type II AV block. Interventions to consider in the management of this patient include
    a. administering oxygen.
    b. administering atropine.
    c. establishing IV access.
    d. obtaining a 12-lead ECG.
    e. obtaining a cardiology consult.
    f. preparing for temporary pacing.

11. ECG characteristics of third-degree AV block include
    a. regular atrial and ventricular rhythms.
    b. a QRS that may appear narrow or wide.
    c. an atrial rate is greater than the ventricular rate.
    d. PR intervals that are constant before each QRS.

12. An ECG rhythm strip shows a regular ventricular rhythm at a rate of 128 beats/min, one upright P wave before each QRS, a regular atrial rate, a constant PR interval of 0.24 second, and a QRS duration of 0.08 second. This rhythm is
    a. third-degree AV block.
    b. second-degree AV block type I.
    c. sinus tachycardia with first-degree AV block.
    d. junctional tachycardia with a first-degree AV block.

AV Blocks—Practice Rhythm Strips

Use the five steps of rhythm interpretation to interpret each of the following rhythm strips. All rhythms were recorded in lead II unless otherwise noted.

13. This rhythm strip is from a 66-year-old man complaining of chest pain.

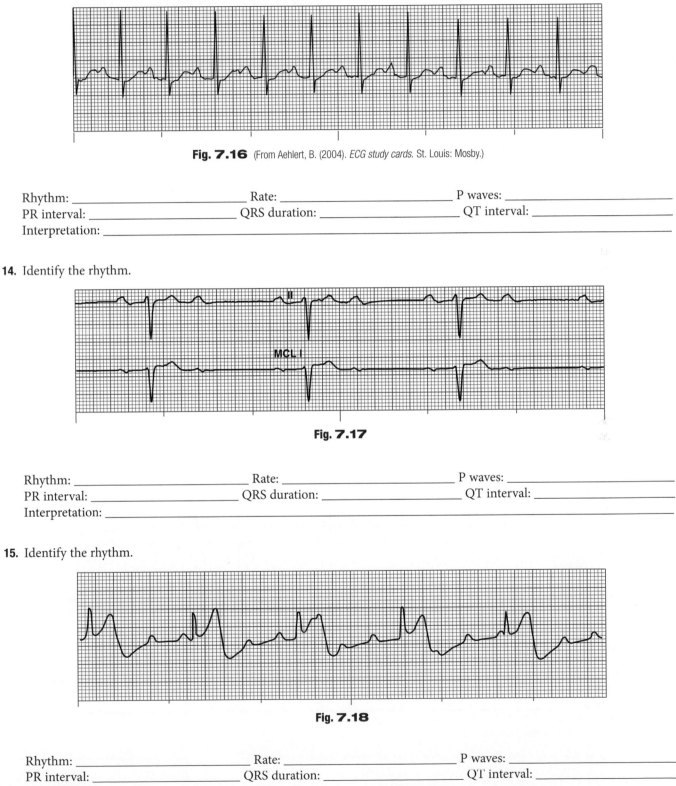

Fig. 7.16 (From Aehlert, B. (2004). *ECG study cards*. St. Louis: Mosby.)

Rhythm: _____ Rate: _____ P waves: _____

PR interval: _____ QRS duration: _____ QT interval: _____

Interpretation: _____

14. Identify the rhythm.

Fig. 7.17

Rhythm: _____ Rate: _____ P waves: _____

PR interval: _____ QRS duration: _____ QT interval: _____

Interpretation: _____

15. Identify the rhythm.

Fig. 7.18

Rhythm: _____ Rate: _____ P waves: _____

PR interval: _____ QRS duration: _____ QT interval: _____

Interpretation: _____

16. Identify the rhythm.

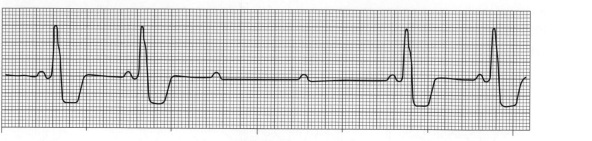

Fig. 7.19

Rhythm: _____ Rate: _____ P waves: _____
PR interval: _____ QRS duration: _____ QT interval: _____
Interpretation: _____

17. Identify the rhythm.

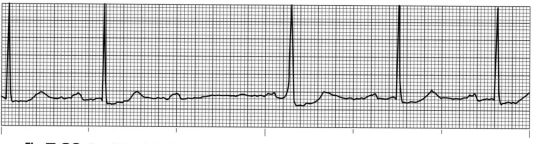
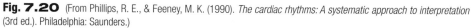

Fig. 7.20 (From Phillips, R. E., & Feeney, M. K. (1990). *The cardiac rhythms: A systematic approach to interpretation* (3rd ed.). Philadelphia: Saunders.)

Rhythm: _____ Rate: _____ P waves: _____
PR interval: _____ QRS duration: _____ QT interval: _____
Interpretation: _____

18. Identify the rhythm.

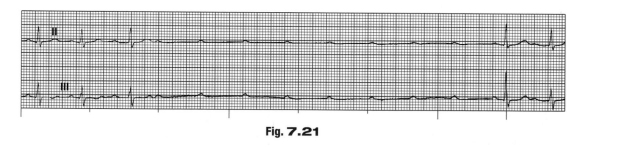

Fig. 7.21

Rhythm: _____ Rate: _____ P waves: _____
PR interval: _____ QRS duration: _____ QT interval: _____
Interpretation: _____

19. Identify the rhythm.

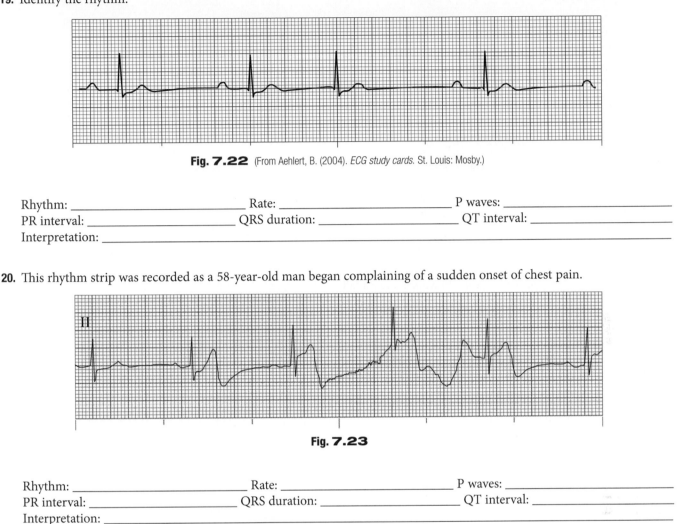

Fig. 7.22 (From Aehlert, B. (2004). *ECG study cards.* St. Louis: Mosby.)

Rhythm: _____ Rate: _____ P waves: _____
PR interval: _____ QRS duration: _____ QT interval: _____
Interpretation: _____

20. This rhythm strip was recorded as a 58-year-old man began complaining of a sudden onset of chest pain.

II

Fig. 7.23

Rhythm: _____ Rate: _____ P waves: _____
PR interval: _____ QRS duration: _____ QT interval: _____
Interpretation: _____

21. This rhythm strip is from a 77-year-old woman who stated that she felt fine. She stopped at a blood pressure machine in Walmart, and the machine would not read her pulse rate. She later went to her physician's office and then to the emergency department.

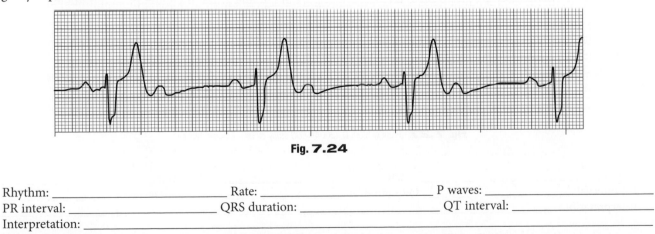

Fig. 7.24

Rhythm: _____ Rate: _____ P waves: _____
PR interval: _____ QRS duration: _____ QT interval: _____
Interpretation: _____

22. Identify the rhythm.

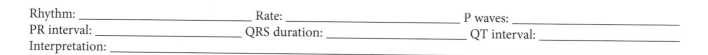

Fig. 7.25 (From Aehlert, B. (2004). *ECG study cards*. St. Louis: Mosby.)

Rhythm: _____ Rate: _____ P waves: _____
PR interval: _____ QRS duration: _____ QT interval: _____
Interpretation: _____

23. This rhythm strip is from a 97-year-old woman after a fall.

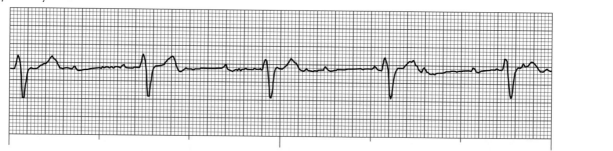

Fig. 7.26 (From Aehlert, B. (2004). *ECG study cards*. St. Louis: Mosby.)

Rhythm: _____ Rate: _____ P waves: _____
PR interval: _____ QRS duration: _____ QT interval: _____
Interpretation: _____

24. Identify the rhythm.

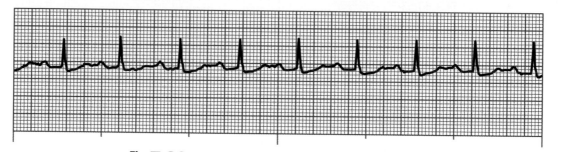

Fig. 7.27 (From Aehlert, B. (2004). *ECG study cards*. St. Louis: Mosby.)

Rhythm: _____ Rate: _____ P waves: _____
PR interval: _____ QRS duration: _____ QT interval: _____
Interpretation: _____

25. Identify the rhythm.

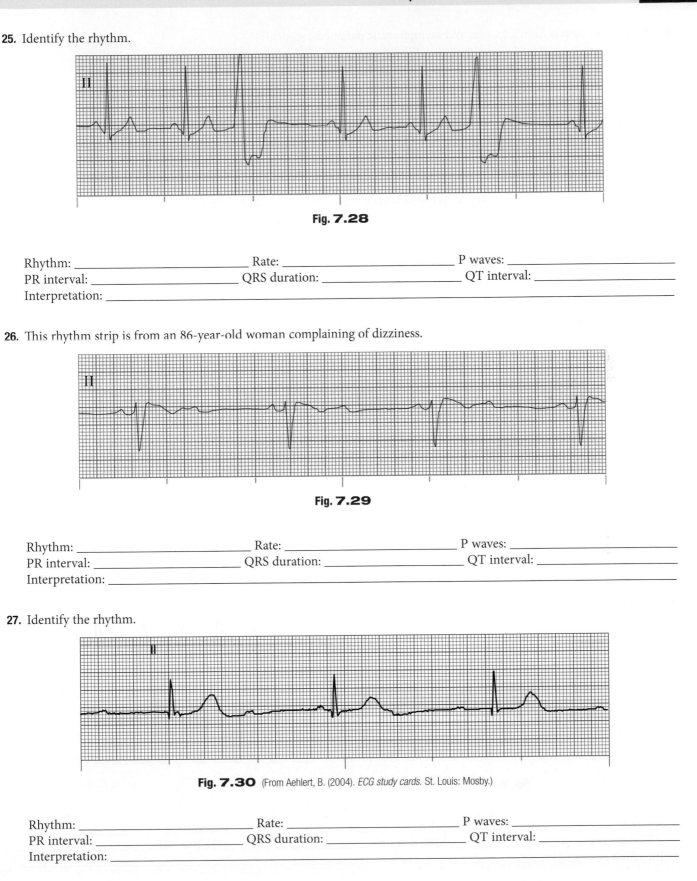

Fig. 7.28

Rhythm: _____ Rate: _____ P waves: _____
PR interval: _____ QRS duration: _____ QT interval: _____
Interpretation: _____

26. This rhythm strip is from an 86-year-old woman complaining of dizziness.

Fig. 7.29

Rhythm: _____ Rate: _____ P waves: _____
PR interval: _____ QRS duration: _____ QT interval: _____
Interpretation: _____

27. Identify the rhythm.

Fig. 7.30 (From Aehlert, B. (2004). *ECG study cards*. St. Louis: Mosby.)

Rhythm: _____ Rate: _____ P waves: _____
PR interval: _____ QRS duration: _____ QT interval: _____
Interpretation: _____

28. This rhythm strip is from a 25-year-old asymptomatic paramedic student.

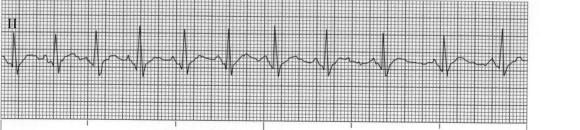

Fig. 7.31 (From Aehlert, B. (2004). *ECG study cards.* St. Louis: Mosby.)

Rhythm: _____ Rate: _____ P waves: _____

PR interval: _____ QRS duration: _____ QT interval: _____

Interpretation: _____

29. This rhythm strip is from an asymptomatic 56-year-old man.

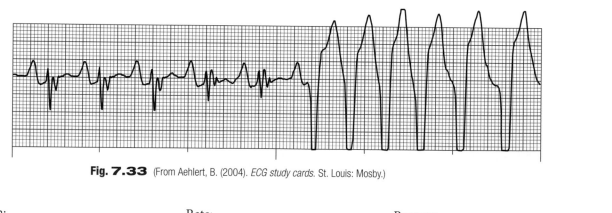

Fig. 7.32 (From Aehlert, B. (2004). *ECG study cards.* St. Louis: Mosby.)

Rhythm: _____ Rate: _____ P waves: _____

PR interval: _____ QRS duration: _____ QT interval: _____

Interpretation: _____

30. Identify the rhythm.

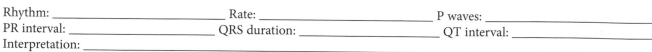

Fig. 7.33 (From Aehlert, B. (2004). *ECG study cards.* St. Louis: Mosby.)

Rhythm: _____ Rate: _____ P waves: _____

PR interval: _____ QRS duration: _____ QT interval: _____

Interpretation: _____

31. Identify the rhythm.

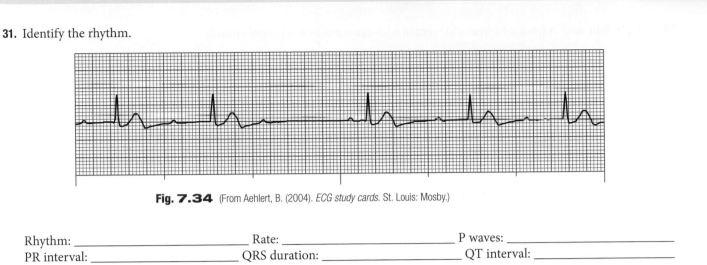

Fig. 7.34 (From Aehlert, B. (2004). *ECG study cards.* St. Louis: Mosby.)

Rhythm: _____ Rate: _____ P waves: _____
PR interval: _____ QRS duration: _____ QT interval: _____
Interpretation: _____

32. These rhythm strips are from a 26-year-old man with end-stage cardiomyopathy. His condition was apparently the result of chronic methamphetamine use.

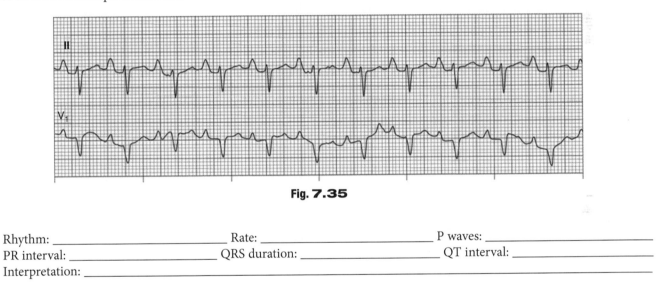

Fig. 7.35

Rhythm: _____ Rate: _____ P waves: _____
PR interval: _____ QRS duration: _____ QT interval: _____
Interpretation: _____

33. This rhythm strip is from a 51-year-old man experiencing dull chest discomfort that he rates 6/10. His symptoms began about 2 hours ago. His blood pressure is 70/48 mm Hg and his skin is cool and diaphoretic.

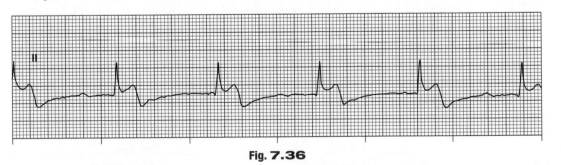

Fig. 7.36

Rhythm: _____ Rate: _____ P waves: _____
PR interval: _____ QRS duration: _____ QT interval: _____
Interpretation: _____

34. This rhythm strip is from a 62-year-old woman who experienced a syncopal episode.

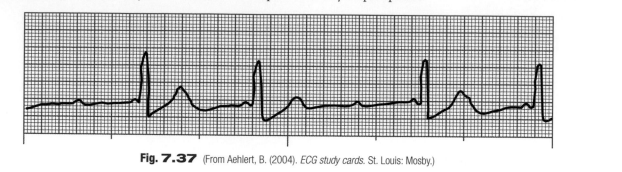

Fig. 7.37 (From Aehlert, B. (2004). *ECG study cards.* St. Louis: Mosby.)

Rhythm: _____ Rate: _____ P waves: _____
PR interval: _____ QRS duration: _____ QT interval: _____
Interpretation: _____

35. This rhythm strip is from a 66-year-old woman with abdominal pain and weakness that began suddenly while she was eating breakfast.

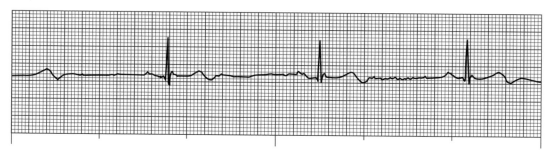

Fig. 7.38 (From Aehlert, B. (2004). *ECG study cards.* St. Louis: Mosby.)

Rhythm: _____ Rate: _____ P waves: _____
PR interval: _____ QRS duration: _____ QT interval: _____
Interpretation: _____

36. Identify the rhythm.

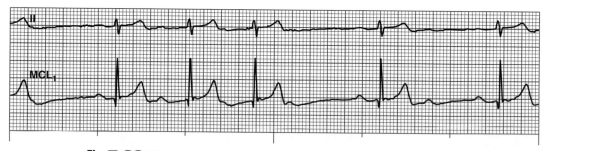

Fig. 7.39 (From Aehlert, B. (2004). *ECG study cards.* St. Louis: Mosby.)

Rhythm: _____ Rate: _____ P waves: _____
PR interval: _____ QRS duration: _____ QT interval: _____
Interpretation: _____

37. Identify the rhythm.

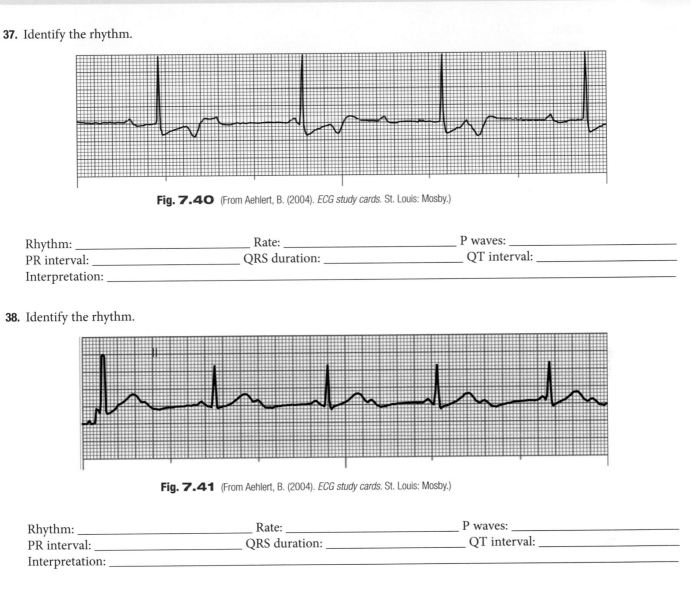

Fig. 7.40 (From Aehlert, B. (2004). *ECG study cards.* St. Louis: Mosby.)

Rhythm: _____ Rate: _____ P waves: _____
PR interval: _____ QRS duration: _____ QT interval: _____
Interpretation: _____

38. Identify the rhythm.

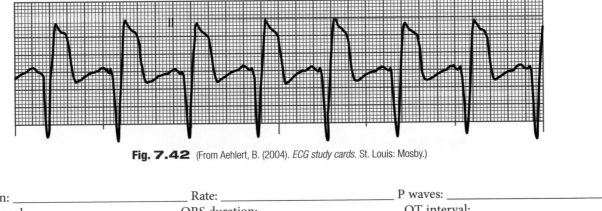

Fig. 7.41 (From Aehlert, B. (2004). *ECG study cards.* St. Louis: Mosby.)

Rhythm: _____ Rate: _____ P waves: _____
PR interval: _____ QRS duration: _____ QT interval: _____
Interpretation: _____

39. This rhythm strip is from a 78-year-old woman complaining of left upper quadrant abdominal pain.

Fig. 7.42 (From Aehlert, B. (2004). *ECG study cards.* St. Louis: Mosby.)

Rhythm: _____ Rate: _____ P waves: _____
PR interval: _____ QRS duration: _____ QT interval: _____
Interpretation: _____

40. Identify the rhythm.

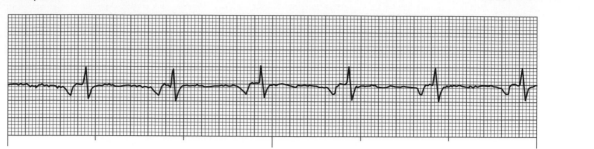

Fig. 7.43 (From Aehlert, B. (2004). *ECG study cards*. St. Louis: Mosby.)

Rhythm: _____ Rate: _____ P waves: _____
PR interval: _____ QRS duration: _____ QT interval: _____
Interpretation: _____

41. Identify the rhythm.

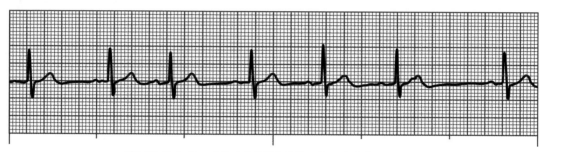

Fig. 7.44 (From Aehlert, B. (2004). *ECG study cards*. St. Louis: Mosby.)

Rhythm: _____ Rate: _____ P waves: _____
PR interval: _____ QRS duration: _____ QT interval: _____
Interpretation: _____

42. Identify the rhythm.

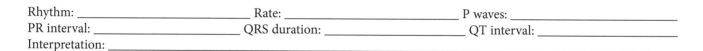
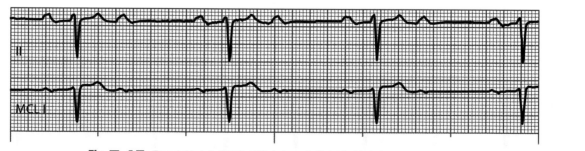

Fig. 7.45 (From Aehlert, B. (2004). *ECG study cards*. St. Louis: Mosby.)

Rhythm: _____ Rate: _____ P waves: _____
PR interval: _____ QRS duration: _____ QT interval: _____
Interpretation: _____

STOP & REVIEW ANSWERS

1. **B**. First-degree AV block may be a normal finding in individuals with no history of cardiac disease, especially in athletes. In some people, mild prolongation of the PR interval may be a normal variant, especially with sinus bradycardia during rest or sleep. Second-degree AV block type I can also occur in athletes, probably related to an increase in resting vagal tone, and in healthy individuals during sleep.

2. **B**. When analyzing a rhythm strip, assess PR intervals to detect AV conduction disturbances.

3. **A, C**. Second-degree AV block type I is also known as type I block, Mobitz I, or Wenckebach.

4. **B, C**. Characteristics of 2:1 AV block can be summarized as follows:
   Rhythm: Ventricular regular; atrial regular
   Rate: Atrial rate is twice the ventricular rate
   P waves: Normal in size and shape; every other P wave is not followed by a QRS complex
   PR interval: Constant
   QRS duration: May be narrow or wide; complexes are absent after every other P wave

5. **D**. With both second-degree type I and type II AV blocks, P waves occur regularly and the ventricular rhythm is irregular. With second-degree type II, the QRS duration is within normal limits if the block occurs above or within the bundle of His and it is greater than 0.11 second if the block occurs below the bundle of His. QRS complexes are periodically absent after P waves. With second-degree AV block type II the PR intervals before and after a blocked P wave are constant; with second-degree AV block type I, the PR interval after a nonconducted P wave is shorter than the interval preceding the nonconducted beat.

6. **B**. Third-degree AV block is characterized by regular P to P intervals (i.e., a regular atrial rhythm) and regular R to R intervals (i.e., a regular ventricular rhythm); however, because there is no relationship between the atrial and ventricular rhythms there is no true PR interval.

7. **B**. Remember that the RCA supplies the AV node in 90% of the population. The RCA also supplies the inferior wall of the left ventricle and the right ventricle in most individuals. Blockage of the RCA, resulting in an inferior myocardial infarction or right ventricular infarction, can also result in conduction delays such as first-degree AV block and second-degree AV block type I.

8. **C**. With second-degree AV block type I, the ventricular rhythm is irregular. There are more P waves than QRS complexes and the P-P interval is regular. P waves are normal in size and shape, but some P waves are not followed by a QRS complex. The PR intervals are inconstant. The PR interval after a nonconducted P wave is shorter than the interval preceding the nonconducted beat. The QRS duration is usually 0.11 second or less and QRS complexes are periodically dropped.

9. **D**. With second-degree AV block type II, the ventricular rhythm is irregular. There are more P waves than QRS complexes and the P-P interval is regular. P waves are normal in size and shape, but some P waves are not followed by a QRS complex. The PR interval may be within normal limits or prolonged, but it is constant for the conducted beats; the PR intervals before and after a blocked P wave are constant. The QRS duration is within normal limits if the block occurs above or within the bundle of His; it is greater than 0.11 second if the block occurs below the bundle of His. QRS complexes are periodically absent after P waves.

10. **A, C, D, E, F**. This patient is clearly symptomatic with this dysrhythmia. Treatment should include applying a pulse oximeter, administering oxygen (when indicated), obtaining the patient's vital signs, and establishing IV access. Obtain a 12-lead ECG and a cardiology consult. Temporary or permanent pacing may be necessary. Reports exist of occasional worsened AV conduction and/or hemodynamic compromise following atropine administration to patients with AV block and wide QRS complexes.

11. **A, B, C**.
    Rhythm: Ventricular regular; atrial regular; no relationship between the atrial and ventricular rhythms
    Rate: The ventricular rate is determined by the origin of the escape pacemaker; the atrial rate is greater than (and independent of) the ventricular rate
    P waves: Normal in size and shape; some P waves are not followed by a QRS complex
    PR interval: None: the atria and the ventricles beat independently of each other, thus there is no true PR interval
    QRS duration: Narrow or wide, depending on the location of the escape pacemaker and the condition of the intraventricular conduction system

12. **C**. A sinus tachycardia is present when there is a 1:1 relationship between P waves and QRS complexes and the ventricular rate is faster than 100 beats/min. A first-degree AV block is present when there is a 1:1 relationship between P waves and QRS complexes and the PR interval is prolonged (i.e., more than 0.20 second) and constant.

Practice Rhythm Strip Answers

Note: The rate and interval measurements provided here were obtained using electronic calipers.

13. Fig. 7.16

Rhythm: Regular

Rate: 110 beats/min

P waves: Positive; 1:1 (P wave to QRS) relationship

PR interval: 0.24 second

QRS duration: 0.07 second

QT interval: 0.30 second

Interpretation: Sinus tachycardia at 110 beats/min with first-degree AV block

14. Fig. 7.17

Rhythm: Regular

Rate: Ventricular 34 beats/min; atrial 65 beats/min

P waves: Positive; 2:1 relationship

PR interval: 0.33 second

QRS duration: 0.12 second

QT interval: 0.38 second

Interpretation: 2:1 AV block at 34 beats/min with a wide QRS

15. Fig. 7.18

Rhythm: Regular

Rate: Ventricular 53 beats/min; atrial 178 beats/min

P waves: Positive; more Ps than QRSs; no relationship to QRSs

PR interval: None

QRS duration: 0.06 second

QT interval: 0.30 second

Interpretation: Third-degree AV block at 53 beats/min with STE

16. Fig. 7.19

Rhythm: Ventricular irregular; atrial regular

Rate: Ventricular about 40 beats/min; atrial 58 beats/min

P waves: Positive; more Ps than QRSs

PR interval: 0.16 second

QRS duration: 0.13 second

QT interval: Unable to determine because T waves are not visible

Interpretation: Advanced second-degree AV block at 40 beats/min with a wide QRS and ST-segment depression

17. Fig. 7.20

Rhythm: Ventricular irregular; atrial regular

Rate: Ventricular about 50 beats/min; atrial 54 beats/min

P waves: Positive; more Ps than QRSs

PR interval: Lengthening

QRS duration: 0.07 second

QT interval: 0.46 second (prolonged)

Interpretation: Second-degree AV block type I at 50 beats/min with ST-segment depression and a prolonged QT interval; baseline artifact is present

18. Fig. 7.21

Rhythm: Ventricular irregular; atrial regular

Rate: Ventricular ranges from less than 20 to 94 beats/min; atrial 94 beats/min

P waves: Positive; more Ps than QRSs

PR interval: Lengthening

QRS duration: 0.07 second

QT interval: 0.36 second

Interpretation: Second-degree AV block type I with a ventricular response ranging from less than 20 to 94 beats/min; note the absence of ventricular activity for slightly more than 5 seconds

19. Fig. 7.22

Rhythm: Irregular

Rate: 40 beats/min

P waves: Positive before the QRS of beats 1, 2 and 4, none visible in beat 3

PR interval: 0.35 second

QRS duration: 0.07 second

QT interval: 036 second

Interpretation: Sinus bradycardia at 40 beats/min with first-degree AV block and a premature junctional complex

20. Fig. 7.23

Rhythm: Regular

Rate: 54 beats/min

P waves: Positive but artifact obscures visibility with some beats

PR interval: 0.20 to 0.23 second

QRS duration: 0.07 second

QT interval: 0.28 second

Interpretation: Sinus bradycardia at 54 beats/min with first-degree AV block and STE; artifact is present

21. Fig. 7.24

Rhythm: Regular

Rate: Ventricular 36 beats/min; atrial 68 beats/min

P waves: Positive; 2:1 relationship

PR interval: 0.30 second

QRS duration: 0.14 second

QT interval: 0.44 second

Interpretation: 2:1 AV block at 36 beats/min with a wide QRS and STE

22. Fig. 7.25

Rhythm: Regular

Rate: Ventricular 54 beats/min; atrial 108 beats/min

P waves: Positive; 2:1 relationship

PR interval: 0.16 second

QRS duration: 0.06 second

QT interval: Unable to determine because T waves are not clearly visible

Interpretation: 2:1 AV block at 54 beats/min with STE

23. Fig. 7.26
  Rhythm: Regular
  Rate: 89 beats/min
  P waves: Positive before each QRS; 1:1 relationship
  PR interval: 0.24 second
  QRS duration: 0.06 second
  QT interval: 0.32 second
  Interpretation: Sinus rhythm at 89 beats/min with
    first-degree AV block and ST-segment depression;
    baseline artifact is present

24. Fig. 7.27
  Rhythm: Regular
  Rate: Ventricular 45 beats/min; atrial 110 beats/min
  P waves: Positive; more Ps than QRSs
  PR interval: None
  QRS duration: 0.14 second
  QT interval: 0.40 to 0.44 second
  Interpretation: Third-degree AV block at 45 beats/min;
    baseline artifact is present

25. Fig. 7.28
  Rhythm: Irregular
  Rate: 70 beats/min
  P waves: Sinus P waves; none with early beats
  PR interval: 0.15 second (sinus beats)
  QRS duration: 0.10 second (sinus beats)
  QT interval: 0.38 second (sinus beats)
  Interpretation: Sinus rhythm at 70 beats/min with uni-
    form premature ventricular complexes (PVCs) and
    ST-segment depression

26. Fig. 7.29
  Rhythm: Regular
  Rate: Ventricular rate 35 beats/min; atrial rate 70 beats/
    min
  P waves: Positive before each QRS; 2:1 relationship
  PR interval: 0.20 second
  QRS duration: 0.13 second
  QT interval: 0.50 second (prolonged)
  Interpretation: 2:1 AV block at 35 beats/min with a
    wide QRS and a prolonged QT interval

27. Fig. 7.30
  Rhythm: Essentially regular
  Rate: Ventricular 32 beats/min; atrial 71 beats/min
  P waves: Positive; more Ps than QRSs
  PR interval: None
  QRS duration: 0.09 second
  QT interval: 0.57 second (prolonged)
  Interpretation: Third-degree AV block at 32 beats/min
    with a prolonged QT interval; baseline artifact is
    present

28. Fig. 7.31
  Rhythm: Irregular
  Rate: 110 beats/min
  P waves: Positive before each QRS; 1:1 relationship
  PR interval: 0.11 to 0.14 second
  QRS duration: 0.11 second
  QT interval: 0.28 second
  Interpretation: Sinus tachyarrhythmia at 110 beats/min;
    artifact is present

29. Fig. 7.32
  Rhythm: Irregular
  Rate: 80 beats/min
  P waves: Positive before each QRS; none with early ven-
    tricular beat
  PR interval: 0.18 second (sinus beats)
  QRS duration: 0.15 second (sinus beats)
  QT interval: 0.36 second (sinus beats)
  Interpretation: Sinus rhythm at 80 beats/min with a
    wide QRS, an R-on-T PVC (beat 3), and STE

30. Fig. 7.33
  Rhythm: Irregular
  Rate: 100 beats/min (sinus beats); 150 beats/min (ven-
    tricular tachycardia [VT])
  P waves: Sinus P waves; none with ventricular beats
  PR interval: 0.24 second (sinus beats)
  QRS duration: 0.09 second (sinus beats)
  QT interval: 0.50 second (prolonged) (sinus beats)
  Interpretation: Sinus rhythm at 100 beats/min with
    first-degree AV block and a prolonged QT interval to
    monomorphic VT at 150 beats/min

31. Fig. 7.34
  Rhythm: Ventricular irregular; atrial regular
  Rate: Ventricular 50 beats/min; atrial 60 beats/min
  P waves: Positive; more Ps than QRSs
  PR interval: Lengthening
  QRS duration: 0.08 second
  QT interval: 0.33 second
  Interpretation: Second-degree AV block type I at 50
    beats/min

32. Fig. 7.35
  Rhythm: Regular
  Rate: 111 beats/min
  P waves: Tall and positive before each QRS; 1:1 relation-
    ship
  PR interval: 0.19 second
  QRS duration: 0.09 second
  QT interval: 0.27 second
  Interpretation: Sinus tachycardia at 111 beats/min; tall
    P waves

33. Fig. 7.36
    Rhythm: Ventricular regular; atrial slightly irregular
    Rate: Ventricular 52 beats/min; atrial 71 beats/min
    P waves: Positive; more Ps than QRSs
    PR interval: None
    QRS duration: 0.07 second
    QT interval: 0.26 second
    Interpretation: Third-degree AV block at 52 beats/min with STE; artifact is present

34. Fig. 7.37
    Rhythm: Ventricular irregular; atrial regular
    Rate: Ventricular 40 beats/min; atrial 100 beats/min
    P waves: Positive; more Ps than QRSs
    PR interval: 0.13 second
    QRS duration: 0.12 second
    QT interval: 0.57 second (prolonged)
    Interpretation: Second-degree AV block type II at 40 beats/min with ST-segment depression and a prolonged QT interval

35. Fig. 7.38
    Rhythm: Regular
    Rate: 37 beats/min
    P waves: Positive; 1:1 relationship
    PR interval: 0.24 second
    QRS duration: 0.08 second
    QT interval: 0.46 second (slightly prolonged)
    Interpretation: Sinus bradycardia at 37 beats/min with first-degree AV block and a slightly prolonged QT interval; artifact is present

36. Fig. 7.39
    Rhythm: Ventricular irregular; atrial regular
    Rate: Ventricular 50 beats/min; atrial 83 beats/min
    P waves: Positive; more Ps than QRSs
    PR interval: Lengthening
    QRS duration: 0.08 second
    QT interval: 0.37 second
    Interpretation: Second-degree AV block type I at 50 beats/min; although the complexes on the right side of the rhythm strip show 2:1 conduction, comparison of the PR intervals of beats 1 through 3 enable a diagnosis of second-degree type I AV block

37. Fig. 7.40
    Rhythm: Ventricular regular; atrial regular
    Rate: Ventricular 38 beats/min; atrial 63 beats/min
    P waves: Positive; more Ps than QRSs
    PR interval: None
    QRS duration: 0.06 second
    QT interval: 0.50 second (prolonged)
    Interpretation: Third-degree AV block at 38 beats/min with ST-segment depression, inverted T waves, and a prolonged QT interval

38. Fig. 7.41
    Rhythm: Ventricular regular; atrial regular
    Rate: Ventricular 47 beats/min; atrial 92 beats/min
    P waves: Positive; more Ps than QRSs; 2:1 relationship
    PR interval: 0.15 second
    QRS duration: 0.09 second
    QT interval: 0.47 second (prolonged)
    Interpretation: 2:1 AV block at 47 beats/min with a prolonged QT interval

39. Fig. 7.42
    Rhythm: Regular
    Rate: 75 beats/min
    P waves: Low amplitude, but positive before each QRS; 1:1 relationship
    PR interval: 0.16 second
    QRS duration: 0.11 second
    QT interval: 0.33 second (estimated; difficult to determine because the ends of the T waves are not clearly visible)
    Interpretation: Sinus rhythm at 75 beats/min with STE

40. Fig. 7.43
    Rhythm: Regular
    Rate: 60 beats/min
    P waves: One inverted P wave precedes each QRS
    PR interval: 0.22 second
    QRS duration: 0.11 second
    QT interval: Unable to determine
    Interpretation: Junctional rhythm at 60 beats/min with first-degree AV block; artifact is present

41. Fig. 7.44
    Rhythm: Irregular
    Rate: 70 beats/min
    P waves: Positive before each QRS; the P wave of beat 3 is early; an early P wave with no QRS after it distorts the T wave of beat 6
    PR interval: 0.20 second (sinus beats)
    QRS duration: 0.09 second (sinus beats)
    QT interval: 0.32 second (sinus beats)
    Interpretation: Sinus rhythm at 70 beats/min with a PAC (beat 3) and a nonconducted PAC

42. Fig. 7.45
    Rhythm: Ventricular regular; atrial regular
    Rate: Ventricular 36 beats/min; atrial 70 beats/min
    P waves: Positive; more Ps than QRSs; 2:1 relationship
    PR interval: 0.32 second
    QRS duration: 0.12 second
    QT interval: 0.38 second
    Interpretation: 2:1 AV block at 36 beats/min with a wide QRS

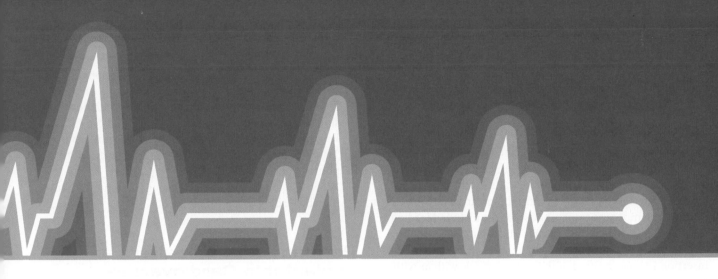

Pacemaker Rhythms 8

LEARNING OBJECTIVES

After reading this chapter, you should be able to:

1. Identify the components of a pacemaker system.
2. Discuss the terms *triggering, inhibition, pacing, capture, electrical capture, mechanical capture,* and *sensitivity.*
3. Describe the appearance of a typical pacemaker spike on the electrocardiogram (ECG).
4. Describe the appearance of the waveform on the ECG produced as a result of atrial pacing and ventricular pacing.

5. Explain the differences between single-chamber and dual-chamber pacemakers.
6. List three types of pacemaker malfunction.
7. Describe how to analyze pacemaker function on the ECG.

KEY TERMS

atrioventricular (AV) interval: In dual-chamber pacing, the length of time between an atrial sensed or atrial paced event and the delivery of a ventricular pacing stimulus; analogous to the PR interval of intrinsic waveforms; also called the artificial or electronic PR interval.

capture: The successful conduction of an artificial pacemaker's impulse through the myocardium, resulting in depolarization.

escape interval: Time measured between a sensed cardiac event and the next pacemaker output.

failure to capture: A pacemaker malfunction that occurs when the artificial pacemaker stimulus is unable to depolarize the myocardium.

failure to pace: A pacemaker malfunction that occurs when the pacemaker fails to deliver an electrical stimulus at its programmed time; also referred to as failure to fire or failure of pulse generation.

oversensing: A pacemaker malfunction that results from inappropriate sensing of extraneous electrical signals.

paced interval: Period between two consecutive paced events in the same cardiac chamber; also known as the automatic interval.

sensitivity: The extent to which an artificial pacemaker recognizes intrinsic cardiac electrical activity.

threshold: The minimum amount of voltage (i.e., milliamperes) needed to obtain consistent capture.

undersensing: A pacemaker malfunction that occurs when the artificial pacemaker fails to recognize spontaneous myocardial depolarization.

PACEMAKER SYSTEMS

A cardiac pacemaker is a battery-powered device that delivers an electrical current to the heart to stimulate depolarization. A pacemaker system consists of a pulse generator and pacing leads. A pacing lead is an insulated wire used to carry an electrical impulse from the pulse generator to the patient's heart. It also carries information about the heart's electrical activity back to the pacemaker. The pulse generator is the power source that houses a battery and electronic circuitry. The circuitry works like a computer, converting energy from the battery into electrical pulses. The pacemaker responds to the information received either by sending a pacing impulse to the heart (i.e., triggering) or by not sending a pacing impulse to the heart (i.e., inhibition).

An artificial pacemaker can be external (a temporary intervention) or implanted.

Temporary Pacing Routes

The pulse generator of a temporary pacemaker is located externally. An external pacemaker may be used to control transient disturbances in heart rate or conduction resulting from drug toxicity or that occur during a myocardial infarction (MI) or after cardiac surgery when increased vagal tone is often present. Temporary pacing can be accomplished through transvenous, epicardial, or transcutaneous means.

TRANSVENOUS PACING

Transvenous pacemakers stimulate the endocardium of the right atrium or ventricle (or both) using an electrode introduced into a central vein, such as the subclavian, femoral, brachial, internal jugular, or external jugular vein. Complications of temporary transvenous pacing include bleeding; infection; pneumothorax; cardiac dysrhythmias; MI; lead displacement; fracture of the pacing lead; hematoma at the insertion site; perforation of the right ventricle with or without pericardial tamponade; and perforation of the inferior vena cava, pulmonary artery, or coronary arteries because of improper placement of the pacing lead.

EPICARDIAL PACING

Epicardial pacing is the placement of pacing leads directly onto or through the epicardium. Epicardial leads may be used when a patient is undergoing cardiac surgery and the heart's outer surface is easy to reach.

TRANSCUTANEOUS PACING

Transcutaneous pacing (TCP), also called temporary external pacing or noninvasive pacing, uses electrical stimulation through two pacing pads positioned on a patient's torso to stimulate contraction of the heart. The electrical stimulus exits from the negative terminal on the machine (and subsequently the negative electrode) and passes through the chest wall to the heart. The range of output current of a transcutaneous pacemaker varies depending on the manufacturer.

TCP is indicated for significant bradycardias unresponsive to atropine therapy or when atropine is not immediately available or indicated. It may also be used as a bridge until transvenous pacing can be accomplished or the cause of the bradycardia is reversed (e.g., drug overdose, hyperkalemia).

🔘 ECG Pearl _____

Standby pacing refers to applying the pacing pads to the patient's chest in anticipation of possible use, but pacing is not yet needed. For example, standby pacing is often warranted when second-degree AV block type II or third-degree AV block is present in the setting of acute MI.

_____

The primary limitation of TCP is patient discomfort that is proportional to the intensity of skeletal muscle contraction and the direct electrical stimulation of cutaneous nerves. Because TCP is uncomfortable, the administration of sedatives or analgesics is usually necessary for responsive patients. Temporary transvenous pacing is indicated when prolonged TCP is needed.

Possible complications of TCP include the following:
- Coughing
- Skin burns
- Interference with sensing from patient agitation or muscle contractions
- Discomfort as a result of the electrical stimulation of the skin and muscles
- Failure to recognize that the pacemaker is not capturing
- Tissue damage, including third-degree burns, with improper or prolonged TCP
- When pacing is prolonged, pacing **threshold** changes, thereby leading to capture failure

Permanent Pacemakers and Implantable Cardioverter-Defibrillators

Patients who have chronic dysrhythmias that are unresponsive to medication therapy and that result in decreased cardiac output may require the surgical implantation of a permanent pacemaker or an implantable cardioverter-defibrillator (ICD). Pacemakers and ICDs are called cardiovascular implantable electronic devices (CIEDs).

A permanent pacemaker is used to treat disorders of the sinoatrial (SA) node (e.g., bradycardias), disorders of the AV conduction pathways (e.g., second-degree AV block type II, third-degree AV block), or both, that produce signs and symptoms as a result of inadequate cardiac output. The pacemaker's pulse generator is usually implanted under local anesthesia into the subcutaneous tissue of the anterior chest just below the right or left clavicle. The patient's handedness, occupation, and hobbies determine whether the pacemaker is implanted on the right or left side.

The circuitry of CIEDs is housed in a sealed case made of titanium that is airtight and impermeable to fluid (Fig. 8.1). These devices store information about the activities of the patient's heart and information about the device itself (e.g., number of dysrhythmia episodes; provoking rhythm; dates of pacing, defibrillation, or both). The stored information is periodically retrieved and reviewed by the patient's physician, and, if necessary, changes in the device's settings are made. Lithium batteries are almost exclusively used in modern CIEDs. Battery life is generally 5 to 15 years but depends on type, programming, the number of times therapies are delivered, the frequency of pacing, and the number of cardiac chambers paced.

An ICD can deliver a range of therapies (also called tiered therapy), including defibrillation, antitachycardia pacing (i.e., overdrive pacing), synchronized cardioversion, and bradycardia pacing, depending on the dysrhythmia detected and how the device is programmed (Fig. 8.2). A physician determines the appropriate ICD therapies for each patient.

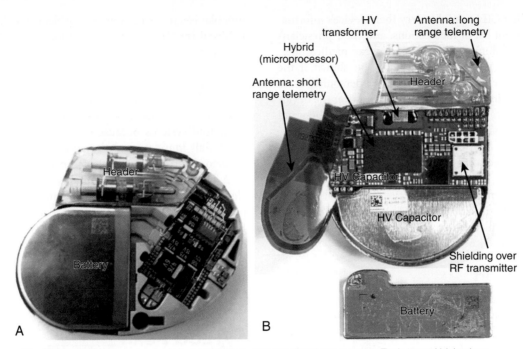

Fig. 8.1 A, Pacemaker generator. B, Implantable cardioverter-defibrillator pulse generator. The battery, which has been removed, fits under electronic components. *HV*, High-voltage; *RF*, radiofrequency. (From Zipes, D. P., Libby, P., Bonow, R. O., Mann, D. L., Tomaselli, G. F., & Braunwald, E. (2019). *Braunwald's heart disease: A textbook of cardiovascular medicine* (11th ed.). Philadelphia: Elsevier.)

ICD: Tiered Therapy

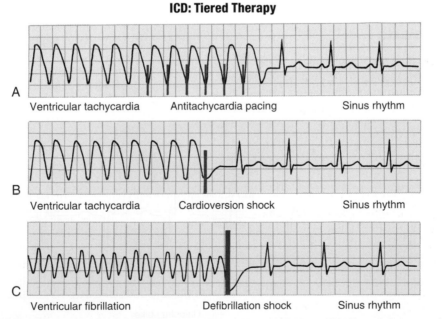

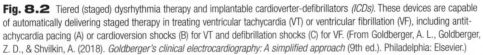

Fig. 8.2 Tiered (staged) dysrhythmia therapy and implantable cardioverter-defibrillators *(ICDs)*. These devices are capable of automatically delivering staged therapy in treating ventricular tachycardia (VT) or ventricular fibrillation (VF), including antitachycardia pacing (A) or cardioversion shocks (B) for VT and defibrillation shocks (C) for VF. (From Goldberger, A. L., Goldberger, Z. D., & Shvilkin, A. (2018). *Goldberger's clinical electrocardiography: A simplified approach* (9th ed.). Philadelphia: Elsevier.)

Examples of ICD indications include patients who have experienced a sudden cardiac arrest due to ventricular tachycardia (VT) or ventricular fibrillation (VF), structural heart disease with sustained VT, or syncope caused by ventricular dysrhythmias. Patients with an ICD should notify their physician after the device fires to have it checked.

Patients should schedule regular appointments with their cardiologist for device function checks (e.g., battery status, system checks). Generally, a CIED's battery does not suddenly fail. Instead, the battery gradually wears out, enabling elective CIED replacement. In some cases, CIED monitoring can be accomplished remotely using a device connected to the patient's phone.

Patients with a CIED should carry their device's information card, a current list of medications, and their physician's name and phone number and have or wear medical alert identification. The information card can be shown if the CIED sets off a metal detector. If security personnel use a metal-detecting wand, it should not be placed over the device for more than a second because the magnet inside the wand may temporarily change the operating mode of the CIED.

Cell phones can interfere with proper CIED function because they send electromagnetic signals. Therefore, the patient should hold a cell phone to the ear farthest from the CIED. Even when turned off, cell phones should not be worn in a shirt pocket on the side of the CIED. Some CIED manufacturers use special filters in their devices to prevent cell phone interference.

⟳ ECG Pearl

Historically, cardiac implanted devices were considered a contraindication to magnetic resonance imaging (MRI). However, many newer implanted devices are classified as *MRI conditional*, a phrase used by the American Society for Testing and Materials to denote a product that poses no hazards to a specified MRI environment with specified conditions of use. In some cases, patients with older devices may safely undergo MRI if they are appropriately screened and their devices are reprogrammed according to standard protocols.

Pacemaker Leads

Pacemaker lead systems may consist of single, double, or multiple leads. A separate lead is used for each heart chamber paced. The exposed portion of the pacing lead—the electrode—is placed in direct contact with the heart. A unipolar electrode has one pacing electrode that is located at its distal tip. The negative electrode is in contact with the cardiac tissue, and the pulse generator (located outside the heart) functions as the positive electrode. The pacemaker spike produced by a unipolar lead system is often large because of the distance between the positive and negative electrodes. Unipolar leads are less commonly used than bipolar lead systems because of the potential for pacing the chest wall muscles, and the susceptibility of the unipolar leads to electromagnetic interference.

A bipolar lead system contains a positive and negative electrode at the distal tip of the pacing lead wire. Most temporary transvenous pacemakers use a bipolar lead system. However, a permanent pacemaker may have either a bipolar or a unipolar lead system. The pacemaker spike produced by a bipolar lead system is smaller than that of a unipolar system because of the shorter distance between the positive and negative electrodes (Fig. 8.3).

⟳ ECG Pearl

A leadless pacemaker consists of a self-contained generator and lead system. It is inserted through the femoral vein and into the right ventricle, eliminating the need for a chest incision and creating a pocket in the patient's chest to house a pulse generator. First-generation leadless pacemakers provide only single-chamber ventricular pacing. The Micra Transcatheter Pacing System (Medtronic PLC, Minneapolis, MN), which is about a large vitamin capsule size, received US Food and Drug Administration (FDA) approval in 2016. The Nanostim Leadless Cardiac Pacemaker (Abbott Laboratories, Abbott Park, IL) is awaiting FDA approval.

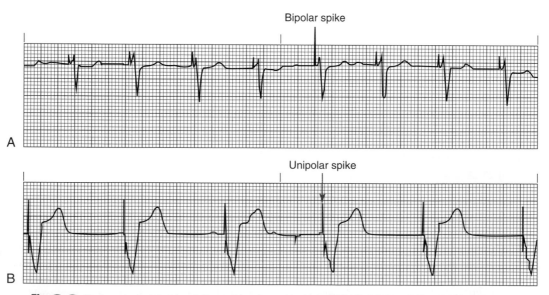

Fig. 8.3 Bipolar and unipolar pacing. A, Pacemaker spike produced by a bipolar lead system. B, Pacemaker spike produced by a unipolar lead system. (From Urden, L. D., Stacy, K. M., & Lough, M. E. (2022). *Critical care nursing: Diagnosis and management* (9th ed.). St. Louis: Elsevier.)

PACING PRINCIPLES

Pacing, also called pacemaker firing, occurs when the pacemaker's pulse generator delivers energy (milliamperes [mA]) through the pacing electrode to the myocardium. As mentioned earlier, a pacemaker responds to the information received either by sending a pacing stimulus to the heart (i.e., triggering) or by not sending a pacing stimulus to the heart (i.e., inhibiting).

A fixed-rate (asynchronous) pacemaker continuously discharges at a preset rate (usually 70 to 80 impulses/min) regardless of the patient's heart rate or metabolic demands. An advantage of the fixed-rate pacemaker is its simple circuitry, reducing the risk of pacemaker failure. However, because this type of pacemaker does not sense the patient's own cardiac rhythm, competition between the patient's cardiac rhythm and that of the pacemaker can result. VT or VF may be induced if the pacemaker were to fire during the T wave (i.e., the vulnerable period) of a preceding patient beat. Therefore, fixed-rate pacemakers are not often used today.

A demand (synchronous) pacemaker discharges when the patient's heart rate drops below the pacemaker's lower rate limit (also called the base rate), which is expressed in paced pulses per minute (ppm). For example, if the demand pacemaker were preset at a lower rate limit of 70 ppm, it would sense the patient's heart rate and allow electrical impulses to flow from the pacemaker through the pacing lead to stimulate the heart only when the rate fell below 70/min.

Evidence of pacing can be seen as a vertical line or spike on the ECG. **Capture** is the successful conduction of an artificial pacemaker's impulse through the myocardium, resulting in depolarization. Capture is obtained after the pacemaker electrode is correctly positioned in the heart; with one-to-one capture, each pacing stimulus depolarizes the appropriate chamber. On the ECG, evidence of *electrical capture* can be seen as a pacemaker spike followed by an atrial or a ventricular complex, depending on the cardiac chamber that is being paced (see Fig. 8.3). *Mechanical capture* is assessed by palpating the patient's pulse or observing right atrial pressure, left atrial pressure, or pulmonary artery or arterial pressure waveforms.

Pacemaker Modes

Pacemaker modes are characterized using a three- to five-letter code that identifies a pacemaker's preprogrammed pacing, sensing, and response functions. The first three letters are the most helpful when providing patient care.

The *first letter* of the code identifies the heart chamber (or chambers) paced: O (none), A (atrial), V (ventricular), or D (dual, both atrium and ventricle). The *second letter* identifies the heart's chamber where patient-initiated (i.e., intrinsic) electrical activity is sensed by the pacemaker. O (none), A (atrial), V (ventricular), or D (dual). The *third*

letter indicates how the pacemaker will respond when it senses patient-initiated electrical activity: O (none), T (triggered, the pacemaker will initiate a pacing stimulus in response to a sensed event), I (inhibited, the pacemaker will not initiate a pacing stimulus if electrical activity is sensed), or D (dual, triggered and inhibited). The *fourth letter* identifies the availability of rate modulation (i.e., the pacemaker's ability to adapt its rate to meet the body's needs caused by increased physical activity and increase or decrease the pacing rate accordingly). A pacemaker's rate modulation capability may also be referred to as rate responsiveness or rate adaptation. Finally, the *fifth letter* denotes multisite pacing (i.e., biventricular pacing or more than one pacing site in one ventricle): O (none), A (atrium), V (ventricle), or D (dual, atrium and ventricle).

Single-Chamber Pacemakers

A pacemaker that paces a single heart chamber, either the atrium or ventricle, has one lead placed in the heart. Atrial pacing, achieved by placing the pacing electrode in the right atrium, may be used when the SA node is diseased or damaged, but conduction through the AV junction and ventricles is normal. This type of pacemaker is ineffective if an AV block develops because it cannot pace the ventricles. An atrial demand pacemaker (AAI) senses atrial activity (i.e., P waves). When spontaneous atrial depolarization does not occur within a preset interval, the pacemaker fires and stimulates atrial depolarization at a preset rate. Atrial stimulation produces a pacemaker spike on the ECG followed by a P wave (Fig. 8.4).

With ventricular demand pacing (VVI), the pacemaker electrode is placed in the right ventricle (V), the ventricle is sensed (V), and the pacemaker is inhibited (I) when spontaneous ventricular depolarization occurs within a preset interval. The pacemaker will fire and stimulate ventricular depolarization at a preset rate if spontaneous ventricular depolarization does not occur within this preset interval. Stimulation of the ventricles produces a pacemaker spike on the ECG followed by a wide QRS, resembling a ventricular ectopic beat (Fig. 8.5). The QRS complex is wide because a paced impulse does not follow the heart's normal conduction pathway. A VVI pacemaker may be used for patients with atrial fibrillation and a slow ventricular response. Because a VVI pacemaker does not coordinate pacing with the patient's intrinsic atrial rate, it can result in asynchronous contraction of the atrium and ventricle (i.e., AV asynchrony). The loss of AV synchrony can result in a loss of the atrial contribution to cardiac output (i.e., atrial kick), decreased stroke volume, and decreased cardiac output, producing a constellation of signs and symptoms known as pacemaker syndrome. Pacemaker syndrome signs and symptoms may include dizziness, acute mental status changes, dyspnea on exertion, orthopnea, fatigue, palpitations, hypotension, syncope or near-syncope, neck vein distention, and lower extremity edema.

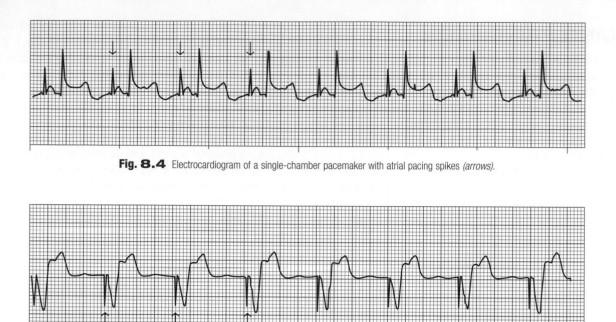

Fig. 8.4 Electrocardiogram of a single-chamber pacemaker with atrial pacing spikes *(arrows)*.

Fig. 8.5 Electrocardiogram of a single-chamber pacemaker with ventricular pacing spikes *(arrows)*.

ECG Pearl

On the ECG, P waves can appear anywhere in the cardiac cycle and have no relationship with the QRS complexes because a ventricular demand pacemaker does not sense or pace atrial activity.

Dual-Chamber Pacemakers

A dual-chamber pacemaker is the most common type of implanted pacemaker. It uses two leads: one lead is placed in the right atrium and the other in the right ventricle.

An atrial synchronous pacemaker (VDD) senses both atrial and ventricular activity but paces only the ventricle when a spontaneous ventricular depolarization does not occur. A VDD pacemaker is used for patients who have impaired AV conduction but an intact SA node. The presence of SA node disease is a contraindication for a VDD pacemaker.

An AV sequential pacemaker (DVI) first stimulates the right atrium and then the right ventricle but senses only the ventricle. It may be used for patients with severe sinus bradycardia. Asynchronous atrial pacing and the potential for AV asynchrony (with possible pacemaker syndrome) can occur with DVI pacing.

An optimal sequential pacemaker (DDD), also called a physiologic or universal pacemaker, is used when the SA node is intact but AV conduction is impaired. In DDD mode, both the atrium and ventricle are paced (D), both chambers are sensed (D), and the pacemaker has both a triggered and inhibited mode of response (D). The pacemaker is programmed to wait between atrial and ventricular stimulation, simulating the usual delay in conduction through the AV node (i.e., the PR interval). The artificial or electronic PR interval is referred to as an **AV interval** (Fig. 8.6). If spontaneous atrial or ventricular depolarization does not occur within a preset interval, the pacemaker fires and stimulates the appropriate chamber at a preset rate. DDD pacemaker functions are summarized in Fig. 8.7. New dual-chamber pacemakers are equipped with programmable features that enable automatic adjustment of the AV interval in response to paced versus sensed P waves and in response to the atrial rate. A DDD pacemaker can be programmed to VVI mode, depending on patient need (e.g., the development of chronic atrial fibrillation).

Biventricular Pacemakers

A biventricular pacemaker has three leads—one lead for each ventricle and one lead for the right atrium. These devices use cardiac resynchronization therapy (CRT) to restore normal simultaneous ventricular contraction, thus improving stroke volume, ejection fraction, cardiac output, and exercise tolerance. CRT, which is indicated for selected patients with moderate to severe heart failure, has been shown to reduce heart failure symptoms and mortality.

PACEMAKER COMPLICATIONS

Complications of permanent pacing associated with the implantation procedure include bleeding, local tissue infection, pneumothorax, cardiac dysrhythmias, air embolism, and catheter-related thrombosis. Long-term complications of permanent pacing may include infection, heart failure, lead displacement or fracture of the pacing lead, externalization of the pacemaker generator, chamber perforation, and

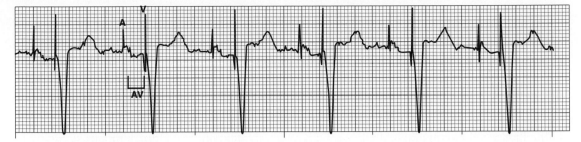

Fig. 8.6 Electrocardiogram of a dual-chamber pacemaker with atrial pacing spikes *(A)*, ventricular pacing spikes *(V)*. *AV, Atrioventricular interval.*

Dual-Chamber (DDD) Pacemaker Functions

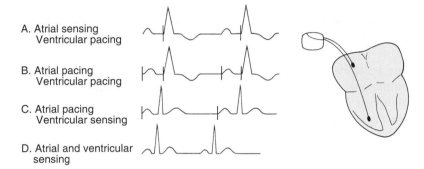

A. Atrial sensing
   Ventricular pacing

B. Atrial pacing
   Ventricular pacing

C. Atrial pacing
   Ventricular sensing

D. Atrial and ventricular
   sensing

Fig. 8.7 A dual-chamber *(DDD)* pacemaker senses and paces in both the atria and ventricles. The pacemaker emits a stimulus (spike) whenever an intrinsic P wave or QRS complex is not sensed within a programmed interval. (From Goldberger, A. L., Goldberger, Z. D., & Shvilkin, A. (2018). *Goldberger's clinical electrocardiography: A simplified approach* (9th ed.). Philadelphia: Elsevier.)

Failure to pace

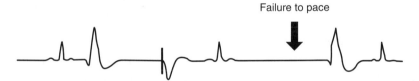

Fig. 8.8 Failure to pace. (From Wiegand, D. L. (2017). *AACN procedure manual for high acuity, progressive, and critical care* (7th ed.). St. Louis: Elsevier.)

pacemaker-induced dysrhythmias. Problems that can occur with pacing include failure to pace, failure to capture, and failure to sense (e.g., undersensing, oversensing).

Failure to Pace

Failure to pace, also referred to as failure to fire or failure of pulse generation, is a pacemaker malfunction that occurs when the pacemaker fails to deliver an electrical stimulus at its programmed time. Failure to pace is recognized on the ECG as an absence of pacemaker spikes, even though the patient's intrinsic rate is less than that of the pacemaker, and a return of the underlying rhythm for which pacing was initiated (Fig. 8.8). Patient signs and symptoms may include bradycardia, chest discomfort, hypotension, and syncope.

Causes of failure to pace are listed in Box 8.1. Treatment may include adjusting the sensitivity setting, replacing the pulse generator battery, replacing the pacing lead, replacing the pulse generator unit, tightening connections between the pulse generator unit, tightening connections between the

| Box 8.1 | Causes of Failure to Pace |

- Battery failure
- Broken or loose connection between the pacing lead and the pulse generator
- Displacement of the electrode tip
- Electromagnetic interference
- Fracture of the pacing lead wire
- Pulse generator failure
- Sensitivity set too high

pacing lead and pulse generator, or removing the source of electromagnetic interference.

Failure to Capture

Failure to capture is the inability of the artificial pacemaker stimulus to depolarize the myocardium. It is recognized on the ECG by visible pacemaker spikes not followed by

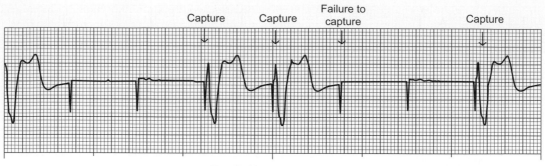

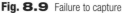

Fig. 8.9 Failure to capture.

P waves (if the electrode is in the atrium) or QRS complexes (if the electrode is in the right ventricle) (Fig. 8.9). Patient signs and symptoms may include bradycardia, fatigue, and hypotension.

Causes of failure to capture are shown in Box 8.2. If the problem results from low output energy, slowly increasing the output setting (mA) until capture occurs may resolve the problem. With transvenous pacing, repositioning the patient to the left side may promote the contact of a transvenous pacing lead with the endocardium and septum.

Failure to Sense

Sensitivity is the extent to which an artificial pacemaker recognizes intrinsic cardiac electrical activity. **Undersensing** occurs when the artificial pacemaker fails to recognize

Box **8.2**	**Causes of Failure to Capture**

- Battery failure
- Displacement of pacing lead wire (common cause)
- Edema or scar tissue formation at the electrode tip
- Faulty connections
- Fracture of the pacing lead wire
- Increased stimulation threshold as a result of medications or electrolyte imbalance
- Output energy (i.e., mA) set too low (common cause)
- Ventricular perforation

spontaneous myocardial depolarization. It is recognized on the ECG by pacemaker spikes that occur within P waves, pacemaker spikes that follow too closely behind the patient's QRS complexes, or pacemaker spikes that appear within T waves (Fig. 8.10). Because pacemaker spikes occur when they should not, this type of pacemaker malfunction may result in pacemaker spikes that fall on T waves (i.e., R-on-T phenomenon), competition between the pacemaker and the patient's intrinsic cardiac rhythm, or both. As a result, the patient may complain of palpitations or skipped beats.

Causes of failure to sense are shown in Box 8.3. Treatment may include increasing the sensitivity setting, replacing the pulse generator battery, or replacing or repositioning the pacing lead.

Oversensing is a pacemaker malfunction that results from inappropriate sensing of extraneous electrical signals. For example, atrial sensing pacemakers may inappropriately sense ventricular activity; ventricular sensing pacemakers may misidentify a tall, peaked intrinsic T wave as a QRS complex. Oversensing is recognized on the ECG as pacemaker spikes at a rate slower than the pacemaker's preset rate or no paced beats even though the pacemaker's preset rate is greater than the patient's intrinsic rate (Fig. 8.11). Treatment includes adjustment of the pacemaker's sensitivity setting or possible insertion of a bipolar lead if oversensing is caused by unipolar lead dysfunction.

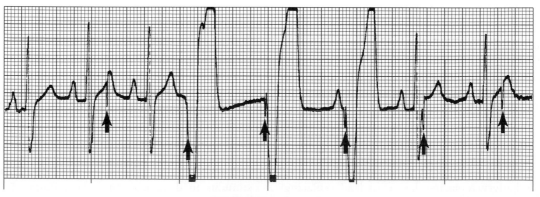

Fig. 8.10 Undersensing.

- Battery failure
- Circuitry dysfunction (e.g., pulse generator unable to process the QRS signal)
- Decreased P wave or QRS voltage
- Displacement of the electrode tip (most common cause)
- Fracture of the pacing lead wire
- Increased sensing threshold from antiarrhythmic medications
- Myocardial perforation
- Sensitivity setting too high
- Severe electrolyte disturbances

ANALYZING PACEMAKER FUNCTION ON THE ELECTROCARDIOGRAM

To practice analyzing pacemaker function on the ECG, let's look at Fig. 8.12. The first step in our analysis of this rhythm strip should include identification of the patient's underlying rhythm and its rate, if possible. Fig. 8.12 provides a look at the patient's rhythm from two leads, and six QRS complexes are visible in each lead. Each QRS complex is preceded by one upright P wave. Based on this information, we know that the underlying rhythm is sinus in origin. The atrial and ventricular rates are regular at 65 beats per minute (beats/min).

Next, let's look for evidence of paced activity (i.e., atrial pacer spikes, ventricular pacer spikes, or both) and evaluate the paced interval. The **paced interval**, also called the automatic interval, is the period between two consecutive paced events in the same cardiac chamber. Measure the distance between two consecutively paced atrial beats using calipers or paper when atrial pacer spikes are present. Because there is no pacemaker spike before any of the P waves in this rhythm strip, there is no evidence of paced atrial activity; however, a pacer spike is visible before each QRS complex.

Because paced ventricular activity is present, we must evaluate the rate and regularity of the ventricular paced interval by measuring the distance between two consecutively paced ventricular beats. The ventricular paced interval is regular at 65 pulses/min. If both atrial and ventricular pacemaker spikes were present, you would know that this patient had a dual-chamber pacemaker. Because only wide-QRS complexes are present and a pacemaker spike precedes each QRS, it is reasonable to conclude that this patient has a ventricular pacemaker. Next, compare the escape interval with the paced interval measured earlier. The **escape interval** is the time measured between a sensed cardiac event and the next pacemaker output. The paced interval and escape interval should measure the same; these intervals are the same in Fig. 8.12.

Next, analyze the rhythm strip for failure to pace, failure to capture, and failure to sense. Remember that the ECG will reveal an absence of pacemaker spikes at their programmed

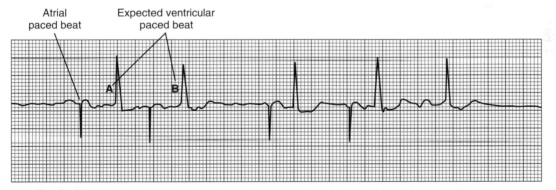

Fig. 8.11 Ventricular oversensing and possibly ventricular pulse generation failure. Ventricular spike expected at 150 msec. Ventricular spike and corresponding ventricular depolarization did not occur at points *A* and *B*. Also, atrial timing reset by oversensed ventricular activity resulted in erratic atrial pacing (suspicious for fracture of ventricular lead). (From Wiegand, D. L. (2017). *AACN procedure manual for high acuity, progressive, and critical care* (7th ed.). St. Louis: Elsevier.)

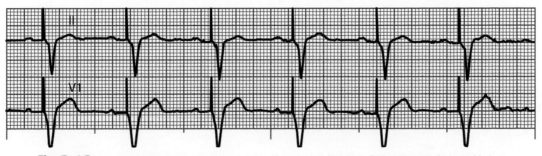

Fig. 8.12 Practice strip, analyzing pacemaker function. (From Aehlert, B. (2004). *ECG study cards.* St. Louis: Mosby.)

time with failure to pace. Because the pacer spikes in Fig. 8.12 occur regularly, we know that failure to pace is not present. When failure to capture occurs, pacer spikes appear regularly, but the waveforms after them are periodically absent (i.e., P waves are periodically absent if the pacing electrode is in the atrium, QRS complexes are periodically absent if the pacing electrode is in the ventricle). Because there is a 1:1 relationship between pacemaker spikes and QRS complexes in this rhythm strip, we know that 100% ventricular capture is present. When failure to sense exists, unexpected paced beats or unexpected pacer spikes are present (i.e., undersensing), or prolonged pauses are present (i.e., oversensing). Evaluation of the waveforms and pacer spikes in Fig. 8.12 reveals no unexpected beats, no unexpected pacer spikes, and no prolonged pauses; thus, failure to sense is not present.

Before we complete our interpretation, we should briefly discuss what looks like ST-segment elevation in this rhythm strip. The QRS complexes are negatively deflected (i.e., a QS configuration), and the ST segments and T waves are in the opposite direction of the last portion of the QRS complex. As you have learned, these findings are expected in ventricular rhythms and left bundle branch block (LBBB). Think of a

ventricular paced beat as a manmade LBBB. When LBBB occurs, the electrical impulse travels down the right bundle branch, depolarizes the right ventricle, and then spreads through the myocardium to depolarize the left ventricle. Pacemakers are most often introduced into the right ventricle. When a pacemaker fires, it sends its impulse into the right ventricle, which depolarizes, and the impulse is spread through the myocardium to depolarize the left ventricle. Therefore, just as with LBBB, ventricular paced rhythms may exhibit ST-segment elevation that is not the result of any infarct-related causes because ventricular depolarization is abnormal.

◑ ECG Pearl

Careful correlation of the patient's ECG, clinical presentation, and the results of other diagnostic studies are essential.

In summary, we will identify the rhythm strip in Fig. 8.12 as a sinus rhythm with a ventricular pacemaker and 100% capture with a paced interval of 65 pulses/min. If the patient's intrinsic rate differed from that of the pacemaker, we would include the paced rate in pulses per minute and the patient's heart rate in beats per minute in our rhythm description.

STOP & REVIEW

Matching

Match the terms below with their descriptions by placing the letter of each correct answer in the space provided.

a. AV interval
b. Oversensing
c. Dual chamber
d. Inhibition
e. Demand
f. Failure to capture
g. Lower rate limit
h. Pacemaker spike

i. Failure to pace
j. Rate modulation
k. Pulse generator
l. Undersensing
m. Threshold
n. Paced interval
o. Fixed rate

_____ **1.** A vertical line on the ECG that indicates the pacemaker has discharged

_____ **2.** A pacemaker malfunction that occurs when the artificial pacemaker fails to recognize spontaneous myocardial depolarization

_____ **3.** A pacemaker malfunction that occurs when the artificial pacemaker stimulus is unable to depolarize the myocardium

_____ **4.** The period between two consecutive paced events in the same cardiac chamber

_____ **5.** This type of pacemaker uses an atrial and ventricular lead

_____ **6.** An artificial PR interval

_____ **7.** This type of pacemaker discharges only when the patient's heart rate drops below the preset rate for the pacemaker

_____ **8.** The ability of a pacemaker to increase the pacing rate in response to physical activity or metabolic demand

_____ **9.** This type of pacemaker continuously discharges at a preset rate regardless of the patient's intrinsic activity

_____ **10.** A pacemaker malfunction that results from inappropriate sensing of extraneous electrical signals

_____ **11.** The power source that houses the battery and circuitry for regulating a pacemaker

_____ **12.** The rate at which the pacemaker's pulse generator initiates impulses when no intrinsic activity is detected; expressed in pulses per minute

_____ **13.** The minimum amount of voltage (i.e., milliamperes) needed to obtain consistent capture

_____ **14.** Pacemaker response in which the output pulse is suppressed when an intrinsic event is sensed

_____ **15.** A pacemaker malfunction that occurs when the pacemaker fails to deliver an electrical stimulus at its programmed time

Pacemaker Rhythms—Practice Rhythm Strips

For each of the following rhythm strips, identify the patient's underlying rhythm (if possible); determine the presence of atrial paced activity, ventricular paced activity, or both; and then analyze the rhythm strip for pacemaker malfunction. All rhythm strips were recorded in lead II unless otherwise noted.

16. These rhythm strips are from a 52-year-old man with syncope.

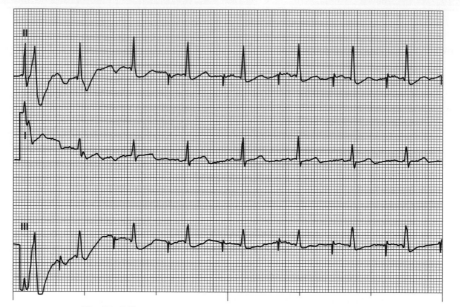

Fig. 8.13 (From Aehlert, B. (2004). *ECG study cards.* St. Louis: Mosby.)

Atrial paced activity? _____ Ventricular paced activity? _____
Pacemaker malfunction? _____ Interpretation: _____

17. Identify the rhythm.

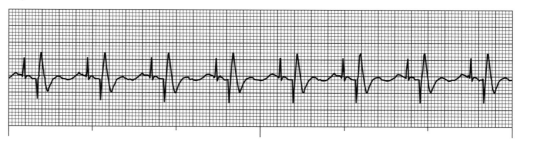

Fig. 8.14 (From Aehlert, B. (2004). *ECG study cards.* St. Louis: Mosby.)

Atrial paced activity? _____ Ventricular paced activity? _____
Pacemaker malfunction? _____ Interpretation: _____

18. Identify the rhythm.

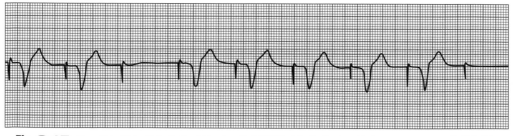

Fig. 8.15 (From Sole, M. L., Klein, D. G., & Moseley, M. J. (2008). *Introduction to critical care nursing* (5th ed.). Philadelphia: Saunders.)

Atrial paced activity? _____ Ventricular paced activity? _____
Pacemaker malfunction? _____ Interpretation: _____

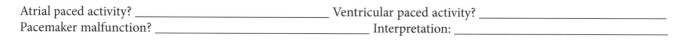

19. These rhythm strips are from a 63-year-old man with epigastric pain.

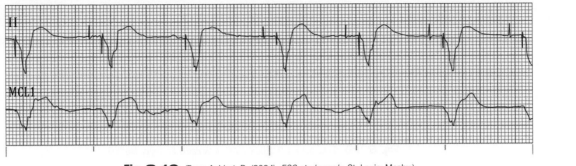

Fig. 8.16 (From Aehlert, B. (2004). *ECG study cards.* St. Louis: Mosby.)

Atrial paced activity? _____ Ventricular paced activity? _____
Pacemaker malfunction? _____ Interpretation: _____

20. This rhythm strip is from a 97-year-old man with chest pain.

Fig. 8.17 (From Aehlert, B. (2004). *ECG study cards.* St. Louis: Mosby.)

Atrial paced activity? _____ Ventricular paced activity? _____
Pacemaker malfunction? _____ Interpretation: _____

21. Identify the rhythm.

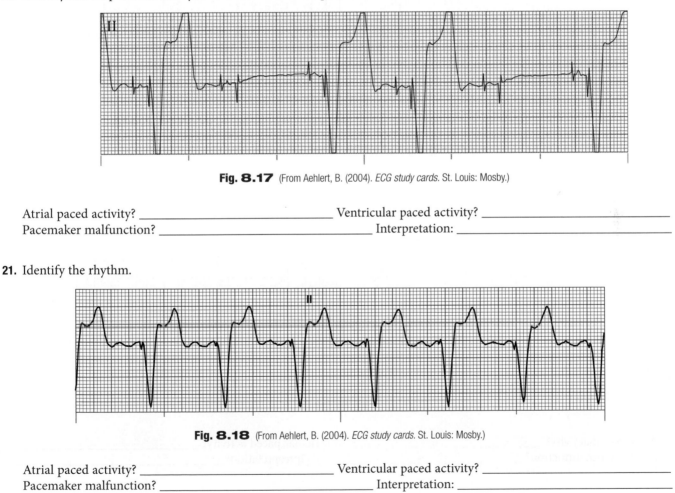

Fig. 8.18 (From Aehlert, B. (2004). *ECG study cards.* St. Louis: Mosby.)

Atrial paced activity? _____ Ventricular paced activity? _____
Pacemaker malfunction? _____ Interpretation: _____

22. Identify the rhythm.

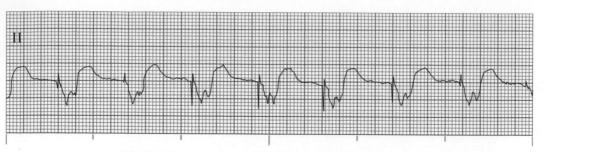

Fig. 8.19 (From Aehlert, B. (2004). *ECG study cards.* St. Louis: Mosby.)

Atrial paced activity? _____ Ventricular paced activity? _____
Pacemaker malfunction? _____ Interpretation: _____

23. Identify the rhythm.

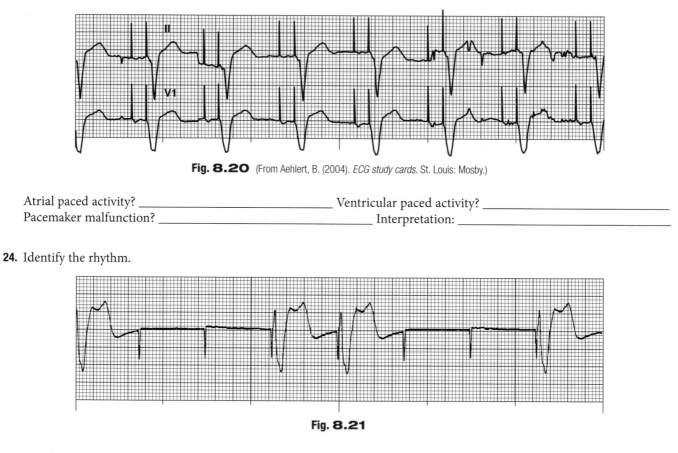

Fig. 8.20 (From Aehlert, B. (2004). *ECG study cards.* St. Louis: Mosby.)

Atrial paced activity? _____ Ventricular paced activity? _____
Pacemaker malfunction? _____ Interpretation: _____

24. Identify the rhythm.

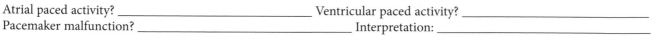

Fig. 8.21

Atrial paced activity? _____ Ventricular paced activity? _____
Pacemaker malfunction? _____ Interpretation: _____

25. This rhythm strip is from a 90-year-old woman with shortness of breath.

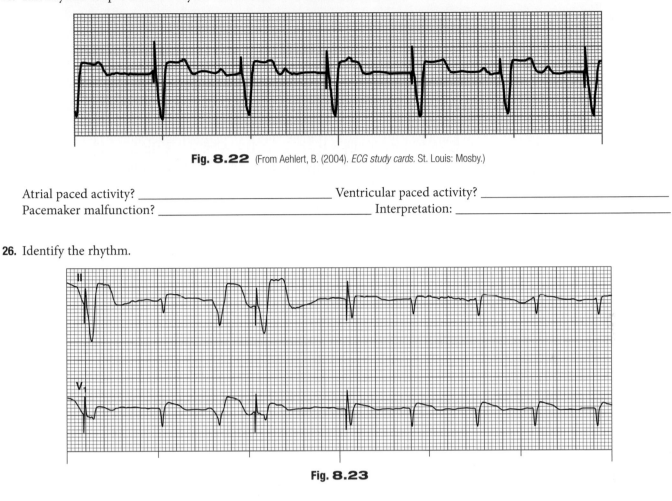

Fig. 8.22 (From Aehlert, B. (2004). *ECG study cards.* St. Louis: Mosby.)

Atrial paced activity? _____ Ventricular paced activity? _____
Pacemaker malfunction? _____ Interpretation: _____

26. Identify the rhythm.

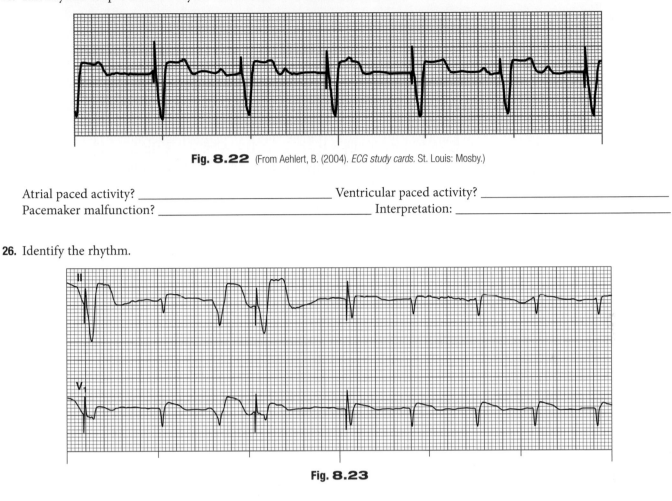

Fig. 8.23

Atrial paced activity? _____ Ventricular paced activity? _____
Pacemaker malfunction? _____ Interpretation: _____

27. Identify the rhythm.

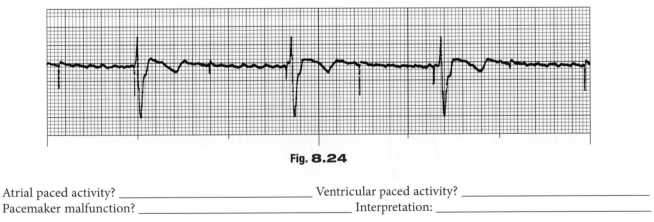

Fig. 8.24

Atrial paced activity? _____ Ventricular paced activity? _____
Pacemaker malfunction? _____ Interpretation: _____

28. Identify the rhythm.

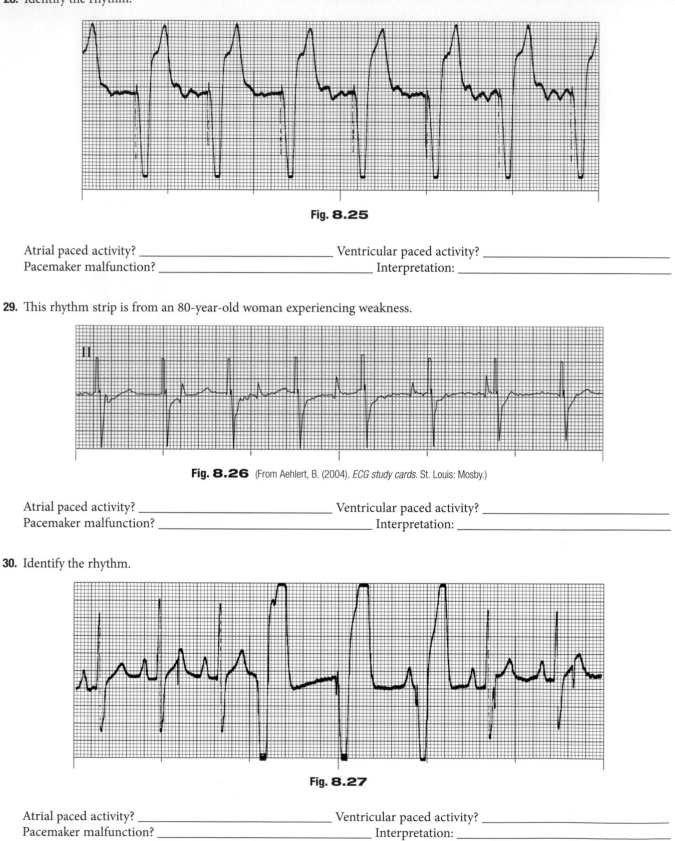

Fig. 8.25

Atrial paced activity? _____ Ventricular paced activity? _____
Pacemaker malfunction? _____ Interpretation: _____

29. This rhythm strip is from an 80-year-old woman experiencing weakness.

Fig. 8.26 (From Aehlert, B. (2004). *ECG study cards.* St. Louis: Mosby.)

Atrial paced activity? _____ Ventricular paced activity? _____
Pacemaker malfunction? _____ Interpretation: _____

30. Identify the rhythm.

Fig. 8.27

Atrial paced activity? _____ Ventricular paced activity? _____
Pacemaker malfunction? _____ Interpretation: _____

STOP & REVIEW ANSWERS

Matching

1. ANS: h
2. ANS: l
3. ANS: f
4. ANS: n
5. ANS: c
6. ANS: a
7. ANS: e
8. ANS: j
9. ANS: o
10. ANS: b
11. ANS: k
12. ANS: g
13. ANS: m
14. ANS: d
15. ANS: i

Practice Rhythm Strip Answers

Note: The rate and interval measurements provided here were obtained using electronic calipers.

16. Fig. 8.13
    Atrial paced activity? Yes
    Ventricular paced activity? No
    Pacemaker malfunction? No
    Interpretation: Atrial paced rhythm with 100% capture at 79 pulses/min

17. Fig. 8.14
    Atrial paced activity? Yes
    Ventricular paced activity? Yes
    Pacemaker malfunction? No
    Interpretation: Dual-chamber pacemaker rhythm with 100% capture at 79 pulses/min

18. Fig. 8.15
    Atrial paced activity? No
    Ventricular paced activity? Yes
    Pacemaker malfunction? Yes—failure to capture; seven of nine paced impulses captured
    Interpretation: Ventricular paced rhythm at 65 pulses/min with failure to capture

19. Fig. 8.16
    Atrial paced activity? Yes
    Ventricular paced activity? Yes
    Pacemaker malfunction? No
    Interpretation: Dual-chamber pacemaker rhythm with 100% capture at 88 pulses/min

20. Fig. 8.17
    Atrial paced activity? Yes
    Ventricular paced activity? Yes
    Pacemaker malfunction? Yes—failure to capture; four of six paced impulses captured
    Interpretation: Dual-chamber pacemaker rhythm at 60 pulses/min with failure to capture

21. Fig. 8.18
    Atrial paced activity? No
    Ventricular paced activity? Yes
    Pacemaker malfunction? No
    Interpretation: Ventricular paced rhythm with 100% capture at 68 pulses/min

22. Fig. 8.19
    Atrial paced activity? No
    Ventricular paced activity? Yes
    Pacemaker malfunction? No
    Interpretation: Ventricular paced rhythm with 100% capture at 80 pulses/min

23. Fig. 8.20
    Atrial paced activity? Yes
    Ventricular paced activity? Yes
    Pacemaker malfunction? No
    Interpretation: Dual-chamber pacemaker rhythm with 100% capture at 71 pulses/min

24. Fig. 8.21
    Atrial paced activity? No
    Ventricular paced activity? Yes
    Pacemaker malfunction? Yes—failure to capture; three of seven paced impulses captured (the first complex is not counted because the pacer spike before the complex is not visible)
    Interpretation: Ventricular paced rhythm at 79 pulses/min with failure to capture

25. Fig. 8.22
    Atrial paced activity? No
    Ventricular paced activity? Yes
    Pacemaker malfunction? No
    Interpretation: Ventricular-paced rhythm with 100% capture at 60 pulses/min; underlying rhythm appears to be a third-degree AV block

26. Fig. 8.23
    Atrial paced activity? No
    Ventricular paced activity? Yes
    Pacemaker malfunction? No
    Interpretation: Ventricular demand pacemaker at 60 pulses/min; underlying rhythm appears to be atrial fibrillation

27. Fig. 8.24
    Atrial paced activity? No
    Ventricular paced activity? Yes
    Pacemaker malfunction? Yes—failure to capture; three of eight paced impulses captured
    Interpretation: Ventricular demand pacemaker rhythm at 72 pulses/min with failure to capture

28. Fig. 8.25

Atrial paced activity? No
Ventricular paced activity? Yes
Pacemaker malfunction? No
Interpretation: Ventricular paced rhythm with 100% capture at 74 pulses/min; underlying rhythm appears to be atrial flutter

29. Fig. 8.26

Atrial paced activity? No
Ventricular paced activity? Yes
Pacemaker malfunction? No
Interpretation: Ventricular paced rhythm with 100% capture at 83 pulses/min

30. Fig. 8.27

Atrial paced activity? No
Ventricular paced activity? Yes
Pacemaker malfunction? Yes—failure to sense (undersensing)
Interpretation: Sinus rhythm at 88 beats/min with a ventricular pacemaker and pacemaker malfunction (undersensing); note the pacer spikes in the T waves of the second and eighth beats from the left

Introduction to the 12-Lead ECG

9

LEARNING OBJECTIVES

After reading this chapter, you should be able to:

1. Give examples of indications for using a 12-lead electrocardiogram (ECG).
2. Explain the term *electrical axis* and its significance.
3. Discuss the determination of electrical axis using leads I and aVF.
4. Recognize the changes on the ECG that may reflect evidence of myocardial ischemia, injury, or infarction.
5. Describe the appearance of right and left bundle branch block as seen in lead V_1.
6. Discuss the ECG changes characteristic of right atrial, left atrial, right ventricular, and left ventricular enlargement.
7. Identify the ECG changes characteristically produced by hyperkalemia, hypokalemia, hypercalcemia, and hypocalcemia.
8. Describe a systematic method for analyzing a 12-lead ECG.

KEY TERMS

bundle branch block (BBB): A disruption in impulse conduction from the bundle of His through the right or left bundle branch to the Purkinje fibers; a BBB may be intermittent or permanent.

electrical axis: Net direction, or angle in degrees, where the main vector of depolarization is pointed.

vector: Quantity having direction and magnitude, usually depicted by a straight arrow whose length represents magnitude and whose head represents direction.

INTRODUCTION

A standard 12-lead electrocardiogram (ECG) provides views of the heart in both the frontal and horizontal planes and views the surfaces of the left ventricle from 12 different angles. Multiple views of the heart can provide helpful information including the following:

- Identification of ST-segment and T-wave changes associated with myocardial ischemia, injury, and infarction
- Identification of ECG changes associated with certain medications and electrolyte imbalances
- Recognition of bundle branch blocks (BBBs)

Indications for obtaining a 12-lead ECG are shown in Box 9.1.

LAYOUT OF THE 12-LEAD ELECTROCARDIOGRAM

Most 12-lead ECGs are displayed in a conventional three-row by four-column format. The standard limb leads are recorded in the first column, the augmented limb leads in the second column, and the chest leads in the third and fourth columns (Table 9.1).

The 12-lead ECG provides a 2.5-second view of each lead because it is assumed that 2.5 seconds is long enough to capture at least one representative complex. Although most 12-lead ECG machines obtain the signals for all leads at the same time, other machines obtain the signals sequentially (i.e., all limb leads, then the augmented limb

Box 9.1	Indications for Obtaining a 12-Lead ECG

- Abdominal or epigastric pain
- Assisting in dysrhythmia interpretation
- Chest pain or discomfort
- Diabetic ketoacidosis
- Dizziness
- Dyspnea
- Electrical injuries
- Known or suspected electrolyte imbalances
- Known or suspected medication overdoses
- Right or left ventricular failure
- Status before and after electrical therapy (e.g., defibrillation, cardioversion, pacing)
- Stroke
- Syncope or near syncope
- Unstable patient, unknown etiology

TABLE 9.1	Layout of a Four-Column 12-Lead ECG		
Limb Leads		**Chest Leads**	
Standard Leads	Augmented Leads	V_1 to V_3	V_4 to V_6
Column I	Column II	Column III	Column IV
I: Lateral	aVR: None	V_1: Septum	V_4: Anterior
II: Inferior	aVL: Lateral	V_2: Septum	V_5: Lateral
III: Inferior	aVF: Inferior	V_3: Anterior	V_6: Lateral

leads followed by leads V_1 through V_3, and finally leads V_4 through V_6). The 12-lead computer's interpretive program provides measurements of intervals and duration in milliseconds (msec). An example of a 12-lead ECG is shown in Fig. 9.1.

VECTORS

Leads have a negative (−) and positive (+) electrode pole that senses the magnitude and direction of the electrical force caused by the spread of waves of depolarization and repolarization throughout the myocardium. A *vector* (arrow) is a symbol representing this force. A vector points in the direction of depolarization. Leads that face the tip or point of a vector record a positive deflection on ECG paper. A mean vector identifies the average of depolarization waves in one portion of the heart. The mean P vector represents the average magnitude and direction of both right and left atrial depolarization. The mean QRS vector represents the average magnitude and direction of both right and left ventricular depolarization. The average direction of a mean vector is called the *mean axis* and is only identified in the frontal plane.

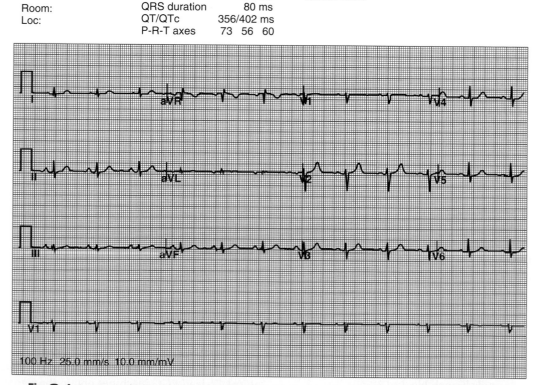

Female Caucasian	Vent. rate	77 bpm	Normal sinus rhythm	
	PR interval	156 ms	Normal ECG	
Room:	QRS duration	80 ms		
Loc:	QT/QTc	356/402 ms		
	P-R-T axes	73 56 60		

100 Hz 25.0 mm/s 10.0 mm/mV

Fig. 9.1 An example of a 12-lead electrocardiogram *(ECG)*. Note the four-column format used on the majority of the page. A continuous recording of lead V_1 is shown at the bottom of the page. (From Phalen, T., & Aehlert, B. J. (2019). *The 12-lead ECG in acute coronary syndromes* (4th ed.). St. Louis: Mosby.)

Axis

An imaginary line joining the positive and negative electrodes of a lead is called the axis of the lead. **Electrical axis** refers to the net direction, or angle in degrees, where the main vector of depolarization is pointed. When *axis* is used by itself, it refers to the QRS axis.

During normal ventricular depolarization, the left side of the interventricular septum is stimulated first. The electrical impulse then crosses the septum to stimulate the right side. The left and right ventricles are then depolarized simultaneously. Because the left ventricle is considerably larger than the right, right ventricular depolarization forces are overshadowed on the ECG. As a result, the mean QRS vector points down (i.e., inferior) and to the left.

The axes of leads I, II, and III form an equilateral triangle with the heart at the center (i.e., Einthoven's triangle) (Fig. 9.2A). Einthoven's law states that the sum of the electrical currents recorded in leads I and III equals the sum of the electrical current recorded in lead II, which can be expressed as lead I + lead III = lead II.

If the augmented limb leads are added to the equilateral triangle, and the axes of the six leads are moved in a way in which they bisect each other, the result is the hexaxial reference system (Fig. 9.2B). The hexaxial reference system represents all of the frontal plane (limb) leads with the heart in the center and is the means used to express the location of the frontal plane axis. This system forms a 360-degree circle surrounding the heart. The positive end of lead I is designated at 0 degrees. The six frontal plane leads divide the circle into segments, each representing 30 degrees. All degrees in the upper hemisphere are labeled as negative degrees, and all degrees in the lower hemisphere are labeled as positive degrees (Fig. 9.2C).

The axes of some leads are perpendicular to each other in the hexaxial reference system. For example, lead I is perpendicular to lead aVF. Lead II is perpendicular to aVL, and lead III is perpendicular to aVR. If the electrical force moves toward a positive electrode, a positive (i.e., upright) deflection will be recorded. If the electrical force moves away from a positive electrode, a negative (i.e., downward) deflection will be recorded. If the electrical force is parallel to a given lead, the largest deflection in that lead will be recorded. If the electrical force is perpendicular to a lead axis, the resulting ECG complex will be isoelectric, equiphasic, or both in that lead. Notice that leads III and aVL are positioned on opposite (i.e., reciprocal) sides of the hexaxial reference system (Fig. 9.3). Axis determination can provide clues in the differential diagnosis of wide QRS tachycardia and localization of accessory pathways.

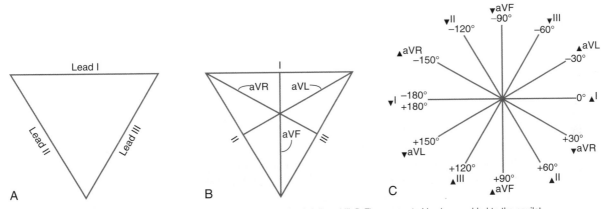

Fig. 9.2 A, Einthoven's equilateral triangle formed by leads I, II, and III. B, The augmented leads are added to the equilateral triangle. C, The hexaxial reference system derived from *B*. (From Chou, I., & Ramaiah, L. S. (1996). *Electrocardiography in clinical practice: Adult and pediatric* (4th ed.). Philadelphia: Saunders.)

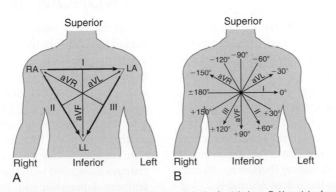

Fig. 9.3 Axis of electrical activation. A, Vectors for the limb leads in the frontal plane. B, Hexaxial reference for determining the frontal plane axis. Note that the vectors for leads I, II, and III are in the same direction as in *A*, but now, similar to the augmented limb leads, these standard limb lead vectors have been moved so that they emanate from the center of the figure. (From Goldman, L., Schafer, A.I., Crow, M.K., Davidson, N.E., Drazen, J.M., Griggs, R.C., Landry, D.W., Levinson, W., Rustgi, A.K., Scheld, W.M., Spiegel, A.M. (2020). *Goldman-Cecil medicine* (26th ed.). Philadelphia: Elsevier.)

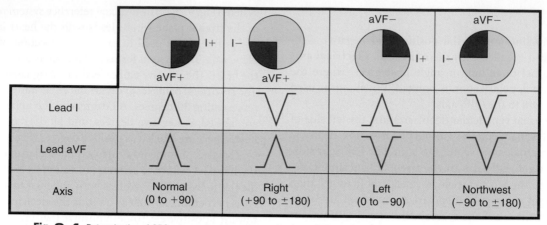

	aVF+	aVF+	aVF− / I+	aVF− / I−
Lead I	Λ	V	Λ	V
Lead aVF	Λ	Λ	V	V
Axis	Normal (0 to +90)	Right (+90 to ±180)	Left (0 to −90)	Northwest (−90 to ±180)

Fig. 9.4 Determination of QRS axis quadrant by noting predominant QRS polarity in leads I and aVF. Normal axis: If the QRS is primarily positive in both I and aVF, the axis falls within the normal quadrant from 0 to 90 degrees. Right axis deviation: If the QRS complex is primarily negative in I and positive in aVF, right axis deviation is present. Left axis deviation: If the QRS complex is predominantly positive in I and negative in aVF, left axis deviation is present. Indeterminate axis: If the QRS is primarily negative in both I and aVF, a markedly abnormal "indeterminate" or "northwest" axis is present. (From Urden, L. D., Stacy, K. M., & Lough, M. E. (2014). *Critical care nursing* (7th ed.). St. Louis: Mosby.)

To determine the electrical axis, look at the 12-lead ECG in Fig. 9.1. Because the hexaxial reference system is derived from the limb leads, we will be focusing on the leads shown in the two columns on the left side of the figure (leads I, II, III, aVR, aVL, and aVF). Look for the most equiphasic or isoelectric QRS complexes in these leads. Lead aVL shows QRS complexes that most closely reflect our criteria. The patient's QRS axis is perpendicular to the positive electrode in lead aVL.

Look at the hexaxial reference system diagram (see Fig. 9.3) to determine which ECG lead is perpendicular to lead aVL. Lead II is perpendicular to lead aVL. Now we know that the patient's QRS axis is moving along the same vector as lead II. Note that the values associated with lead II in the hexaxial reference system diagram are −120 degrees and +60 degrees. To determine if the QRS axis is moving positively or negatively, look at lead II in Fig. 9.1 and determine if the QRS complex is primarily positive or negative in this lead. You will see that the QRS is primarily positive in lead II; therefore, this patient's QRS axis is about +60 degrees. At the top of Fig. 9.1, you will see the computer's calculation of the patient's P-QRS-T axes. The computer calculated the patient's QRS axis at +56 degrees. Our estimate of +60 degrees was very close!

In adults, the normal QRS axis is considered to be between −30 and +90 degrees in the frontal plane. Current flow to the right of normal is called *right axis deviation* (between +90 and ±180 degrees). Current flow in the direction opposite of normal is called *indeterminate*, "no man's land," *northwest*, or *extreme right axis deviation* (between −90 and ±180 degrees). Current flow to the left of normal is called *left axis deviation* (between −30 and −90 degrees).

Shortcuts exist to determine axis deviation. Leads I and aVF divide the heart into four quadrants. These two leads can be used to quickly estimate the electrical axis. In leads I and aVF, the QRS complex is normally positive. If the QRS complex in either or both of these leads is negative, axis deviation is present (Fig. 9.4).

Right axis deviation may be a normal variant, particularly in the young and in thin individuals. Other causes of right axis deviation include mechanical shifts associated with inspiration or emphysema, right ventricular hypertrophy (RVH), chronic obstructive pulmonary disease (COPD), Wolff-Parkinson-White syndrome, and pulmonary embolism.

Left axis deviation may be a normal variant, particularly in older and obese individuals. Other causes of left axis deviation include mechanical shifts associated with expiration; a high diaphragm caused by pregnancy, ascites, or abdominal tumors; hyperkalemia; emphysema; left atrial hypertrophy; and dextrocardia.

ACUTE CORONARY SYNDROMES

Recall that acute coronary syndromes (ACSs) are conditions caused by an abrupt reduction in coronary artery blood flow. Partial or intermittent blockage of a coronary artery may result in no clinical signs and symptoms (silent ischemia), unstable angina (UA), non–ST-elevation MI (NSTEMI), or possibly, sudden death. Complete blockage of a coronary artery may result in ST-elevation MI (STEMI) or sudden death. UA and NSTEMI are often grouped as non–ST-elevation acute coronary syndromes (NSTE-ACS) because ECG changes associated with these conditions usually include ST-segment depression and T-wave inversion in the leads that face the affected area. Cardiac biomarkers (e.g., troponins) are elevated when an infarction is present. Biomarkers are not elevated in patients with UA because there is no tissue death.

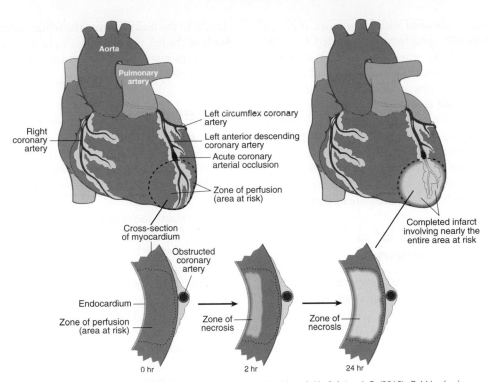

Fig. 9.5 Progression of a myocardial infarction. (From Kumar, V., Abbas, A. K., & Aster, J. C. (2018). *Robbins basic pathology* (10th ed.). Philadelphia: Elsevier.)

The diagnosis of an ACS is made based on the patient's clinical presentation, history, ECG findings, and cardiac biomarker results. If ST segments are elevated in two contiguous leads, and elevated cardiac biomarkers are present, the diagnosis is STEMI. If ST-segment elevation (STE) is not present, but biomarker levels are elevated, the diagnosis is NSTEMI. If the ST segments and cardiac biomarkers are not elevated, the diagnosis is UA.

Time is muscle when caring for any patient with an ACS. The region of the heart supplied by the blocked artery is called the *area at risk* (Fig. 9.5). The longer the area at risk is deprived of oxygen and nutrients, the greater the likelihood of permanent damage. Therefore, if myocardium is to be saved, the blockage must be removed before irreversible tissue death occurs. If blood flow is quickly restored, the area at risk can potentially be salvaged. Of the patients experiencing ACSs, those experiencing a STEMI are most likely to benefit from reperfusion therapy. The benefits of reperfusion therapy are often time dependent. The primary choices for reperfusion therapy are fibrinolysis and percutaneous coronary intervention (PCI). Fibrinolytics are medications that are administered to break up blood clots. A PCI is a procedure in which a catheter is used to open a coronary artery blocked or narrowed by coronary artery disease.

The area supplied by a blocked coronary artery goes through a sequence of events that have been identified as zones of ischemia, injury, and infarction. Each zone is associated with characteristic ECG changes that affect the shape of the QRS complex, the ST segment, and the T wave (Fig. 9.6).

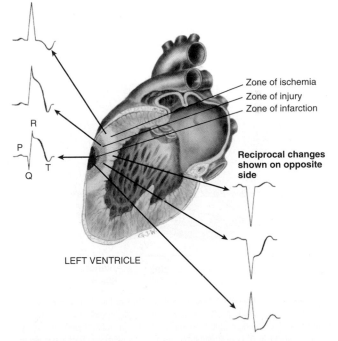

Fig. 9.6 Zones of ischemia, injury, and infarction showing indicative electrocardiogram changes and reciprocal changes corresponding to each zone. (Modified from Urden, L. D., Stacy, K. M., & Lough, M. E. (2014). *Critical care nursing* (7th ed.). St. Louis: Mosby.)

Because most infarctions occur in the left ventricle and a standard 12-lead ECG views the surfaces of the left ventricle from multiple angles, obtaining and reviewing a 12-lead ECG are essential components of the initial care provided to a patient presenting with ischemic chest discomfort. The first

12-lead ECG should be obtained with 10 minutes of patient contact in all patients with symptoms of suspected ACS. Obtain a repeat 12-lead ECG when the patient's condition changes and as often as necessary. After the 12-lead ECG has been obtained, carefully review it for signs of ischemia, injury, and infarction. Look closely at each lead for STE or ST-segment depression. If present, compare the ST segment deviation to the isoelectric line using the TP segment for this comparison and document the degree of displacement in millimeters. Examine the T waves for any changes in orientation, shape, and size. Next, look at each lead for the presence of a Q wave. If a Q wave is present, measure its duration.

Anatomic Location of a Myocardial Infarction

The left ventricle has been divided into regions where a myocardial infarction (MI) may occur: septal, anterior, lateral, inferior, and inferobasal (i.e., posterior). You will recall that ECG changes are considered significant if viewed in two or more anatomically contiguous leads (Fig. 9.7). Color has been added to Table 9.2 so you can quickly recognize contiguous lead groups.

In the standard 12-lead ECG, leads II, III, and aVF view the inferior wall of the left ventricle, which is supplied by the right coronary artery (RCA) in most people. Therefore, if an ECG shows STE in these leads, it is reasonable to suppose that these ECG changes are caused by a partial or complete blockage of the RCA. Likewise, when indicative changes

appear in the leads viewing the septal, anterior, and/or lateral walls of the left ventricle (i.e., V_1 to V_6, I, and aVL), it is reasonable to suspect that the left coronary artery is partially or entirely blocked.

ECG Pearl

I See **A**ll **L**eads is a commonly used mnemonic to recall the lead groupings when localizing an infarction and predicting which coronary artery is occluded. **I** (inferior) = II, III, aVF; **S** (septal) = V_1, V_2; **A** (anterior) = V_3, V_4; **L** (lateral) = I, aVL, V_5, V_6.

To evaluate the relative extent or size of an infarction, determine how many leads show indicative changes. An ECG showing changes in only a few leads suggests a smaller infarction than one that produces changes in many leads. In general, the more proximal the blockage in the vessel, the larger the infarction and the greater the number of leads showing indicative changes. Table 9.3 summarizes the pattern in which coronary arteries most commonly supply the myocardium.

It is important to emphasize that the approach discussed here concerning the localization of an infarction (i.e., determining which and how many coronary arteries are affected) works reasonably well for STEMI. However, ST-segment depression and T-wave changes that suggest the presence of myocardial ischemia, as in NSTE-ACS, are less reliable in localizing the culprit vessel because these ECG changes reflect subendocardial rather than transmural ischemia (Halim et al., 2010). Furthermore, recognition of STEMI can be tricky in the presence of right BBBs (RBBBs) and left BBBs (LBBBs), left ventricular hypertrophy (LVH), pericarditis, and paced

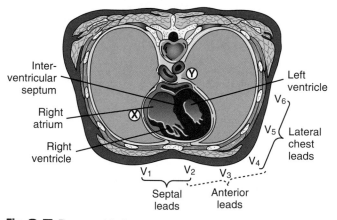

Fig. 9.7 The areas of the heart as seen by the chest leads. Leads V_1, V_2, and V_3 are contiguous. Leads V_3, V_4, and V_5 are contiguous, as well as V_4, V_5, and V_6. Note that neither the right ventricular wall *(X)* nor the inferobasal (posterior) surface of the left ventricle *(Y)* is well visualized by any of the usual six chest leads. (From Grauer, K. (1998). *A practical guide to ECG interpretation* (2nd ed.). St. Louis: Mosby.)

TABLE 9.2	Localizing ECG Changes		
I: Lateral	aVR: None	V_1: Septum	V_4: Anterior
II: Inferior	aVL: Lateral	V_2: Septum	V_5: Lateral
III: Inferior	aVF: Inferior	V_3: Anterior	V_6: Lateral

TABLE 9.3	Localizing a Myocardial Infarction	
MI Location	**ECG Leads**	**Probable Culprit Coronary Artery**
Anterior wall	Indicative changes: V_3, V_4 Reciprocal changes: III, aVF	LAD
Ventricular septum	Indicative changes: V_1, V_2	LAD
Lateral wall	Indicative changes: I, aVL, V_5, V_6 Reciprocal changes: II, III, aVF (if high lateral MI)	Cx, LAD, or RCA
Inferior wall	Indicative changes: II, III, aVF Reciprocal changes: I, aVL	RCA (most common) or Cx
Inferobasal (posterior) wall	Indicative changes: V_7, V_8, V_9 Reciprocal changes: V_1, V_2, V_3	RCA or Cx
Right ventricle	Indicative changes: V_1R to V_6R Reciprocal changes: I, aVL	RCA

Cx, Circumflex artery; *ECG,* electrocardiogram; *LAD,* left anterior descending artery; *MI,* myocardial infarction; *RCA,* right coronary.

ventricular rhythms because these conditions can cause STE, mimicking STEMI. Factors including the anatomic position and size of the heart, the patient's unique pattern of coronary artery distribution, the location of the occlusion along the length of the coronary artery, the presence of collateral circulation, previous infarctions, and related drug- and electrolyte-related ECG changes may also affect the perceived location of an infarction versus its actual location.

⊘ ECG Pearl

It is important to remember that some areas of the heart are not shown on a standard 12-lead ECG. It is also essential to recall that some infarctions do not show changes on the 12-lead ECG. Therefore, if infarct changes are seen on the 12-lead ECG, the greater the number of leads showing indicative changes, the larger the infarction. But if the patient presents with signs and symptoms suggestive of an ACS and the 12-lead ECG does not show indicative changes, an MI cannot be ruled out based solely on the ECG findings.

ANTERIOR INFARCTION

The left main coronary artery supplies the left anterior descending (LAD) artery and the circumflex (Cx) artery (Fig. 9.8). Blockage of the proximal portion of the LAD artery (i.e., the "widow maker") often leads to cardiogenic shock and death if reperfusion does not occur promptly.

An anterior myocardial infarction occurs when the blood supply to the LAD artery is disrupted (Fig. 9.9). Evidence of an anterior MI can be seen in leads V_3 and V_4, which face the anterior wall of the left ventricle. Septal involvement is evidenced by changes in leads V_1 and V_2 (Fig. 9.10). If an infarction involves the anterior wall and septum, ECG changes will be visible in V_1, V_2, V_3, and V_4, and the descriptive name *anteroseptal MI* is used (Fig. 9.11).

Because the LAD artery supplies a large portion of the left ventricle, a blockage in this area can lead to more widespread myocardial damage and complications (e.g., heart failure, cardiogenic shock) than infarctions involving other areas of the heart. Increased sympathetic nervous system activity is common with anterior MIs with resulting sinus

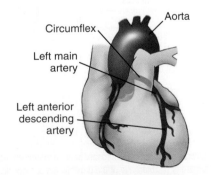

Fig. 9.8 The left main coronary artery supplies the left anterior descending artery and the circumflex artery. (From Phalen, T., & Aehlert, B. J. (2019). *The 12-lead ECG in acute coronary syndromes* (4th ed.). St. Louis: Mosby.)

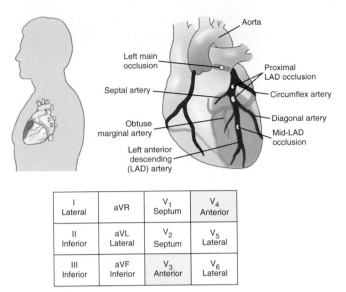

I Lateral	aVR	V₁ Septum	V₄ Anterior
II Inferior	aVL Lateral	V₂ Septum	V₅ Lateral
III Inferior	aVF Inferior	V₃ Anterior	V₆ Lateral

Fig. 9.9 Anterior infarction. Occlusion of the midportion of the left anterior descending *(LAD)* artery results in an anterior infarction. Proximal occlusion of the LAD may become an anteroseptal infarction if the septal branch is involved or an anterolateral infarction if the marginal branch is involved. An extensive anterior infarction will result if the occlusion occurs proximal to both the septal and diagonal branches. (From Phalen, T., & Aehlert, B. J. (2019). *The 12-lead ECG in acute coronary syndromes* (4th ed.). St. Louis: Mosby.)

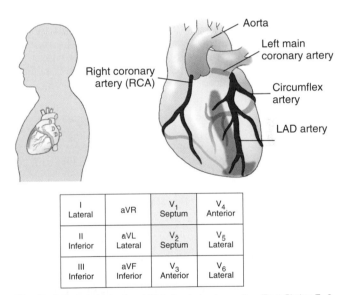

I Lateral	aVR	V₁ Septum	V₄ Anterior
II Inferior	aVL Lateral	V₂ Septum	V₅ Lateral
III Inferior	aVF Inferior	V₃ Anterior	V₆ Lateral

Fig. 9.10 Septal infarction. *LAD*, Left anterior descending. (From Phalen, T., & Aehlert, B. J. (2019). *The 12-lead ECG in acute coronary syndromes* (4th ed.). St. Louis: Mosby.)

tachycardia, hypertension, or both. A blockage in the septal area may result in BBBs, second-degree atrioventricular (AV) block type II, and third-degree AV block. BBBs are discussed later in this chapter.

R-Wave Progression

The wave of ventricular depolarization in the major portions of the ventricles is normally from right to left and in an anterior to posterior direction. When viewing the chest leads in a normal heart, the R wave becomes taller (i.e., increases

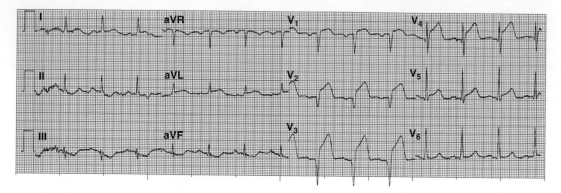

Fig. 9.11 Anteroseptal infarction. Note the ST-segment elevation in leads V_1 through V_4. (From Phalen, T., & Aehlert, B. J. (2019). *The 12-lead ECG in acute coronary syndromes* (4th ed.). St. Louis: Mosby.)

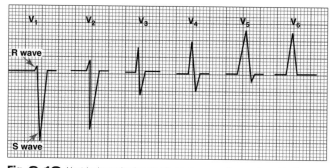

Fig. 9.12 Ventricular activation and R-wave progression as viewed in the chest leads. In normal R-wave progression, the QRS complex is negative in V_1, positive in V_6, and switches from negative to positive in the V_3 to V_4 transition zone. (From Sole, M. L., Klein, D. G., & Moseley, M. J. (2017). *Introduction to critical care nursing* (7th ed.). St. Louis: Elsevier.)

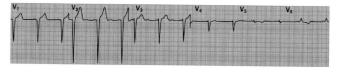

Fig. 9.13 Poor R-wave progression in V_1 through V_4; QRS greater than 0.12 second; and left bundle branch block. (From Khan, M. (1997). *Rapid ECG interpretation*. Philadelphia: Saunders.)

in amplitude), and the S wave becomes smaller as the electrode is moved from right to left (Fig. 9.12). This pattern is called R-wave progression. In V_1 and V_2, the QRS deflection is predominantly negative (i.e., moving away from the positive chest electrode), reflecting depolarization of the septum and right ventricle (small R wave) and the left ventricle (large S wave). As the chest electrode is placed farther left, the wave of depolarization is moving toward the positive electrode. The *transition zone* is where the R wave amplitude begins to exceed the amplitude of the S wave. Transition usually occurs in the area of leads V_3 and V_4. The phrase *early transition* is used when the transition is seen in V_2. *Late transition* describes a delay in transition until leads V_4 and V_5. Electrode placement in the correct intercostal space is critical when evaluating R-wave progression.

Poor R-wave progression, a phrase used to describe R waves that decrease in size from V_1 to V_4 (Fig. 9.13), may be

a nonspecific indicator of an anterior infarction or a normal variant in young people, particularly in young women. Other causes of poor R-wave progression include LBBB, RVH or LVH, and severe COPD (particularly emphysema).

LATERAL INFARCTION

Leads I, aVL, V_5, and V_6 view the lateral wall of the left ventricle. Because the lateral wall of the left ventricle may be supplied by the Cx artery, the LAD artery, or a branch of the RCA, a lateral infarction may be associated with an anterior, inferior, or posterior infarction (Fig. 9.14). An example of an infarction involving the lateral wall is shown in Fig. 9.15.

INFERIOR INFARCTION

Leads II, III, and aVF view the inferior surface of the left ventricle. In most individuals, the inferior wall of the left ventricle is supplied by the posterior descending branch of the RCA (Fig. 9.16). Increased parasympathetic nervous system activity is common with inferior MIs, resulting in

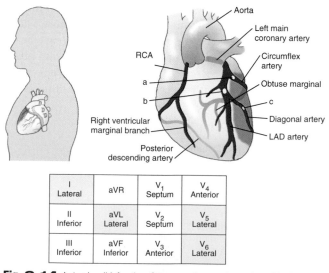

I Lateral	aVR	V_1 Septum	V_4 Anterior
II Inferior	aVL Lateral	V_2 Septum	V_5 Lateral
III Inferior	aVF Inferior	V_3 Anterior	V_6 Lateral

Fig. 9.14 Lateral wall infarction. Coronary artery anatomy shows blockage of the circumflex (Cx) artery (*a*), blockage of the proximal left anterior descending artery (*b*), and blockage of the diagonal artery (*c*). *LAD,* Left anterior descending; *RCA,* right coronary artery. (From Phalen, T., & Aehlert, B. J. (2019). *The 12-lead ECG in acute coronary syndromes* (4th ed.). St. Louis: Mosby.)

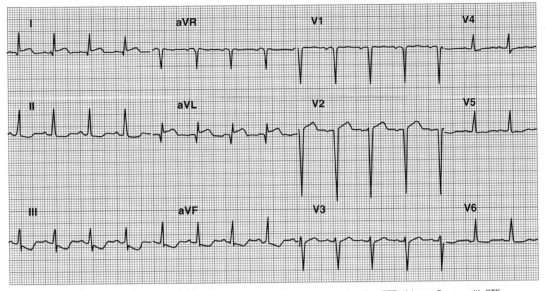

Fig. 9.15 Lateral infarction. Lead I shows a small Q wave with ST-segment elevation (STE). A larger Q wave with STE can be seen in lead aVL. This patient had an anterior non–ST-segment elevation infarction 4 days earlier with STE and T-wave inversion in leads V_2 through V_6. A coronary arteriogram at that time showed a blocked left anterior descending artery distal to its first large septal perforator. The STE evolved, and the T waves in all of the chest leads had become upright the day before this tracing was recorded. The patient then had another episode of chest pain associated with the appearance of signs of acute lateral infarction, as shown in this tracing. A repeat coronary arteriogram showed new blockage of the obtuse marginal branch of the circumflex (Cx) artery. (From Surawicz, B., & Knilans, T. K. (2001). *Chou's electrocardiography in clinical practice: adult and pediatric* (5th ed.). Philadelphia: Saunders.)

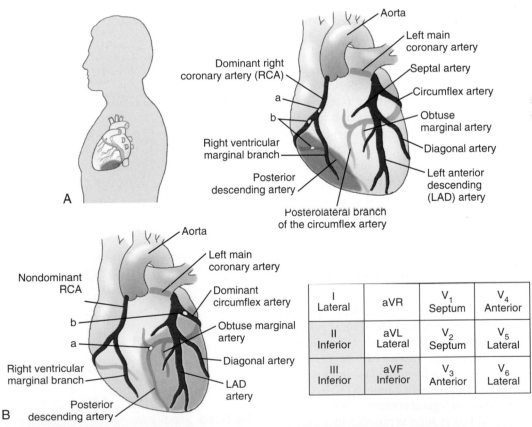

I Lateral	aVR	V_1 Septum	V_4 Anterior
II Inferior	aVL Lateral	V_2 Septum	V_5 Lateral
III Inferior	aVF Inferior	V_3 Anterior	V_6 Lateral

Fig. 9.16 A, Inferior wall infarction. Coronary anatomy shows a dominant right coronary artery *(RCA)*. A blockage at point *A* results in an inferior infarction and right ventricular infarction. A blockage at point *B* involves only the inferior wall, sparing the right ventricle. B, Inferior wall infarction. Coronary anatomy shows a dominant circumflex artery. A blockage at point *A* results in an inferior infarction. A blockage at point *B* may result in a lateral and inferobasal infarction. *LAD,* Left anterior descending. (From Phalen, T., & Aehlert, B. J. (2019). *The 12-lead ECG in acute coronary syndromes* (4th ed.). St. Louis: Mosby.)

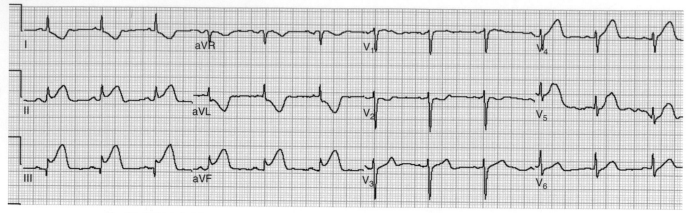

Fig. 9.17 Inferior infarction. Marked ST-segment elevation in leads II, III, and aVF with reciprocal ST-segment depression in leads I and aVL. (From Walls, R. M., Hockberger, R. S., & Gausche-Hill, M. (2018). *Rosen's emergency medicine: Concepts and clinical practice* (9th ed.). Philadelphia: Elsevier.)

bradydysrhythmias. Conduction delays (e.g., first-degree AV block, second-degree AV block type I) are common and are usually transient. An example of an infarction involving the inferior wall is shown in Fig. 9.17.

INFEROBASAL INFARCTION

Inferobasal (i.e., posterior) infarctions usually occur in conjunction with an inferior or lateral infarction. The inferobasal wall of the left ventricle is supplied by the Cx artery in most patients; however, in some patients, it is supplied by the RCA (Fig. 9.18). Because no leads of a standard 12-lead ECG directly view the posterior wall of the left ventricle, additional chest leads (V_7 to V_9) may be used to view the heart's posterior surface. Indicative changes of a posterior wall infarction include STE in these leads. If the placement of posterior chest leads is not feasible, the mirror test may be helpful in recognizing the ECG changes suggesting an inferobasal MI (Fig. 9.19).

Complications of a posterior wall MI may include left ventricular dysfunction. In addition, if the RCA supplies the posterior wall, complications may include dysrhythmias involving the sinoatrial (SA) node, the AV node, and the bundle of His. An example of an inferobasal MI is shown in Fig. 9.20.

RIGHT VENTRICULAR INFARCTION

A right ventricular infarction (RVI) is usually the result of an RCA occlusion (Fig. 9.21). However, the Cx artery supplies a significant proportion of the right ventricle in some patients. Although RVI may occur by itself, it has been estimated that about one-third of patients with inferior MI experience an RVI (O'Gara et al., 2013). Use right-sided chest leads to look for evidence of RVI in all patients with inferior STEMI. Of the right chest leads, V_4R has the highest sensitivity. It is essential to record leads V_3R and V_4R as soon as possible after the patient's onset of ischemic symptoms. In addition, leads aVR or V_1 may show STE of 1 mm or more in patients with inferior and suspected RVI (Thygesen et al., 2018). An example of an infarction involving the right ventricle is shown in Fig. 9.22.

Because patients experiencing an RVI are often preload sensitive, they can develop hypotension of varying degrees in response to medications that reduce preload, such as nitrates and diuretics. Other complications associated with RVI include bradycardias, AV blocks, and ventricular dysrhythmias.

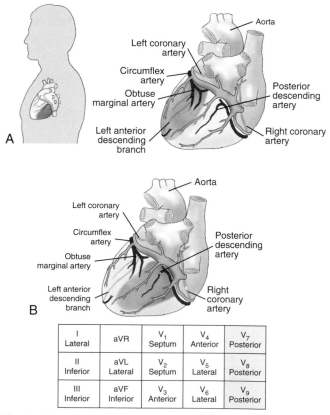

I Lateral	aVR	V_1 Septum	V_4 Anterior	V_7 Posterior
II Inferior	aVL Lateral	V_2 Septum	V_5 Lateral	V_8 Posterior
III Inferior	aVF Inferior	V_3 Anterior	V_6 Lateral	V_9 Posterior

Fig. 9.18 Inferobasal infarction. A, Coronary anatomy shows a dominant right coronary artery (RCA). Occlusion of the RCA commonly results in an inferior and inferobasal infarction. B, Coronary anatomy shows a dominant circumflex artery. Occlusion of a marginal branch is the cause of most isolated inferobasal infarctions. (From Phalen, T., & Aehlert, B. J. (2019). *The 12-lead ECG in acute coronary syndromes* (4th ed.). St. Louis: Mosby.)

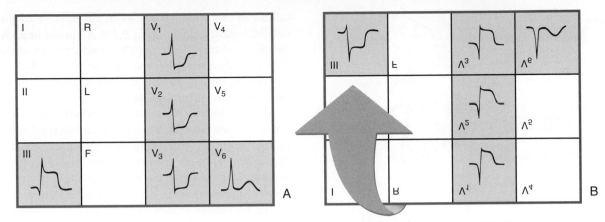

Fig. 9.19 Application of the mirror test. This test is most helpful in assessing a patient with an acute inferior infarction, in whom you suspect an acute inferobasal infarction. A, Schematic 12-lead ECG with indicative changes of inferior infarction in lead III. Note the tall R wave in lead V₁ and the ST-segment depression in leads V₁, V₂, and V₃. B, The tracing in *A* is now flipped over. Looking through the paper (as it is held up to the light), you now see Q waves and ST-segment elevation in leads V₁, V₂, and V₃. This positive mirror test suggests that the lead changes observed in A may reflect associated acute inferobasal infarction. (From Grauer, K. (1998). *A practical guide to ECG interpretation* (2nd ed.). St. Louis: Mosby.)

I	II	III	aVR	aVL	aVF	V₁	V₂	V₃	V₄	V₅	V₆

Control

2 hours later

24 hours later

48 hours later

8 days later

6 months later

Fig. 9.20 Evolutionary changes in a posteroinferior myocardial infarction. Control tracing is normal. The tracing recorded 2 hours after onset of chest pain demonstrated development of early Q waves; marked ST-segment elevation; and hyperacute T waves in leads II, III, and aVF. In addition, a larger R wave, ST-segment depression, and negative T waves have developed in leads V₁ and V₂. These are early changes indicating acute posteroinferior myocardial infarction. The 24-hour tracing demonstrates evolutionary changes. In leads II, III, and aVF, the Q wave is larger, the ST segments have almost returned to baseline, and the T wave has begun to invert. In leads V₁ to V₂, the duration of the R wave now exceeds 0.04 second, the ST segment is depressed, and the T wave is upright. (In this example, electrocardiogram [ECG] changes of true posterior involvement extend past lead V₂; ordinarily, only leads V₁ and V₂ may be involved.) Only minor further changes occur through the 8-day tracing. Finally, 6 months later, the ECG illustrates large Q waves, isoelectric ST segments, and inverted T waves in leads II, III, and aVF and large R waves, isoelectric ST segment, and upright T waves in leads V₁ and V₂, indicative of an old posteroinferior myocardial infarction. (From Wing, E. J., & Schiffman, F. J. (2022). *Cecil essentials of medicine* (10th ed.). Philadelphia: Elsevier.)

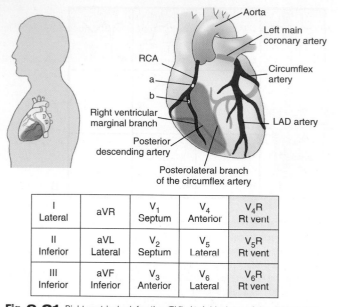

I Lateral	aVR	V₁ Septum	V₄ Anterior	V₄R Rt vent
II Inferior	aVL Lateral	V₂ Septum	V₅ Lateral	V₅R Rt vent
III Inferior	aVF Inferior	V₃ Anterior	V₆ Lateral	V₆R Rt vent

Fig. 9.21 Right ventricular infarction (RVI). At *A*, blockage of the right coronary artery proximal to the right ventricular marginal branch results in an inferior infarction and RVI. At *B*, blockage of the right ventricular marginal branch results in an isolated RVI. *LAD*, Left anterior descending; *RCA*, right coronary artery. (From Phalen, T., & Aehlert, B. J. (2019). *The 12-lead ECG in acute coronary syndromes* (4th ed.). St. Louis: Mosby.)

INTRAVENTRICULAR CONDUCTION DELAYS

Structures of the Intraventricular Conduction System

After passing through the AV node, the electrical impulse enters the bundle of His, which is normally the only electrical connection between the atria and the ventricles. The bundle of His conducts the electrical impulse to the right and left bundle branches (Fig. 9.23). A **bundle branch block (BBB)** is a disruption in impulse conduction from the bundle of His through either the right or left bundle branch to the Purkinje fibers. A BBB may be intermittent or permanent, complete or incomplete.

The right bundle branch travels down the right side of the interventricular septum to conduct the electrical impulse to the right ventricle. Structurally, the right bundle branch is long, thin, and more fragile than the left. Because of its structure, a relatively small lesion in the right bundle branch can result in delays or interruptions in electrical impulse transmission.

The left bundle branch begins as a single structure that is short and thick and then divides into two subdivisions called the anterior fascicle and the posterior fascicle. The anterior fascicle spreads the electrical impulse to the anterior portions of the left ventricle. This fascicle is thin and vulnerable to disruptions in electrical impulse transmission. The posterior fascicle relays the impulse to the posterior portions of the left ventricle. It is short, thick, and rarely disrupted because of its structure and dual blood supply from both the LAD artery and the RCA. In some people, a third fascicle, called the medial fascicle or septal fascicle, emerges from the left bundle itself or its posteroinferior division (Latcu & Nadir, 2010).

Bundle Branch Activation

The wave of normal ventricular depolarization moves from the endocardium to the epicardium. The left side of the interventricular septum, which is stimulated by the left posterior fascicle, is stimulated first. The electrical impulse (i.e., wave of depolarization) then traverses the septum to stimulate the right side. The left and right ventricles are then depolarized at the same time (Fig. 9.24).

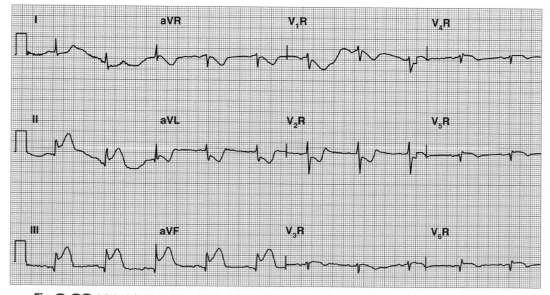

Fig. 9.22 Inferior infarction, right ventricular infarction. (From Goldberger, A. L. (2006). *Clinical electrocardiography: A simplified approach* (7th ed). St. Louis: Mosby.)

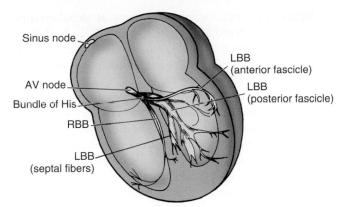

Fig. 9.23 Cardiac conduction system. *AV,* Atrioventricular; *LBB,* left bundle branch; *RBB,* right bundle branch. (From Conover, M. B. (1995). *Understanding electrocardiography* (7th ed.). St. Louis: Mosby.)

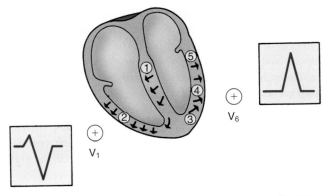

Fig. 9.24 Sequence of normal ventricular depolarization and resulting QRS complex, as seen in leads V_1 and V_6. (From Urden, L. D., Stacy, K. M., & Lough, M. E. (2022). *Critical care nursing: diagnosis and management* (9th ed.). St. Louis: Elsevier.)

A delay or block can occur in any part of the intraventricular conduction system. If a delay or block occurs in one of the bundle branches, the ventricles will not be depolarized simultaneously. Instead, the electrical impulse travels first down the unblocked branch and stimulates that ventricle. Because of the block, the impulse must then travel from cell to cell through the myocardium, rather than through the normal conduction pathway, to stimulate the other ventricle. Thus, the ventricle with the blocked bundle branch is the last to be depolarized.

How Do I Recognize It?

Essentially, two conditions must exist to suspect BBB. First, the QRS complex must have an abnormal duration (i.e., 0.12 second or more in duration if a complete BBB). Second, the QRS complex must arise due to supraventricular activity (this excludes paced beats and beats originating from the ventricles). If these two conditions are met, delayed ventricular conduction is assumed to be present, and BBB is the most common (but not the only) cause of this abnormal conduction.

When one of the bundles becomes blocked, the impulse that is normally conducted by that bundle branch is interrupted, and it does not depolarize the intended ventricle. Meanwhile, the other bundle branch is conducting its impulse and depolarizing its respective ventricle. For the second ventricle to depolarize, the electrical impulses must trudge through myocardial cells, which are not specialized for electrical conduction. Thus, the impulses from one ventricle must be transmitted, cell by cell, to the other ventricle. Because the impulses are not traveling down the normal conduction pathway, ventricular depolarization takes longer to occur. This delay is evidenced in the form of a wide QRS complex.

Variation in QRS duration from lead to lead is often seen and may produce confusion about whether the complex is or is not wide. As a rule, use the widest QRS complex to determine width. However, trying to pinpoint the exact beginning and end of the QRS complex can be challenging and sometimes impossible. Therefore, *when measuring for BBB, select the widest QRS complex with a discernible beginning and end.*

The criteria for BBB recognition may be identified in any lead of the ECG. However, in differentiating RBBB from LBBB, pay particular attention to the QRS morphology (i.e., shape) in specific leads. Lead V_1 is probably the single best lead to use in differentiating between RBBB and LBBB.

⊙ ECG Pearl

To be considered a BBB, the following ECG criteria must be met:

- QRS duration of 0.12 second or more in adults (if a *complete* RBBB or LBBB); if a BBB pattern is discernible and the QRS duration is between 0.11 and 0.119 second in adults, it is called an *incomplete* RBBB or LBBB (Surawicz et al., 2009). (If the QRS is wide but there is no BBB pattern, the term *wide QRS* or *intraventricular conduction delay* is used to describe the QRS)
- Visible QRS complexes are produced by supraventricular activity (i.e., the QRS complex is not a paced beat and does not originate in the ventricles).

DIFFERENTIATING RIGHT BUNDLE BRANCH BLOCK FROM LEFT BUNDLE BRANCH BLOCK

When BBB is suspected, an examination of V_1 can reveal whether the block affects the right or the left bundle branch. Following are descriptions of how each type of block affects the direction of electrical current and produces its own, distinct QRS morphology (Phalen & Aehlert, 2019).

Right Bundle Branch Block

With RBBB, the electrical impulse travels through the AV node and down the left bundle branch into the interventricular septum. The septum is activated by the left posterior fascicle and is depolarized in a left-to-right direction (Fig. 9.25),

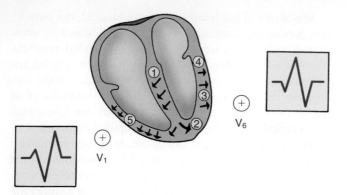

Fig. 9.25 Sequence of ventricular depolarization for a right bundle branch block and resulting QRS complex, as seen in leads V₁ and V₆. (From Urden, L. D., Stacy, K. M., & Lough, M. E. (2022). *Critical care nursing: Diagnosis and management* (9th ed.). St. Louis: Elsevier.)

which is toward V₁, producing an initial small R wave. As the left bundle continues to conduct impulses, the entire left ventricle is depolarized from right to left, producing movement away from V₁ and resulting in a negative deflection (i.e., an S wave). Now the impulses that depolarized the left ventricle conduct through the myocardial cells and depolarize the right ventricle. This depolarization creates a movement of electrical activity in the direction of V₁, so a second positive deflection is recorded (R′). The rSR′ pattern is characteristic of RBBB. The rSR′ pattern is sometimes referred to as an "M" or "rabbit ear" pattern.

Left Bundle Branch Block

With LBBB, the septum is depolarized by the right bundle branch, as is the right ventricle. The septum is part of the left ventricle and is normally depolarized by the left bundle branch. Because the left bundle branch is blocked, depolarization of the septum by the right bundle branch occurs in an abnormal direction (i.e., from right to left); thus, the wave of myocardial depolarization begins with the net movement of current going away from V₁ and is recorded as an initial negative deflection (Fig. 9.26). The right ventricle

is depolarized next. Because the wave of depolarization moves briefly toward the positive electrode in lead V₁, a small upright notch in the QRS complex is seen on the ECG. As the remainder of the left ventricle is depolarized, the QRS complex is inscribed in lead V₁ as a deep, negative deflection (i.e., an S wave), reflecting the left ventricle's large muscle mass. Sometimes depolarization of the left ventricle overshadows that of the right ventricle on the ECG. When this occurs, a QS deflection is inscribed in lead V₁, and the small upright notch that is usually seen with right ventricular depolarization is absent.

Unfortunately, not every BBB presents a clear pattern as previously described, making the differentiation between RBBB and LBBB less clear. Variant patterns of BBB as seen in lead V₁ appear in Fig. 9.27.

An Easier Way

Remember that in the setting of BBB, the ventricles are not depolarized in their usual simultaneous manner. Instead, they are depolarized sequentially. The last ventricle to be depolarized is, of course, the ventricle with the blocked bundle branch. Therefore, if it is possible to determine which ventricle was depolarized last, it becomes possible to determine which bundle branch was blocked. For example, if the right ventricle was depolarized last, the impulse traveled down the left bundle branch, depolarized the left ventricle first, and then marched through and depolarized the right ventricle. Thus, it stands to reason that if one ventricle is depolarized late, its depolarization makes up the last portion of the QRS complex.

The final portion of the QRS complex is referred to as the terminal force. Examination of the terminal force of the QRS complex reveals the ventricle that was depolarized last and the bundle that was blocked. To identify the terminal force, first locate the J point. Then, from the J point, move backward into the QRS and determine whether the

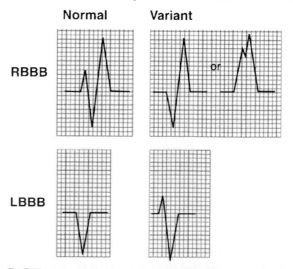

Fig. 9.27 Variant patterns of bundle branch block as seen in lead V₁. *LBBB*, Left bundle branch block; *RBBB*, right bundle branch block. (From Phalen, T., & Aehlert, B. J. (2019). *The 12-lead ECG in acute coronary syndromes* (4th ed.). St. Louis: Mosby.)

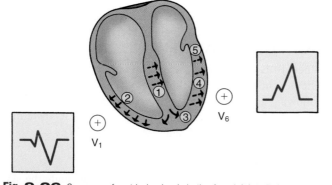

Fig. 9.26 Sequence of ventricular depolarization for a left bundle branch block and resulting QRS complex, as seen in leads V₁ and V₆. (From Urden, L. D., Stacy, K. M., & Lough, M. E. (2022). *Critical care nursing: Diagnosis and management* (9th ed.). St. Louis: Elsevier.)

last electrical activity produced an upward or downward deflection.

An example of the terminal force in both RBBB and LBBB is illustrated in Fig. 9.28. If the right bundle branch is blocked, then the right ventricle will be depolarized last. As a result, the current will be moving from the left ventricle to the right, creating a positive deflection of the terminal force of the QRS complex in V_1. On the other hand, if the left bundle branch is blocked, the left ventricle will be depolarized last. As a result, the current will flow from right to left, producing a negative deflection of the terminal force of the QRS complex seen in V_1. Therefore, to differentiate RBBB from LBBB, look at V_1 and determine whether the terminal force of the QRS complex is a positive or negative deflection. If it is directed upward, an RBBB is present (i.e., the current is moving toward the right ventricle and toward V_1). Conversely, an LBBB is present when the terminal force of the QRS complex is directed downward (i.e., the current is moving away from V_1 and toward the left ventricle). This rule is beneficial when rSR′ and QS variants are present.

A simple way to remember this rule has been suggested by Mike Taigman and Syd Canan and is demonstrated in Fig. 9.29. They recognized the similarity between this rule and the turn signal on a car. For example, to indicate a right turn, you lift the arm of the turn signal. Likewise, when an RBBB is present, the terminal force of the QRS complex points up. Conversely, left turns and LBBB move downward.

EXCEPTIONS

Two notable exceptions must be mentioned to complete the discussion of BBB. The first involves the criteria used to recognize BBB, and the second relates to differentiating LBBB from RBBB.

The criteria used to recognize BBB are valid but lack some sensitivity and specificity. The sensitivity can be limited by junctional rhythms because there may be no discernible P waves when the AV junction is the pacemaker site. The AV junction is a supraventricular pacemaker, but this presents an exception to the two-part rule of BBB recognition. Specificity is limited by Wolff-Parkinson-White (WPW) syndrome and other conditions that produce wide QRS complexes resulting from atrial activity. If the characteristic delta wave and shortened PR interval are recognized, WPW syndrome should be suspected.

As for differentiating LBBB from RBBB, a third category exists: nonspecific intraventricular conduction delay (NSIVCD). These blocks do not display the typical V_1 morphologies generally produced by BBB. Their origin may not result from a complete BBB but are often the result of several factors, of which incomplete BBB may be one. Atypical patterns of BBB can be attributed to NSIVCD.

What Causes It?

RBBB can occur in individuals with no underlying heart disease, but it occurs more commonly in the presence of organic heart disease, with coronary artery disease being the most common cause. Acute RBBB may occur secondary to an RVI. LBBB may result from an anteroseptal or inferior MI, conduction system degeneration, acute heart failure, acute pericarditis or myocarditis, or following cardiac procedures (Tan et al., 2020).

Other causes of BBBs include aortic valve disease; congenital, hypertensive, and rheumatic heart disease; and trauma (e.g., cardiac surgery). Sometimes the ECG will show occasional QRS complexes that have an RBBB or LBBB morphology interspersed with normal QRS complexes. When a BBB occurs intermittently and is related to the patient's heart rate, it is referred to as a rate-related BBB. Nonischemic diseases are also capable of producing a BBB.

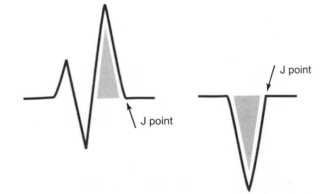

Fig. 9.28 Determining the direction of the terminal force. In lead V_1, move from the J point into the QRS complex and determine whether the terminal portion (last 0.04 second) of the QRS complex is a positive (upright) or negative (downward) deflection. (From Phalen, T., & Aehlert, B. J. (2019). *The 12-lead ECG in acute coronary syndromes* (4th ed.). St. Louis: Mosby.)

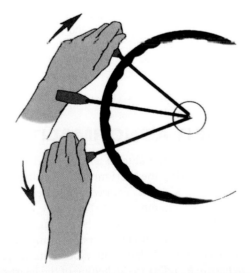

Fig. 9.29 Differentiating between right and left bundle branch blocks. The "turn signal" theory is that right is up and left is down. (From Phalen, T., & Aehlert, B. J. (2019). *The 12-lead ECG in acute coronary syndromes* (4th ed.). St. Louis: Mosby.)

What Do I Do About It?

Because the LAD artery supplies much of the bundle branches, patients experiencing septal and anteroseptal infarctions are most likely to develop BBB. Of course, a patient experiencing an infarction and presenting with BBB may have had it as a preexisting condition. Unless a previous ECG is available for comparison or the BBB develops during the infarction, it can be challenging to determine which came first, the infarction or the BBB. BBB in the setting of infarction also identifies patients with a higher likelihood of developing third-degree AV block.

The presence of a BBB in an asymptomatic patient requires no specific treatment. RBBB generally requires no specific treatment; however, when RBBB occurs in the setting of an acute MI, close ECG monitoring for the development of symptomatic AV conduction system disturbances is essential.

For the patient experiencing chest discomfort, the presence of LBBB can complicate the diagnosis of an acute MI because LBBB can produce STE and wide Q waves that look remarkably similar to infarction. Therefore, close ECG monitoring and frequent patient reassessment are essential. Because of its association with organic heart disease, patients with LBBB should be evaluated for cardiomyopathies, coronary disease, hypertension, valvular heart disease, and other conditions associated with LBBB. Insertion of a permanent pacemaker is generally required for patients with LBBB who develop second-degree AV block type II or third-degree AV block.

◎ ECG Pearl

When BBB is present, STE is often seen in leads with negatively deflected QRS complexes. RBBB rarely produces STE because most of the leads remain positively deflected. Occasionally, when the inferior leads (II, III, and aVF) happen to be negatively deflected, an RBBB may produce STE in those leads and may occasionally mimic an inferior wall infarction. Although this combination is possible, LBBB is by far the more common cause of STE.

CHAMBER ABNORMALITIES

Cardiomyopathy is a general term used to describe different heart diseases involving the heart muscle, resulting in abnormal enlargement. *Cardiac enlargement* refers to either dilation of a heart chamber or hypertrophy of the heart muscle (Goldberger et al., 2018). With dilation, stretching of a chamber of the heart muscle occurs, resulting in enlargement of that chamber. Dilation may be acute or chronic. *Cardiac hypertrophy* refers to thickening of the heart muscle, with resultant enlargement of a heart chamber. Hypertrophy is commonly accompanied by dilation. When evaluating the ECG for indications of chamber enlargement, it is essential

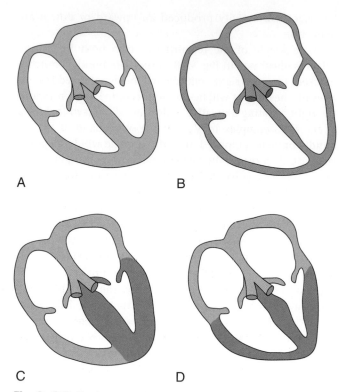

Fig. 9.30 The three types of cardiomyopathy. A, Normal heart. B, Dilated cardiomyopathy demonstrating enlargement of all four chambers. C, Hypertrophic cardiomyopathy showing a thickened left ventricle. D, Restrictive cardiomyopathy characterized by a small left ventricular volume. (From Copstead-Kirkhorn, L. E., & Banasik, J. L. (2013). *Pathophysiology* (5th ed.). St. Louis: Saunders.)

to check the calibration marker to ensure that it is 10 mm (1 mV) tall.

Cardiomyopathies can be classified into three physiologic categories: (1) dilated cardiomyopathy (DCM) (most common), (2) hypertrophic cardiomyopathy (HCM), and (3) restrictive cardiomyopathy (least common) (Fig. 9.30).

DCM is characterized by enlargement of all heart chambers with progressive dilation of both the right and left ventricles, resulting in impaired contractile (systolic) function. As a result, patients may present with fatigue, dyspnea, jugular venous distention, pedal edema, and pulmonary congestion. Possible causes of DCM include poorly controlled hypertension, ischemic heart disease, valvular disease, diabetes, alcohol or drug abuse, renal failure, hyperthyroidism, exposure to heavy metals (e.g., lead, arsenic, cobalt, mercury), or infection. Peripartum cardiomyopathy occurs in previously healthy women in the last month of pregnancy or within 5 months after delivery.

HCM is characterized by thickening of the septal wall without ventricular dilation, resulting in a reduced stroke volume because of impaired diastolic filling. Patients with HCM may be asymptomatic or present with dysrhythmias, syncope on exertion, angina, palpitations, left heart failure, or sudden death. Because most cases have a genetic origin, screening of first-degree family members of patients with HCM is recommended.

Restrictive cardiomyopathy is characterized by increased ventricular wall stiffness that impedes ventricular filling, reduced diastolic volume of either or both ventricles, and normal or nearly normal systolic function. Although the ventricles are typically of normal size or are only slightly enlarged, dilation of both atria is common because of poor ventricular filling and pressure overload (Kumar et al., 2018). Restrictive cardiomyopathy may be caused by amyloidosis, myocardial fibrosis, scleroderma, or an unknown cause. Patients often present with signs and symptoms that are consistent with progressive left- and right-sided heart failure.

Atrial Abnormalities

The first half of the P wave is recorded when the electrical impulse that originated in the SA node stimulates the right atrium and reaches the AV node. The downslope of the P wave reflects stimulation of the left atrium. The appearance of abnormal P waves on the ECG may be caused by delayed intra-atrial conduction, elevated atrial pressure, atrial dilation, and atrial muscular hypertrophy, among other causes. In the past, terms used to describe atrial abnormalities have included P-mitrale, P-pulmonale, left atrial enlargement, right atrial enlargement, atrial hypertrophy, and atrial overload. Today, experts recommend that the terms *left atrial abnormality* (LAA) and *right atrial abnormality* (RAA) be used because a combination of several factors that may not be distinguishable can result in abnormal P waves (Hancock et al., 2009).

You will recall that the normal P wave results from atrial depolarization. The initial portion of the P wave represents depolarization of the right atrium, and the middle and end portions represent left atrial depolarization. Because these events normally occur nearly at the same time, they fuse into a single, smooth rounded waveform.

RAA produces changes in the initial part of the P wave. The P wave is tall (more than 2.5 mm in height), peaked, and usually of normal duration (Hancock et al., 2009) (Fig. 9.31). The abnormal P waves characteristic of RAA are usually best seen in leads II, III, aVF, and sometimes V_1 (Goldberger et al., 2018). Lead V_1 may reveal a biphasic P wave. Examples of conditions that may cause RAA include COPD with or without pulmonary hypertension, congenital heart disease, and right ventricular failure.

With LAA, the middle and end of the P wave are prolonged because depolarization of the left atrium begins and ends later than right atrial depolarization (Surawicz & Knilans, 2008). Notched P waves are usually visible and correspond with the delay in left atrial activation because the right and left atrial peaks that are usually nearly simultaneous and fused into a single peak become more widely separated (Hancock et al., 2009) (see Fig. 9.31). Notched P waves are generally most easily seen in the limb leads. The P wave may be biphasic in lead V_1 with a slight initial positive deflection and a prominent, wide negative deflection (Goldberger et al., 2018). Examples of conditions in which LAA may occur include coronary artery disease, cardiomyopathies, hypertensive heart disease, and valvular heart disease. When the ECG reflects both RAA and LAA, the term *combined atrial abnormality* is used.

Ventricular Abnormalities

With RVH, current travels between hypertrophied cells and moves through the enlarged right ventricle, producing higher-than-normal voltages on the body surface (Mirvis & Goldberger, 2019) (Fig. 9.32). Because the right ventricle usually is considerably smaller than the left, it must become significantly enlarged before changes are visible on the ECG. Characteristic ECG changes associated with

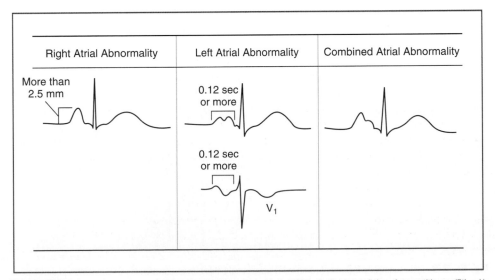

Fig. 9.31 Criteria for atrial abnormalities. (Modified from Park, M. K. (2008). *Pediatric cardiology for practitioners* (5th ed.). St. Louis: Mosby.)

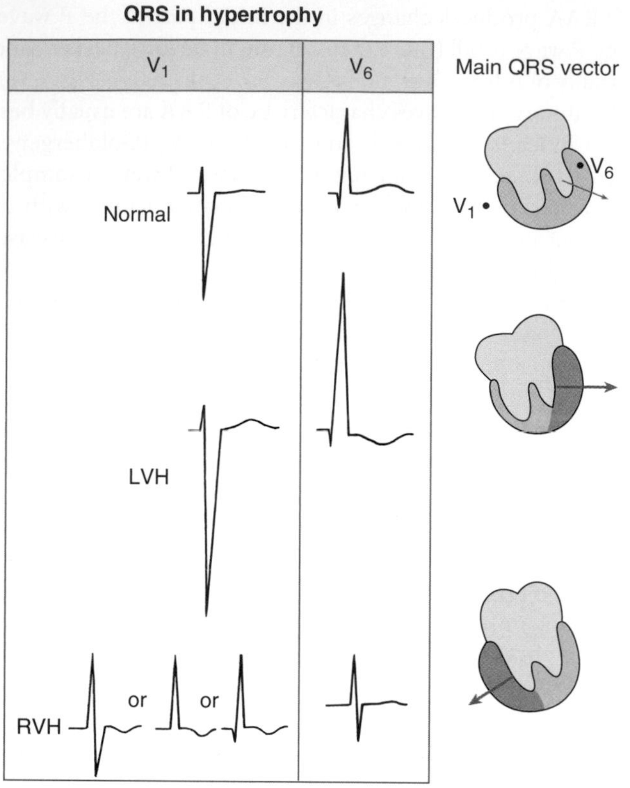

QRS in hypertrophy

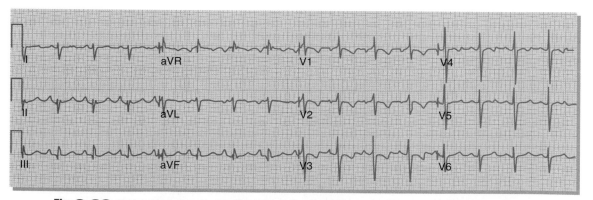

Fig. 9.32 Left ventricular hypertrophy (*LVH*) increases the amplitude of electrical forces directed to the left and posteriorly. In addition, repolarization abnormalities can cause ST-segment depression and T-wave inversion in leads with a prominent R wave. Right ventricular hypertrophy (*RVH*) can shift the QRS vector to the right, usually with an R, RS, or qR complex in lead V_1, especially when caused by severe pressure overload. T-wave inversion may be present in the right chest leads. (From Goldberger, A. L., Goldberger, Z. D., & Shvilkin, A. (2018). *Goldberger's clinical electrocardiography* (9th ed.). Philadelphia: Elsevier.)

chronic pulmonary diseases, valvular heart disease, and congenital heart disease.

LVH is recognized on the ECG by increased QRS amplitude and changes in the ST segment and T wave (see Fig. 9.32). Typically, R waves in leads I, aVL, V_5, and V_6 are taller than usual, and S waves in leads V_1 through V_2 are deeper than normal (Mirvis & Goldberger, 2019). The QRS duration is often increased in LVH and may be attributed to the longer time required to activate the thickened wall of the left ventricle (Hancock et al., 2009) and the slower-than-normal conduction within the working myocardium (Mirvis & Goldberger, 2019). Causes of LVH include systemic hypertension, HCM, aortic stenosis, and aortic insufficiency. In addition, LVH may be accompanied by left axis deviation.

The Cornell voltage criterion is often used to check for the presence of LVH. This formula adds the S wave amplitude in lead V_3 and the R wave amplitude in lead aVL. A total greater than 20 mm (2 mV) in women and 28 mm or more (2.8 mV) in men suggests that LVH is present (Ganz & Link, 2019). A 12-lead ECG's interpretive algorithm checks for the presence of LVH using preprogrammed criteria, including formulas, to measure voltage. If the 12-lead machine determines that an ECG meets the criteria for LVH, a message is displayed, such as "Meets voltage criteria for left ventricular hypertrophy."

An example of LVH is shown in Fig. 9.34. Note that the ST segment in Fig. 9.34 is elevated in V_1, V_2, and V_3. Also note the ST-segment depression shown in leads V_5 and V_6. Recall that when the QRS complexes of LBBBs, ventricular rhythms, and ventricular paced rhythms are negatively deflected (i.e., a QS configuration), the ST segments and T waves are in the opposite direction of the last portion of the QRS complex. Similarly, when the QRS complex of LVH is negatively deflected, these ECG findings are shared by LVH, making the identification of ECG changes associated with acute MI complicated. Therefore, careful correlation of the patient's ECG, clinical presentation, and the results of other diagnostic studies are essential.

RVH include tall R waves in leads V_1 through V_3 and deeper than normal S waves in leads I, aVL, V_5, and V_6 (Sharma & Morrison, 2022) (Fig. 9.33). Right axis deviation is usually present, and evidence of RAA may be seen. Causes of RVH include pulmonary hypertension and

Fig. 9.33 Right ventricular hypertrophy with tall R wave in right chest leads, downsloping ST depression in the chest leads, right axis deviation, and evidence of right atrial enlargement. (From Wing, E. J., & Schiffman, F. J. (2022). *Cecil essentials of medicine* (10th ed.). Philadelphia: Elsevier.)

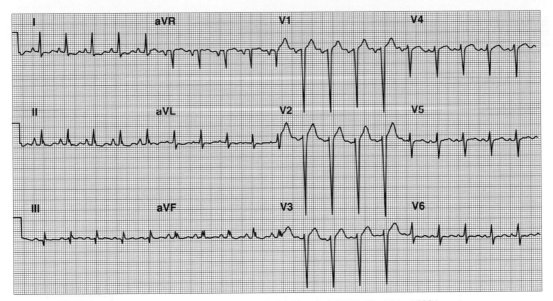

Fig. 9.34 Left ventricular hypertrophy. (From Phalen, T., & Aehlert, B. J. (2019). *The 12-lead ECG in acute coronary syndromes* (4th ed.). St. Louis: Mosby.)

ELECTROLYTE DISTURBANCES

Because electrolyte imbalances may increase cardiac irritability and cause cardiac dysrhythmias, a patient's ECG can be evaluated for evidence of electrolyte disturbances. ECG changes associated with electrolyte imbalances can vary widely from patient to patient.

Sodium

Sodium is the most abundant electrolyte in the body. It is vital in maintaining water balance, is necessary for the normal conduction of impulses in nerve and muscle fibers (in conjunction with potassium and calcium), and plays an essential role in the voltage of action potentials. Food and drink are the primary sources of sodium. In healthy individuals, sodium is primarily excreted in sweat and urine.

HYPERNATREMIA

Hypernatremia (sodium excess) may result from several factors, including dehydration due to vomiting, severe watery diarrhea, excessive sweating, heat stroke, prolonged high fever, or Cushing syndrome. In addition, possible causes of hypernatremia because of the retention of relatively more sodium than water include excess aldosterone secretion, excess secretion of adrenocorticotropic hormone (ACTH), hypertonic parenteral fluid administration, inadequate fluid intake, or ingestion of abnormal amounts of sodium.

The patient may present with restlessness, irritability, confusion, thirst, dry and flushed skin, dry mucous membranes, decreased urine output, seizures, and coma. Hypernatremia does not cause any significant ECG changes.

HYPONATREMIA

Hyponatremia (sodium deficit) may result from inadequate sodium intake, prolonged diuretic therapy, excessive diaphoresis, excessive loss of sodium from trauma (e.g., burns), adrenal insufficiency, renal disease, severe gastrointestinal (GI) fluid losses from gastric suctioning or lavage, and prolonged vomiting or diarrhea. In addition, some medications may impair water excretion and contribute to hyponatremia.

The patient may present with irritability, fatigue, headache, nausea and vomiting, abdominal cramps, and muscle weakness. Hyponatremia does not cause any significant ECG changes.

Potassium

Potassium is the primary intracellular fluid cation. It is essential for many cell functions, including cardiac and neuromuscular activity, resting membrane potential, growth, enzyme function, and regulation of fluid volume and pH (Stanton & Koeppen, 2018).

HYPERKALEMIA

Hyperkalemia (potassium excess) may occur because of acute or chronic renal failure, excessive administration of intravenous (IV) potassium, metabolic acidosis, ingestion of excessive amounts of salt substitutes, medications (e.g., spironolactone, angiotensin-converting enzyme inhibitors, nonsteroidal antiinflammatory drugs), or widespread cell damage (e.g., crush injuries, burns). The patient may present with anxiety, restlessness, cardiac dysrhythmias, skeletal muscle weakness, abdominal muscle cramping, and diarrhea.

The effects of hyperkalemia depend on the tissue involved. The atrial myocardium is the most sensitive, the ventricular myocardium less sensitive, and the SA node and bundle of His the least sensitive (El-Sherif et al., 2012).

- Tall, peaked (tented), narrow, symmetric T waves
- P waves decrease in amplitude as potassium level increases
- PR interval and QRS duration increase as potassium level increases

- ST-segment depression
- Decrease in T wave amplitude
- Prominent U waves; the amplitude of U waves may exceed that of T waves in the same lead with marked hypokalemia
- P wave amplitude and duration are usually increased
- Slight prolongation of the PR interval
- Increased QRS duration with severe hypokalemia

When the potassium level exceeds 5.5 mEq/L, tall, peaked (tented), narrow, symmetric T waves may be seen on the ECG (Box 9.2). However, 50% of patients with potassium levels higher than 6.5 mEq/L will not manifest any ECG changes (El-Sherif et al., 2012). As the potassium level rises, PR intervals lengthen and the QRS duration increases, reflecting slowed conduction. When the potassium level nears 10 mEq/L, intraventricular conduction delays and dysrhythmias such as ventricular tachycardia, ventricular fibrillation, and asystole may develop. Examples of the effects of hyperkalemia on the ECG are shown in Fig. 9.35.

HYPOKALEMIA

Hypokalemia (potassium deficit) is one of the most common electrolyte disorders (Stanton & Koeppen, 2018). It may occur because of prolonged diuretic therapy with thiazide diuretics or furosemide, an inadequate dietary intake of potassium, administration of potassium-deficient parenteral fluids, starvation, severe GI fluid losses from gastric suctioning or lavage, prolonged vomiting or diarrhea, or laxative use without potassium replacement. It has been estimated that as many as 10% to 40% of patients taking thiazide diuretics and almost 50% of patients resuscitated from out-of-hospital ventricular fibrillation have low potassium levels (El-Sherif et al., 2012).

The patient may present with skeletal muscle weakness, fatigue, paresthesias, and cardiac dysrhythmias (e.g., sinus bradycardia, AV blocks). The electrophysiologic effects of hypokalemia include increased automaticity, decreased conduction velocity, shortening of the effective refractory

period, and prolongation of the relative refractory period (El-Sherif et al., 2012). Possible ECG manifestations of hypokalemia are shown in Box 9.3 and Fig. 9.36.

Calcium

Calcium is essential in bone formation, nerve and muscle function, and blood clotting.

HYPERCALCEMIA

Causes of hypercalcemia (calcium excess) include hyperparathyroidism, chronic and acute renal failure, excessive vitamin D or vitamin A intake, hyperthyroidism, adrenal insufficiency, cancer (e.g., breast, lung, multiple myeloma), excessive use of calcium-containing antacids, and an excessive intake of calcium supplements.

The patient may present with nausea, vomiting, acute mental status changes ranging from mild confusion to coma, fatigue, skeletal muscle weakness, constipation, and cardiac dysrhythmias. ECG changes associated with hypercalcemia include shortening of the ST segment and decreased QT interval duration.

HYPOCALCEMIA

Hypocalcemia (calcium deficit) may result from renal disease, dietary deficiency of calcium and vitamin D, pancreatic disease, malabsorption because of small bowel disease, hypoparathyroidism, and certain medications.

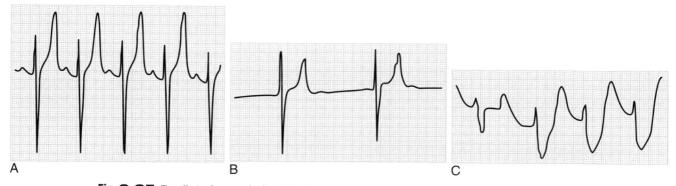

A   B   C

Fig. 9.35 The effects of progressive hyperkalemia on the electrocardiogram. All of the illustrations are from lead V_3. A, Serum potassium concentration (K^+) was 6.8 mEq/L; note the peaked T waves together with sinus rhythm. B, Serum K^+ was 8.9 mEq/L; note the peaked T waves and absent P waves. C, Serum K^+ was greater than 8.9 mEq/L; note the classic sine wave with absent P waves, marked prolongation of the QRS complex, and peaked T waves. (From Goldman, L., Schafer, A.I., Crow, M.K., Davidson, N.E., Drazen, J.M., Griggs, R.C., Landry, D.W., Levinson, W., Rustgi, A.K., Scheld, W.M., Spiegel, A.M. (2020). *Goldman-Cecil medicine* (26th ed.). Philadelphia: Elsevier.)

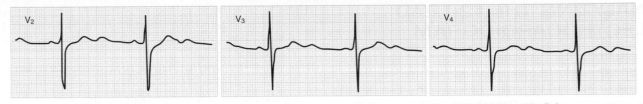

Fig. 9.36 The electrocardiographic manifestations of hypokalemia. The serum potassium concentration was 2.2 mEq/L. The ST segment is prolonged, primarily because of a U wave after the T wave, and the T wave is flattened. (From Goldman, L., Schafer, A.I., Crow, M.K., Davidson, N.E., Drazen, J.M., Griggs, R.C., Landry, D.W., Levinson, W., Rustgi, A.K., Scheld, W.M., Spiegel, A.M. (2020). *Goldman-Cecil medicine* (26th ed.). Philadelphia: Elsevier.)

Symptoms may range from mild to severe, including irritability and confusion, tingling of the nose, mouth, ears, fingers, or toes; nausea, vomiting, and diarrhea; cardiac dysrhythmias; hyperactive deep tendon reflexes; carpal spasms (Trousseau sign); facial muscle contraction (Chvostek sign); and pathologic fractures. ECG changes associated with hypocalcemia include lengthening of the ST segment and increased QT interval duration. Possible ECG manifestations of calcium disturbances are shown in Fig. 9.37.

Magnesium

Magnesium has an essential role in membrane stability, skeletal muscle contraction, respiratory smooth muscle function, and enzyme reactions contributing to cardiovascular function.

HYPERMAGNESEMIA

Causes of hypermagnesemia (magnesium excess) include hypothyroidism, Addison disease, excessive parenteral magnesium (e.g., eclampsia), or excessive use of magnesium-containing antacids, laxatives, or enemas in patients with impaired renal function. Signs and symptoms include drowsiness, hypotension, muscle weakness, impaired breathing, and diminished deep tendon reflexes. In addition, hypermagnesemia depresses AV and intraventricular conduction, increasing the potential for bradycardia and AV blocks.

HYPOMAGNESEMIA

Hypomagnesemia (magnesium deficit) may occur because of prolonged or excessive diuretic therapy, excessive calcium or vitamin D intake, administration of IV fluids or total parenteral nutrition without magnesium replacement, hypercalcemia, malabsorption associated with disease of the small intestine, malnutrition, and alcohol use disorder.

Early signs and symptoms may include fatigue, nausea and vomiting, and a loss of appetite. As hypomagnesemia worsens, the patient may experience acute mental status changes, cardiac dysrhythmias, paresthesias, and muscle weakness and cramps. Hypomagnesemia does not generally produce significant ECG changes; however, it may cause or increase the severity of hypokalemia. In addition, hypomagnesemia has been associated with a prolonged QT interval and implicated as a possible cause of torsades de pointes.

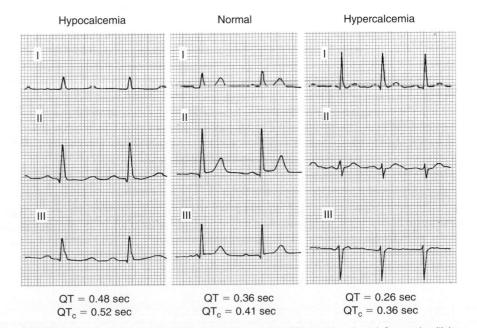

Hypocalcemia	Normal	Hypercalcemia
QT = 0.48 sec	QT = 0.36 sec	QT = 0.26 sec
QT_c = 0.52 sec	QT_c = 0.41 sec	QT_c = 0.36 sec

Fig. 9.37 With hypocalcemia, the ST segment is lengthened, and the QT interval is prolonged. Conversely, with hypercalcemia, the ST segment is shortened, and the duration of the QT interval is decreased. (From Goldberger, A. L., Goldberger, Z. D., & Shvilkin, A. (2018). *Goldberger's clinical electrocardiography* (9th ed.). Philadelphia: Elsevier.)

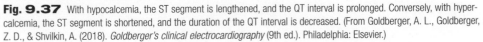

ANALYZING THE 12-LEAD ELECTROCARDIOGRAM

It is essential to use a systematic method when analyzing a 12-lead ECG. Before beginning an in-depth review, take a moment to "take in" the entire 12-lead and get an overall impression of the tracing. Does the rate look as if it is normal, fast, or slow? Do the ST segments look markedly elevated or depressed? Is there evidence of premature beats, pauses, baseline wander, or artifact? If baseline wander or artifact is present to any significant degree, note it. If the presence of either of these conditions interferes with the assessment of any lead, use a modifier such as "possible" or "apparent" in your interpretation. After initially surveying the tracing, consider using the following approach when reviewing a 12-lead ECG:

1. Identify the rate and underlying rhythm. Identify any premature beats and pauses, if present.
2. Estimate the QRS axis using leads I and aVF.
3. Analyze waveforms, segments, and intervals. Before examining waveforms, quickly look at the calibration marker and determine if it is standard, half-standard, or twice the standard. Next, examine each lead, selecting one good representative waveform or complex in each lead. Inspect each waveform, noting any changes in orientation, shape, size, and duration.
4. Examine for evidence of ischemia, injury, and infarction. Look for the presence of ST-segment displacement (i.e., STE or ST-segment depression).
5. Look for evidence of other conditions. Is there evidence of chamber enlargement, electrolyte imbalances, or conditions that mimic MI (e.g., LVH, LBBB, ventricular rhythm, ventricular paced rhythm)?
6. Interpret your findings.

REFERENCES

El-Sherif, N., Turitto, G., & Robotis, D. (2012). Arrhythmias and electrolyte disorders. In S. Saksena & A. J. Camm (Eds.), *Electrophysiological disorders of the heart* (2nd ed., pp. 865–874). Philadelphia: Saunders.

Ganz, L., & Link, M. S. (2020). Electrocardiography. In L. Goldman & A. I. Schafer (Eds.), *Goldman-Cecil medicine* (26th ed., pp. 246–253). Philadelphia: Elsevier.

Goldberger, A. L., Goldberger, Z. D., & Shvilkin, A. (2018). Atrial and ventricular enlargement. In *Goldberger's clinical electrocardiography* (9th ed., pp. 50–60). Philadelphia: Elsevier.

Halim, S. A., Newby, K., & Ohman, E. M. (2010). Diagnosis of acute myocardial ischemia and infarction. In M. H. Crawford, J. P. DiMarco, & W. J. Paulus (Eds.), *Cardiology* (3rd ed., pp. 345–360). Philadelphia: Elsevier.

Hancock, E. W., Drew, B. J., Mirvis, D. M., Okin, P., Kligfield, P., & Gettes, L. S. (2009). AHA/ACCF/HRS recommendations for the standardization and interpretation of the electrocardiogram: Part V: Electrocardiogram changes associated with cardiac chamber hypertrophy. *J Am Coll Cardiol, 53*(11), 992–1002.

Kumar, V., Abbas, A. K., & Aster, J. C. (2018). Heart. In *Robbins Basic Pathology* (10th ed., pp. 399–441). Philadelphia: Elsevier.

Latcu, D., & Nadir, S. (2010). Atrioventricular and intraventricular conduction disorders. In M. H. Crawford, J. P. DiMarco, & W. J. Paulus (Eds.), *Cardiology* (3rd ed., pp. 725–739). Philadelphia: Elsevier.

Mirvis, D. M., & Goldberger, A. L. (2019). Electrocardiography. In D. P. Zipes, P. Libby, R. O. Bonow, D. L. Mann, G. F. Tomaselli, & E. Braunwald (Eds.), *Braunwald's heart disease: A textbook of cardiovascular medicine* (11th ed., pp. 117–153). Philadelphia: Elsevier.

O'Gara, P. T., Kushner, F. G., Ascheim, D. D., Casey Jr., D. E., Chung, M. K., de Lemos, J. A., & Zhao, D. X. (2013). 2013 ACCF/AHA guideline for the management of ST-elevation myocardial infarction. *J Am Coll Cardiol, 61*(4), e78–e140.

Otto, C. M. (2018). Cardiomyopathies, hypertensive and pulmonary heart disease. In *Textbook of clinical echocardiography* (6th ed., pp. 235–267). Philadelphia: Elsevier.

Phalen, T., & Aehlert, B. (2019). ST-elevation variants. In *The 12-lead ECG in acute coronary syndromes* (4th ed., pp. 78–97). St. Louis: Elsevier.

Sharma, E., & Morrison, A. R. (2022). Diagnostic tests and procedures in the patient with cardiovascular disease. In E. J. Wing, & F. J. Schiffman (Eds.), *Cecil essentials of medicine* (10th ed., pp. 24–42). Philadelphia: Elsevier.

Stanton, B. A., & Koeppen, B. M. (2018). Potassium, calcium, and phosphate homeostasis. In B. M. Koeppen & B. A. Stanton (Eds.), *Berne & Levy physiology* (7th ed., pp. 647–669). Philadelphia: Elsevier.

Surawicz, B., Childers, R., Deal, B. J., & Gettes, L. S. (2009). AHA/ACCF/HRS recommendations for the standardization and interpretation of the electrocardiogram: Part III: Intraventricular conduction disturbances: A scientific statement from the American Heart Association Electrocardiography and Arrhythmias Committee. *J Am Coll Cardiol, 53*(11), 976–981.

Surawicz, B., & Knilans, T. K. (2008). Atrial abnormalities. In *Chou's electrocardiography in clinical practice* (6th ed., pp. 29–44). Philadelphia: Saunders.

Tan, N. Y., Witt, C. M., Oh, J. K., & Cha, Y.-M. (2020). Left bundle branch block: Current and future perspectives. *Circ Arrhythm Electrophysiol, 13*(4), e008239.

Thygesen, K., Alpert, J. S., Jaffe, A. S., Chaitman, B. R., Bax, J. J., Morrow, D. A., & White, H. D. (2018). Fourth universal definition of myocardial infarction. *J Am Coll Cardiol, 72*(18), 2231–2264.

STOP & REVIEW

Multiple Response

Identify one or more choices that best complete the statement or answer the question.

1. A 66-year-old man presents with persistent chest pain that has been present for 1 hour. His 12-lead ECG reveals STE in leads V_2, V_3, and V_4, and his cardiac biomarkers are elevated. You suspect
   a. stable angina.
   b. unstable angina.
   c. ST-elevation myocardial infarction (STEMI).
   d. non-ST-elevation myocardial infarction (NSTEMI).

2. Which of the following is probably the single best lead to use when differentiating between right and left bundle branch blocks?
   a. Lead II
   b. Lead V_1
   c. Lead V_4
   d. Lead aVR

3. When leads I and aVF are used to determine the electrical axis, left axis deviation is present if the QRS is
   a. positive in lead I and positive in lead aVF.
   b. positive in lead I and negative in lead aVF.
   c. negative in lead I and negative in lead aVF.
   d. negative in lead I and positive in lead aVF.

4. When evaluating the ECG for the presence of chamber enlargement, an ECG machine's sensitivity must be calibrated so that a 1-millivolt electrical signal will produce a deflection measuring exactly _____ mm tall.
   a. 0.5
   b. 1
   c. 5
   d. 10

5. Which of the following ECG changes is one of the earliest to occur during a STEMI but may have resolved by the time the patient seeks medical assistance?
   a. Pathologic Q waves
   b. Hyperacute T waves
   c. Horizontal ST segments
   d. Lengthening of the QT interval

6. Although a right ventricular infarction may occur by itself, it is more commonly associated with a(n) _____ wall myocardial infarction.
   a. septal
   b. lateral
   c. inferior
   d. anterior

7. Which of the following are possible ECG signs of hyperkalemia?
   a. Peaked P waves
   b. Prominent U waves
   c. Tall, peaked T waves
   d. Elevated ST segments
   e. Shortened PR intervals
   f. Increased QRS duration

8. Which of the following are possible ECG signs of sodium disturbances?
   a. Prominent U waves
   b. Low P wave amplitude
   c. Prolonged PR intervals
   d. ST-segment depression
   e. Sodium disturbances do not cause any significant changes on the ECG.

9. Patients experiencing ___and ___ infarctions are most likely to develop bundle branch blocks.
   a. septal
   b. lateral
   c. inferior
   d. anterior
   e. inferobasal
   f. anteroseptal

10. Normal electrical axis lies between____ in the frontal plane.
    a. −30 and +90 degrees
    b. −30 and −90 degrees
    c. −90 and ±180 degrees
    d. +90 and ±180 degrees

11. In a patient experiencing an acute coronary syndrome, T-wave inversion suggests the presence of
    a. injury
    b. ischemia
    c. infarction
    d. cardiogenic shock

12. Lead II is perpendicular to lead
    a. II.
    b. III.
    c. aVF.
    d. aVL.

13. Which of the following statements is true regarding ventricular hypertrophy?
    a. Hypertrophy increases the QRS amplitude.
    b. Hypertrophy increases the duration of the QRS complex.
    c. Leads I, V_5, and V_6 are the best leads to use when looking for ECG evidence of hypertrophy.
    d. ECG evidence of right ventricular hypertrophy is usually more readily evident than left ventricular hypertrophy.

Matching

Match the terms below with their descriptions by placing the letter of each correct answer in the space provided.

a. Left anterior descending artery
b. STEMI
c. Cardiac enlargement
d. V_1, V_2
e. Positive
f. Dilated cardiomyopathy
g. I and aVF
h. Terminal force
i. Right atrial abnormality
j. QS
k. I, aVL, V_5, V_6
l. rSR′

m. Right coronary artery
n. Negative
o. Tall R waves in leads V_1 through V_3 and deeper than normal S waves in leads I, aVL, V_5, and V_6
p. Left bundle branch block
q. Non-ST elevation acute coronary syndromes
r. Intraventricular conduction delay
s. Hypertrophic cardiomyopathy
t. Increased QRS amplitude and changes in the ST segment and T wave
u. Left atrial abnormality

_____ **14.** This can produce ST-segment elevation and wide Q waves that look remarkably similar to infarction

_____ **15.** Term that refers to either dilation of a heart chamber or hypertrophy of the heart muscle

_____ **16.** Leads commonly used to determine axis deviation

_____ **17.** Non-ST elevation myocardial infarction and unstable angina

_____ **18.** Cardiac biomarkers and ST segments are elevated when this is present

_____ **19.** Leads that view the septum

_____ **20.** QRS pattern that is characteristic of right bundle branch block

_____ **21.** Most common form of cardiomyopathy

_____ **22.** Term used to describe a wide QRS that is not associated with a bundle branch block pattern

_____ **23.** The P wave is tall, peaked, and usually of normal duration

_____ **24.** Vessel that is usually blocked with an inferior myocardial infarction

_____ **25.** Deflection of the terminal force of the QRS complex in V_1 in right bundle branch block

_____ **26.** Vessel that is usually blocked with an anterior myocardial infarction

_____ **27.** Characteristic ECG changes associated with right ventricular hypertrophy

_____ **28.** Leads that view the lateral wall of the left ventricle

_____ **29.** The final portion of the QRS complex

_____ **30.** Characteristic ECG changes associated with left ventricular hypertrophy

_____ **31.** QRS pattern that is characteristic of left bundle branch block

_____ **32.** Type of cardiomyopathy characterized by significant myocardial hypertrophy without ventricular dilation that results in a markedly reduced stroke volume because of impaired diastolic filling

_____ **33.** Associated with prolongation of the middle and end of the P wave

12-Lead Electrocardiograms—Practice

34. Analyze this 12-lead ECG and record your findings below.

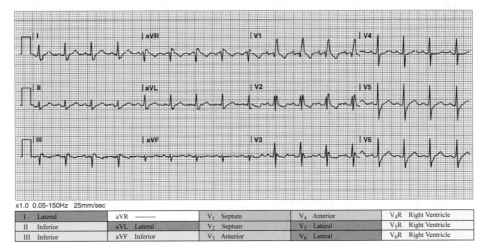

x1.0 0.05-150Hz 25mm/sec

I	Lateral	aVR	---------	V₁	Septum	V₄	Anterior	V₄R	Right Ventricle
II	Inferior	aVL	Lateral	V₂	Septum	V₅	Lateral	V₅R	Right Ventricle
III	Inferior	aVF	Inferior	V₃	Anterior	V₆	Lateral	V₆R	Right Ventricle

Fig. 9.38 (From Phalen, T., & Aehlert, B. J. (2019). *The 12-lead ECG in acute coronary syndromes* (4th ed.). St. Louis: Mosby.)

Rhythm: _____ Rate: _____ P waves: _____

PR interval: _____ QRS duration: _____ QT interval: _____

ST depression: _____ ST elevation: _____ Other findings: _____

Interpretation: _____

35. Analyze this 12-lead ECG and record your findings below.

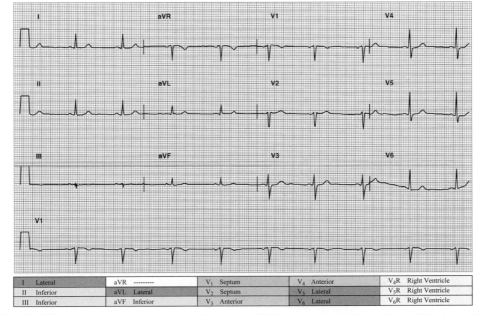

I	Lateral	aVR	---------	V₁	Septum	V₄	Anterior	V₄R	Right Ventricle
II	Inferior	aVL	Lateral	V₂	Septum	V₅	Lateral	V₅R	Right Ventricle
III	Inferior	aVF	Inferior	V₃	Anterior	V₆	Lateral	V₆R	Right Ventricle

Fig. 9.39 (From Phalen, T., & Aehlert, B. J. (2019). *The 12-lead ECG in acute coronary syndromes* (4th ed.). St. Louis: Mosby.)

Rhythm: _____ Rate: _____ P waves: _____

PR interval: _____ QRS duration: _____ QT interval: _____

ST depression: _____ ST elevation: _____ Other findings: _____

Interpretation: _____

36. Analyze this 12-lead ECG and record your findings below.

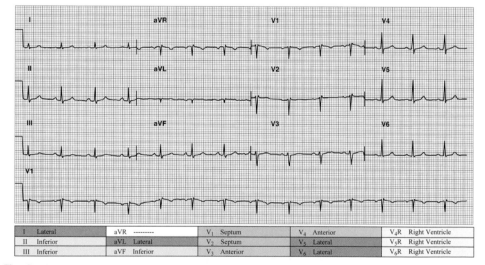

x1.0 0.05-150Hz 25mm/sec

I	Lateral	aVR	---------	V₁	Septum	V₄	Anterior	V₄R	Right Ventricle
II	Inferior	aVL	Lateral	V₂	Septum	V₅	Lateral	V₅R	Right Ventricle
III	Inferior	aVF	Inferior	V₃	Anterior	V₆	Lateral	V₆R	Right Ventricle

Fig. 9.40 (From Phalen, T., & Aehlert, B. J. (2019). *The 12-lead ECG in acute coronary syndromes* (4th ed.). St. Louis: Mosby.)

Rhythm: _____ Rate: _____ P waves: _____
PR interval: _____ QRS duration: _____ QT interval: _____
ST depression: _____ ST elevation: _____ Other findings: _____
Interpretation: _____

37. Analyze this 12-lead ECG and record your findings below.

I	Lateral	aVR	---------	V₁	Septum	V₄	Anterior	V₄R	Right Ventricle
II	Inferior	aVL	Lateral	V₂	Septum	V₅	Lateral	V₅R	Right Ventricle
III	Inferior	aVF	Inferior	V₃	Anterior	V₆	Lateral	V₆R	Right Ventricle

Fig. 9.41 (From Phalen, T., & Aehlert, B. J. (2019). *The 12-lead ECG in acute coronary syndromes* (4th ed.). St. Louis: Mosby.)

Rhythm: _____ Rate: _____ P waves: _____
PR interval: _____ QRS duration: _____ QT interval: _____
ST depression: _____ ST elevation: _____ Other findings: _____
Interpretation: _____

38. Analyze this 12-lead ECG and record your findings below.

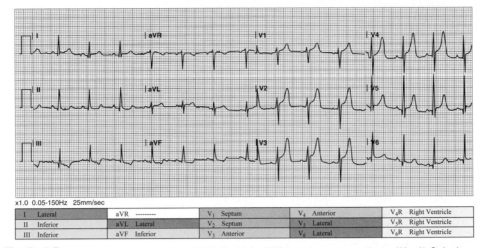

Fig. 9.42 (From Phalen, T., & Aehlert, B. J. (2019). *The 12-lead ECG in acute coronary syndromes* (4th ed.). St. Louis: Mosby.)

Rhythm: _____ Rate: _____ P waves: _____

PR interval: _____ QRS duration: _____ QT interval: _____

ST depression: _____ ST elevation: _____ Other findings: _____

Interpretation: _____

39. Analyze this 12-lead ECG and record your findings below.

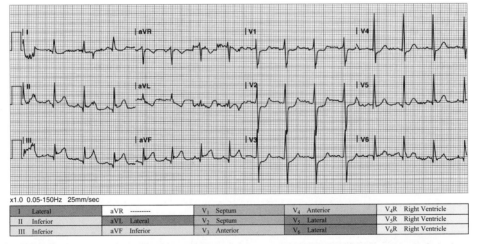

Fig. 9.43 (From Phalen, T., & Aehlert, B. J. (2019). *The 12-lead ECG in acute coronary syndromes* (4th ed.). St. Louis: Mosby.)

Rhythm: _____ Rate: _____ P waves: _____

PR interval: _____ QRS duration: _____ QT interval: _____

ST depression: _____ ST elevation: _____ Other findings: _____

Interpretation: _____

40. Analyze this 12-lead ECG and record your findings below.

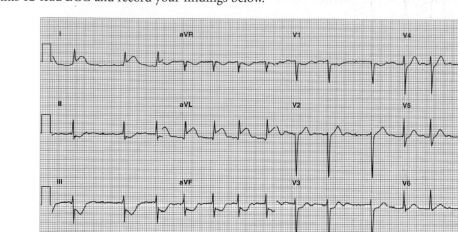

I	Lateral	aVR	---------	V₁	Septum	V₄	Anterior	V₄R	Right Ventricle
II	Inferior	aVL	Lateral	V₂	Septum	V₅	Lateral	V₅R	Right Ventricle
III	Inferior	aVF	Inferior	V₃	Anterior	V₆	Lateral	V₆R	Right Ventricle

Fig. 9.44 (From Phalen, T., & Aehlert, B. J. (2019). *The 12-lead ECG in acute coronary syndromes* (4th ed.). St. Louis: Mosby.)

Rhythm: _____ Rate: _____ P waves: _____

PR interval: _____ QRS duration: _____ QT interval: _____

ST depression: _____ ST elevation: _____ Other findings: _____

Interpretation: _____

41. Analyze this 12-lead ECG and record your findings below.

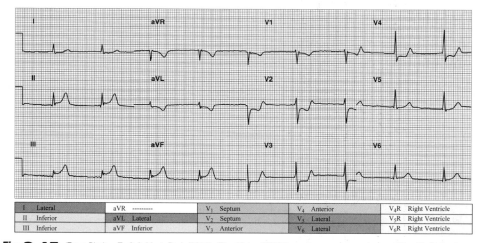

I	Lateral	aVR	---------	V₁	Septum	V₄	Anterior	V₄R	Right Ventricle
II	Inferior	aVL	Lateral	V₂	Septum	V₅	Lateral	V₅R	Right Ventricle
III	Inferior	aVF	Inferior	V₃	Anterior	V₆	Lateral	V₆R	Right Ventricle

Fig. 9.45 (From Phalen, T., & Aehlert, B. J. (2019). *The 12-lead ECG in acute coronary syndromes* (4th ed.). St. Louis: Mosby.)

Rhythm: _____ Rate: _____ P waves: _____

PR interval: _____ QRS duration: _____ QT interval: _____

ST depression: _____ ST elevation: _____ Other findings: _____

Interpretation: _____

42. Analyze this 12-lead ECG and record your findings below.

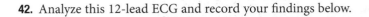

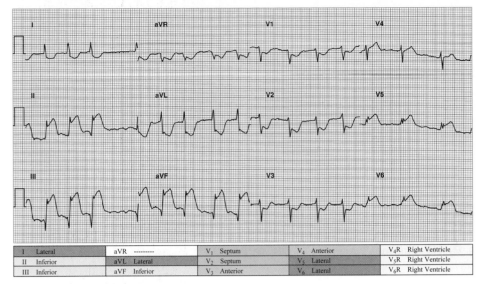

I	Lateral	aVR	---------	V₁	Septum	V₄	Anterior	V₄R	Right Ventricle
II	Inferior	aVL	Lateral	V₂	Septum	V₅	Lateral	V₅R	Right Ventricle
III	Inferior	aVF	Inferior	V₃	Anterior	V₆	Lateral	V₆R	Right Ventricle

Fig. 9.46 (From Phalen, T., & Aehlert, B. J. (2019). *The 12-lead ECG in acute coronary syndromes* (4th ed.). St. Louis: Mosby.)

Rhythm: _____ Rate: _____ P waves: _____
PR interval: _____ QRS duration: _____ QT interval: _____
ST depression: _____ ST elevation: _____ Other findings: _____
Interpretation: _____

43. Analyze this 12-lead ECG and record your findings below.

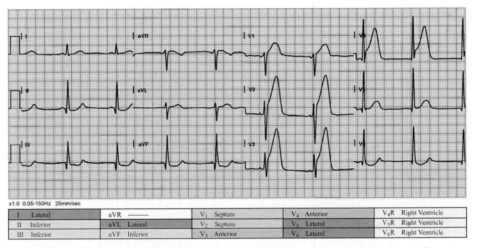

x1.0 0.05-150Hz 25mm/sec

I	Lateral	aVR	---------	V₁	Septum	V₄	Anterior	V₄R	Right Ventricle
II	Inferior	aVL	Lateral	V₂	Septum	V₅	Lateral	V₅R	Right Ventricle
III	Inferior	aVF	Inferior	V₃	Anterior	V₆	Lateral	V₆R	Right Ventricle

Fig. 9.47 (From Phalen, T., & Aehlert, B. J. (2019). *The 12-lead ECG in acute coronary syndromes* (4th ed.). St. Louis: Mosby.)

Rhythm: _____ Rate: _____ P waves: _____
PR interval: _____ QRS duration: _____ QT interval: _____
ST depression: _____ ST elevation: _____ Other findings: _____
Interpretation: _____

44. Analyze this 12-lead ECG and record your findings below.

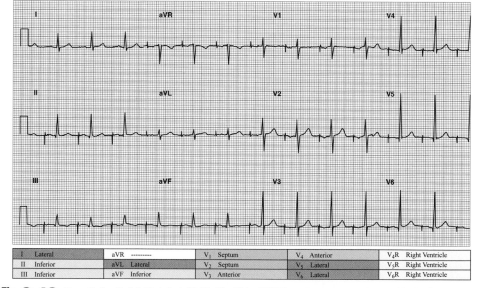

x1.0 0.05-150Hz   25mm/sec

I Lateral	aVR ---------	V₁ Septum	V₄ Anterior	V₄R Right Ventricle
II Inferior	aVL Lateral	V₂ Septum	V₅ Lateral	V₅R Right Ventricle
III Inferior	aVF Inferior	V₃ Anterior	V₆ Lateral	V₆R Right Ventricle

Fig. 9.48 (From Phalen, T., & Aehlert, B. J. (2019). *The 12-lead ECG in acute coronary syndromes* (4th ed.). St. Louis: Mosby.)

Rhythm: _____ Rate: _____ P waves: _____

PR interval: _____ QRS duration: _____ QT interval: _____

ST depression: _____ ST elevation: _____ Other findings: _____

Interpretation: _____

45. Analyze this 12-lead ECG and record your findings below.

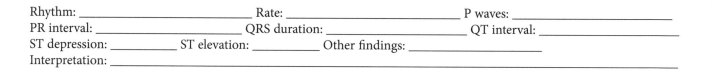

I Lateral	aVR ---------	V₁ Septum	V₄ Anterior	V₄R Right Ventricle
II Inferior	aVL Lateral	V₂ Septum	V₅ Lateral	V₅R Right Ventricle
III Inferior	aVF Inferior	V₃ Anterior	V₆ Lateral	V₆R Right Ventricle

Fig. 9.49 (From Phalen, T., & Aehlert, B. J. (2019). *The 12-lead ECG in acute coronary syndromes* (4th ed.). St. Louis: Mosby.)

Rhythm: _____ Rate: _____ P waves: _____

PR interval: _____ QRS duration: _____ QT interval: _____

ST depression: _____ ST elevation: _____ Other findings: _____

Interpretation: _____

46. Analyze this 12-lead ECG and record your findings below.

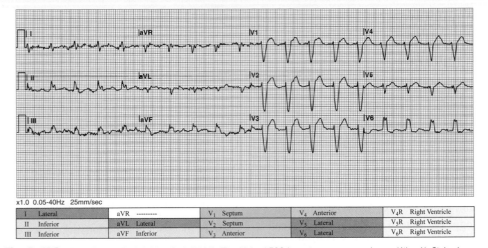

x1.0 0.05-40Hz 25mm/sec

I	Lateral	aVR	---------	V₁	Septum	V₄	Anterior	V₄R	Right Ventricle
II	Inferior	aVL	Lateral	V₂	Septum	V₅	Lateral	V₅R	Right Ventricle
III	Inferior	aVF	Inferior	V₃	Anterior	V₆	Lateral	V₆R	Right Ventricle

Fig. 9.50 (From Phalen, T., & Aehlert, B. J. (2019). *The 12-lead ECG in acute coronary syndromes* (4th ed.). St. Louis: Mosby.)

Rhythm: _____ Rate: _____ P waves: _____

PR interval: _____ QRS duration: _____ QT interval: _____

ST depression: _____ ST elevation: _____ Other findings: _____

Interpretation: _____

STOP & REVIEW ANSWERS

1. **C.** An acute coronary syndrome diagnosis is based on the patient's clinical presentation, history, ECG findings, and cardiac biomarker results. If ST segments are elevated in two contiguous leads, and elevated cardiac biomarkers are present, the diagnosis is STEMI. If ST elevation is not present, but biomarker levels are elevated, the diagnosis is NSTEMI. If the ST segments are not elevated, and cardiac biomarkers are not elevated, the diagnosis is unstable angina.

2. **B.** The criteria for bundle branch block recognition may be found in any lead of the ECG. However, when differentiating RBBB from LBBB, pay particular attention to the QRS morphology (i.e., shape) in specific leads. Lead V_1 is probably the single best lead to use when differentiating between RBBB and LBBB.

3. **B.** Current flow to the left of normal is called left axis deviation (between −30 and −90 degrees). If the QRS complex is predominantly positive in I and negative in aVF, left axis deviation is present.

4. **D.** When evaluating the ECG for chamber enlargement, it is essential to check the calibration marker to ensure that it is 10 mm (1 mV) tall.

5. **B.** Hyperacute (i.e., tall) T waves are sometimes called "tombstone" T waves and typically measure more than 50% of the preceding R wave. In addition to an increase in height, the T wave becomes more symmetric and may become pointed. These changes are often not recorded on the ECG because they have typically resolved by the time the patient seeks medical assistance.

6. **C.** The right ventricle is supplied by the right ventricular marginal branch of the RCA. Occlusion of the right ventricular marginal branch results in an isolated right ventricular infarction (RVI). Occlusion of the RCA proximal to the right ventricular marginal branch results in an inferior and right ventricular infarction. RVI should be suspected when ECG changes suggesting an inferior infarction are seen.

7. **C, F.** ECG signs of hyperkalemia may include:
Tall, peaked (tented), narrow, symmetric T waves
QRS duration increases as potassium level increases
P waves decrease in amplitude as potassium level increases
PR interval duration increases as potassium level increases

8. **E.** Sodium disturbances do not cause any significant changes on the ECG.

9. **A, F.** The septum, which contains the bundle of His and bundle branches, is usually supplied by the left anterior descending coronary artery. ECG changes of infarction are seen in leads V_1 and V_2 if the site of infarction is limited to the septum. If the entire anterior wall is involved, ECG changes will be visible in V_1, V_2, V_3, and V_4. A blockage in this area may result in both right and left bundle branch blocks, second-degree atrioventricular (AV) block type II, and third-degree AV block.

10. **A.** In adults, the normal QRS axis is considered to be between −30 and +90 degrees in the frontal plane. Current flow to the right of normal is called right axis deviation (between +90 and ±180 degrees). Current flow in the direction opposite of normal is called indeterminate, "no man's land," northwest, or extreme right axis deviation (between −90 and ±180 degrees). Current flow to the left of normal is called left axis deviation (between −30 and −90 degrees).

11. **B.** In a patient experiencing an acute coronary syndrome, T-wave inversion suggests the presence of myocardial ischemia.

12. **D.** In the hexaxial reference system, the axes of some leads are perpendicular to each other. For example, lead II is perpendicular to aVL, lead I is perpendicular to lead aVF, and lead III is perpendicular to lead aVR.

13. **A, C.** Ventricular muscle thickens (i.e., hypertrophies) when it sustains a persistent pressure overload. Dilatation occurs because of persistent volume overload. The two often go hand in hand. Hypertrophy increases the QRS amplitude and is often associated with ST-segment depression and asymmetric T-wave inversion. Because the right ventricle is normally considerably smaller than the left, it must become significantly enlarged before changes are visible on the ECG. Leads V_1, V_5, and V_6 are used when looking for ECG evidence of hypertrophy.

Matching

14. ANS: p
15. ANS: c
16. ANS: g
17. ANS: q
18. ANS: b
19. ANS: d
20. ANS: l
21. ANS: f
22. ANS: r
23. ANS: i
24. ANS: m
25. ANS: e
26. ANS: a
27. ANS: o
28. ANS: k
29. ANS: h
30. ANS: t
31. ANS: j
32. ANS: s
33. ANS: u

Practice 12-Lead Electrocardiograms Answers

Note: The rate and interval measurements provided here were obtained using electronic calipers.

34. Fig. 9.38
Rhythm and rate: Sinus tachycardia at 101 beats/min
QRS axis: Left
PR interval: 0.16 second
QRS duration: 0.13 second
QT interval: 0.35 second
ST depression/elevation: Depression in I, II, aVL, V_1 to V_2
Other findings: T waves inverted in V_1 to V_2
Interpretation: Sinus tachycardia at 101 beats/min with RBBB

35. Fig. 9.39
Rhythm and rate: Sinus bradycardia at 56 beats/min
QRS axis: Normal
PR interval: 0.12 second
QRS duration: 0.10 second
QT interval: 0.43 second
ST depression/elevation:
Other findings: T waves inverted in V_1
Interpretation: Sinus bradycardia at 56 beats/min, otherwise normal ECG

36. Fig. 9.40
Rhythm and rate: Sinus rhythm at 60 beats/min
QRS axis: Left
PR interval: 0.16 second
QRS duration: 0.14 second
QT interval: 0.42 second
ST depression/elevation: Elevation V_1 to V_4; depression in I, aVL, V_5, V_6
Other findings: T waves inverted in I, aVL, V_5, V_6
Interpretation: Sinus rhythm at 60 beats/min; possible STEMI/new-onset LBBB; consider clinical presentation

37. Fig. 9.41
Rhythm and rate: Sinus rhythm at 84 beats/min
QRS axis: Normal
PR interval: 0.16 second
QRS duration: 0.08 second
QT interval: 0.34 second
ST depression/elevation:
Other findings:
Interpretation: Normal ECG

38. Fig. 9.42
Rhythm and rate: Sinus rhythm at 86 beats/min
QRS axis: Normal
PR interval: 0.14 second
QRS duration: 0.09 second
QT interval: 0.35 second
ST depression/elevation: Elevation noted in V_1 to V_4
Other findings: T waves inverted in III; tall, peaked in V_2 to V_4; baseline wander in V_6
Interpretation: Sinus rhythm at 86 beats/min. Anteroseptal infarction; STE noted in V_1 to V_4. Tall, peaked T waves in V_2 to V_4. Reciprocal changes noted in III, subtle changes in II and aVF.

39. Fig. 9.43
Rhythm and rate: Sinus rhythm at 92 beats/min
QRS axis: Normal
PR interval: 0.15 second
QRS duration: 0.11 second
QT interval: 0.36 second
ST depression/elevation: Elevation in II, III, aVF; depression in I, aVL, V_1 to V_4
Other findings: Pathologic Q waves in II, III, aVF; baseline wander in I, II, III
Interpretation: Sinus rhythm at 92 beats/min. Inferior STEMI; STE noted in II, III, and aVF. Reciprocal change noted in aVL. ST depression in V_1 to V_4 suggests possible posterior involvement; consider obtaining posterior leads. Obtain V_4R to assess for right ventricular infarction.

40. Fig. 9.44
Rhythm and rate: Atrial fibrillation at 81 beats/min
QRS axis: Left
PR interval: None
QRS duration: 0.09 second
QT interval: 0.39 second
ST depression/elevation: Elevation in I, aVL; depression in II, III, aVF
Other findings:
Interpretation: Atrial fibrillation at 81 beats/min. Lateral STEMI; reciprocal changes noted in II, III, and aVF.

41. Fig. 9.45
Rhythm and rate: Junctional rhythm at 55 beats/min
QRS axis: Normal
PR interval: None
QRS duration: 0.10 second
QT interval: 0.45 second
ST depression/elevation: Elevation in II, III, aVF; depression in I, aVL, V_1 to V_4
Other findings: T waves inverted in aVL, V_1
Interpretation: Junctional rhythm at 55 beats/min. Inferior STEMI; reciprocal changes noted in aVL. Obtain V_4R to assess for right ventricular infarction.

42. Fig. 9.46
Rhythm and rate: Atrial fibrillation at 115 beats/min
QRS axis: Normal
PR interval:
QRS duration: 0.10 second
QT interval: 0.36 second
ST depression/elevation: Elevation in II, III, aVF, V_5, V_6; depression in I, aVL, V_1 to V_3

Other findings: T waves inverted in V_1, V_2
Interpretation: Atrial fibrillation at 115 beats/min. Inferolateral STEMI; reciprocal changes in I and aVL. Obtain V_4R to assess for right ventricular infarction. ST-segment depression in V_1 to V_3 suggests possible posterior involvement; consider obtaining posterior leads.

43. Fig. 9.47
Rhythm and rate: Sinus bradycardia at 56 beats/min
QRS axis: Normal
PR interval: 0.11 second
QRS duration: 0.10 second
QT interval: 0.46 second
ST depression/elevation: Elevation in V_1 to V_4; depression in II, III, aVF
Other findings: Tall T waves in V_2 to V_4
Interpretation: Sinus bradycardia at 56 beats/min. Suspected anteroseptal STEMI; reciprocal changes noted in II, III, aVF. Short PR interval.

44. Fig. 9.48
Rhythm and rate: Supraventricular bradycardia at 42 beats/min
QRS axis: Normal
PR interval: None
QRS duration: 0.09 second
QT interval: 0.52 second
ST depression/elevation: Elevation in II, III, aVF, V_5 to V_6; depression in I, aVL
Other findings: Tall T waves in II, III, aVF
Interpretation: Supraventricular bradycardia at 42 beats/min. Inferolateral STEMI; reciprocal changes in I and aVL. Prolonged QT interval. Obtain V_4R to assess for right ventricular infarction.

45. Fig. 9.49
Rhythm and rate: Electronic atrial pacemaker at 80 pulses/min
QRS axis: Normal
PR interval: 0.26 second
QRS duration: 0.09 second
QT interval: 0.36 second
ST depression/elevation:
Other findings:
Interpretation: Atrial paced rhythm at 80 pulses/min; no ECG evidence of STEMI

46. Fig. 9.50
Rhythm and rate: Sinus tachycardia at 113 beats/min with first-degree AV block and LBBB
QRS axis: Normal
PR interval: 0.33 second
QRS duration: 0.15 second
QT interval: 0.33 second
ST depression/elevation: Elevation in V_1 to V_3
Other findings: Artifact in limb leads
Interpretation: Sinus tachycardia at 113 beats/min with first-degree AV block. Possible anteroseptal STEMI; however, wide QRS and LBBB pattern are also present. Consider clinical presentation and obtain serial ECGs.

Identify one or more choices that best complete the statement or answer the question.

1. The middle layer of the heart wall that contains the atrial and ventricular muscle fibers necessary for contraction is the
   a. epicardium.
   b. pericardium.
   c. myocardium.
   d. endocardium.

2. The _____ supplies the right atrium and right ventricle with blood.
   a. circumflex (Cx) artery
   b. right coronary artery (RCA)
   c. left main coronary artery
   d. left anterior descending (LAD) artery

3. The contribution of blood that is added to the ventricles and results from atrial contraction is called
   a. afterload.
   b. atrial kick.
   c. cardiac output.
   d. peripheral resistance.

4. The right atrium receives deoxygenated blood from which of the following vessels?
   a. Aorta
   b. Coronary sinus
   c. Inferior vena cava
   d. Superior vena cava

5. Which of the following are semilunar valves?
   a. Aortic
   b. Mitral
   c. Pulmonic
   d. Tricuspid

6. Stimulation of parasympathetic nerve fibers typically results in which of the following actions?
   a. Constriction of coronary blood vessels
   b. Increased strength of cardiac muscle contraction
   c. Increased rate of discharge of the sinoatrial (SA) node
   d. Slowed conduction through the atrioventricular (AV) node

7. Which of the following are primary branches of the left main coronary artery?
   a. Cx branch
   b. LAD branch.
   c. Marginal branch
   d. Posterior descending branch

8. _____ cells are specialized cells of the electrical conduction system responsible for the spontaneous generation and conduction of electrical impulses.
   a. Working
   b. Contractile
   c. Pacemaker
   d. Mechanical

9. The absolute refractory period:
   a. begins with the onset of the P wave and terminates with the end of the QRS complex.
   b. begins with the onset of the QRS complex and terminates at approximately the apex of the T wave.
   c. begins with the onset of the QRS complex and terminates with the end of the T wave.
   d. begins with the onset of the P wave and terminates with the beginning of the QRS complex.

10. The ST segment is measured from the
    a. end of the QRS complex to the end of the T wave.
    b. beginning of the QRS complex to the end of the T wave.
    c. end of the QRS complex to the beginning of the T wave.
    d. beginning of the QRS complex to the beginning of the T wave.

11. Which of the following statements is true regarding the QT interval?
    a. The QT interval represents atrial depolarization, followed immediately by atrial systole.
    b. The QT interval corresponds to atrial depolarization and impulse delay in the AV node.
    c. The QT interval represents ventricular depolarization, followed immediately by ventricular systole.
    d. The QT interval represents the time from initial depolarization of the ventricles to the end of ventricular repolarization.

12. Where is the positive electrode placed in lead III?
    a. Left arm
    b. Right arm
    c. Left leg/foot
    d. Right leg/foot

13. A junctional escape rhythm occurs because of
    a. severe chronic obstructive pulmonary disease.
    b. multiple irritable sites firing within the AV junction.
    c. slowing of the rate of the heart's primary pacemaker.
    d. intrathoracic pressure changes associated with the respiratory cycle.

14. How do you determine whether the atrial rhythm on an electrocardiogram (ECG) tracing is regular or irregular?
    a. Compare QT intervals
    b. Compare PR intervals
    c. Compare P to P intervals
    d. Compare R to R intervals

15. Which of the following ECG leads use two distinct electrodes, one of which is positive and the other negative?
    a. Lead I
    b. Lead II
    c. Lead V_1
    d. Lead V_6
    e. Lead aVF

16. Leads II, III, and aVF view the heart's __ surface.
    a. lateral
    b. anterior
    c. inferior
    d. inferobasal

17. An ECG rhythm strip shows a ventricular rate of 46, a regular rhythm, a PR interval of 0.14 second, a QRS duration of 0.06 second, and one positive P wave before each QRS. This rhythm is
    a. sinus arrest.
    b. sinus rhythm.
    c. SA block.
    d. sinus bradycardia.

18. In sinus arrhythmia, a gradual decreasing of the heart rate is usually associated with
    a. expiration.
    b. inspiration.
    c. excessive caffeine intake.
    d. early signs of heart failure.

19. SA block is a disorder of impulse _____ and sinus arrest is a disorder of impulse _____.
    a. formation, conduction
    b. conduction, formation

20. Signs and symptoms experienced during a tachydysrhythmia are usually primarily related to
    a. atrial irritability.
    b. vasoconstriction.
    c. slowed conduction through the AV node.
    d. decreased ventricular filling time and stroke volume.

21. Which of the following are ectopic (latent) pacemakers?
    a. The SA node
    b. The ventricles
    c. The AV junction
    d. The left bundle branch
    e. The right bundle branch

22. A wandering atrial pacemaker rhythm with a ventricular rate of 60 to 100 beats per minute (beats/min) may also be referred to as
    a. atrial flutter.
    b. atrial fibrillation (AFib).
    c. multiformed atrial rhythm.
    d. multifocal atrial tachycardia.

23. The most common type of supraventricular tachycardia (SVT) is
    a. atrial flutter.
    b. atrial tachycardia.
    c. AV reentrant tachycardia (AVRT).
    d. AV nodal reentrant tachycardia (AVNRT).

24. Which of the following is true with regard to treatment of a symptomatic patient with AFib?
    a. With rate control, the patient remains in AFib, but the ventricular rate is reduced (controlled) to decrease acute symptoms.
    b. With rate control, measures are taken (either pharmacologic or electrical) to reestablish sinus rhythm.

25. If the onset or end of paroxysmal atrial tachycardia or paroxysmal supraventricular tachycardia (PSVT) is not observed on the ECG, the dysrhythmia is called
    a. SVT.
    b. sinus tachycardia.
    c. junctional tachycardia.
    d. multifocal atrial tachycardia.

26. Which of the following is the most common sustained dysrhythmia in adults?
    a. AFib
    b. Sinus bradycardia
    c. Junctional rhythm
    d. Ventricular tachycardia (VT)

27. Which of the following statements are true regarding premature atrial complexes (PACs) and premature junctional complexes (PJCs) when viewed in leads II, III, and aVF?
    a. A PJC has a wide QRS complex.
    b. A PAC has a narrow QRS complex.
    c. A P wave may or may not be present with a PJC.
    d. A P wave may or may not be present with a PAC.
    e. A PAC has a positive P wave before the QRS complex.
    f. A PJC has a positive P wave before each QRS complex.

28. Which of the following are characteristics of Wolff-Parkinson-White pattern?
    a. Delta wave
    b. Flutter waves
    c. Long PR interval
    d. Short PR interval
    e. Wide QRS complex
    f. Narrow QRS complex

29. Which of the following ECG characteristics distinguishes atrial flutter from other atrial dysrhythmias?
    a. The presence of fibrillatory waves
    b. The presence of delta waves before the QRS
    c. Clearly identifiable P waves of varying size and amplitude
    d. The "saw-tooth" or "picket-fence" appearance of waveforms before the QRS

30. When a junctional rhythm is viewed in lead II, where is the location of the P wave on the ECG if atrial depolarization and ventricular depolarization occur simultaneously?
    a. Before the QRS complex
    b. Within the QRS complex
    c. After the QRS complex

31. The usual rate of nonparoxysmal junctional tachycardia is
    a. 50 to 80 beats/min.
    b. 80 to 120 beats/min.
    c. 101 to 140 beats/min.
    d. 150 to 300 beats/min.

32. Junctional (or ventricular) complexes may appear early (before the next expected sinus beat) or late (after the next expected sinus beat). If the complex is *early* it is called a(n) _____. If the complex is *late* it is called a(n) _____.
    a. Escape beat; premature complex
    b. Premature complex; escape beat

33. Depending on the severity of the patient's signs and symptoms, management of slow rhythms may require therapeutic intervention including
    a. defibrillation.
    b. vagal maneuvers.
    c. administration of atropine.
    d. administration of adenosine.
    e. synchronized cardioversion.

34. Which statements are correct regarding junctional dysrhythmias?
    a. The QRS complex of a junctional rhythm is usually narrow.
    b. A junctional rhythm is a potentially life-threatening dysrhythmia.
    c. The ventricular rhythm associated with a junctional rhythm is usually very regular.
    d. A compensatory (incomplete) pause often follows a premature junctional complex (PJC).

35. The term for three or more premature ventricular complexes (PVCs) occurring in a row at a rate of more than 100/min is
    a. a run of VT.
    b. ventricular trigeminy.
    c. ventricular fibrillation (VF).
    d. a run of ventricular escape beats.

36. PVCs that look alike in the same lead and begin from the same anatomic site (i.e., focus) are called _____ PVCs.
    a. uniform
    b. isolated
    c. multiform
    d. interpolated

37. Which of the following dysrhythmias has QRS complexes that vary in shape and amplitude from beat to beat and appear to twist from upright to negative or negative to upright and back, resembling a spindle?
    a. AFib
    b. Monomorphic VT
    c. Idioventricular rhythm (IVR)
    d. Polymorphic ventricular tachycardia (PMVT)

38. When a delay or interruption in impulse conduction from the atria to the ventricles occurs as a result of a transient or permanent anatomic or functional impairment, the resulting dysrhythmia is called a(n)
    a. SA block.
    b. AV block.
    c. sinus arrest.
    d. bundle branch block (BBB).

39. Whenever the criteria for BBB have been met and lead V_1 displays an rSR' pattern, you should suspect a
    a. left bundle branch block (LBBB).
    b. right bundle branch block (RBBB).

40. The PR interval of a first-degree AV block
    a. is constant and less than 0.12 second in duration.
    b. is constant and more than 0.20 second in duration.
    c. is generally progressive until a P wave appears without a QRS complex.
    d. gradually decreases in duration until a P wave appears without a QRS complex.

41. Which of the following is an example of a complete AV block?
    a. First-degree AV block
    b. Second-degree AV block type I
    c. Second-degree AV block type II
    d. Third-degree AV block

42. Identify the correct statements regarding 2:1 AV block.
    a. The PR interval is constant.
    b. The atrial rhythm is irregular.
    c. The ventricular rate is twice the atrial rate.
    d. Every other P wave is not followed by a QRS.
    e. The level of the block is located within the SA node.

43. Which lead is probably the best to use when differentiating between RBBB and LBBB?
    a. II
    b. V_1
    c. V_4
    d. aVR

44. The term *capture*, as it pertains to pacing, refers to
    a. a vertical line on the ECG that indicates the pacemaker has discharged.
    b. the extent to which an artificial pacemaker recognizes intrinsic cardiac electrical activity.
    c. a pacemaker response in which the output pulse is suppressed when an intrinsic event is sensed.
    d. the successful conduction of an artificial pacemaker's impulse through the myocardium, resulting in depolarization.

45. The 12-lead ECG only provides a _____-second view of each lead.
    a. 1
    b. 2.5
    c. 4.5
    d. 6

46. Although a right ventricular infarction (RVI) may occur by itself, it is more commonly associated with a(n) _____ wall myocardial infarction (MI).
    a. septal
    b. lateral
    c. inferior
    d. anterior

47. Poor R-wave progression is a phrase used to describe R waves that decrease in size from V_1 to V_4. This is often seen in an _____ infarction.
    a. inferobasal
    b. anteroseptal
    c. anterolateral
    d. inferoposterior

48. A rapid, wide-QRS rhythm associated with pulselessness, shock, or heart failure should be presumed to be
    a. VF.
    b. VT.
    c. AFib.
    d. AVRT.

49. Which of the following are characteristics of IVR?
    a. Ventricular rate 20 to 40 beats/min
    b. Rapid, chaotic rhythm with no pattern or regularity
    c. P waves may occur before, during, or after the QRS
    d. QRS complexes measure 0.12 second or greater; atrial rate not discernible

50. The first letter of a pacemaker identification code represents
    a. the chamber paced.
    b. the chamber sensed.
    c. the mode of response.
    d. programmable functions.

Posttest Rhythm Strips

Use the five steps of rhythm interpretation to interpret each of the following rhythm strips. All rhythms were recorded in lead II unless otherwise noted.

51. This rhythm strip is from a 62-year-old woman with renal failure.

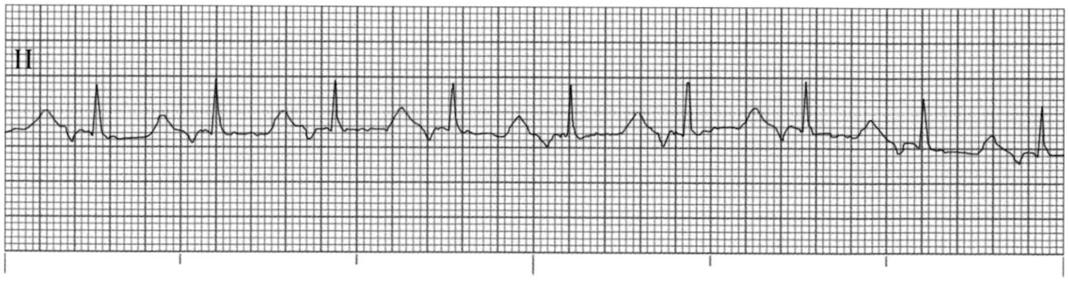

Fig. 10.1

Rhythm: _____ Rate: _____ P waves: _____
PR interval: _____ QRS duration: _____ QT interval: _____
Interpretation: _____

52. Identify the rhythm.

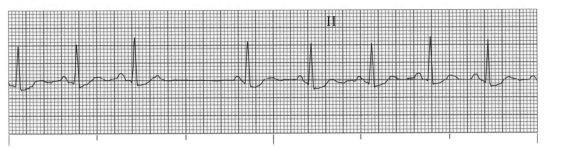

Fig. 10.2 (Modified from Aehlert, B. (2004). *ECG study cards.* St. Louis: Mosby.)

Rhythm: _____ Rate: _____ P waves: _____
PR interval: _____ QRS duration: _____ QT interval: _____
Interpretation: _____

53. Identify the rhythm.

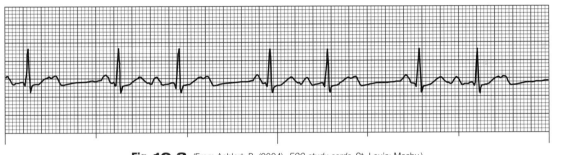

Fig. 10.3 (From Aehlert, B. (2004). *ECG study cards.* St. Louis: Mosby.)

Rhythm: _____ Rate: _____ P waves: _____
PR interval: _____ QRS duration: _____ QT interval: _____
Interpretation: _____

54. Identify the rhythm.

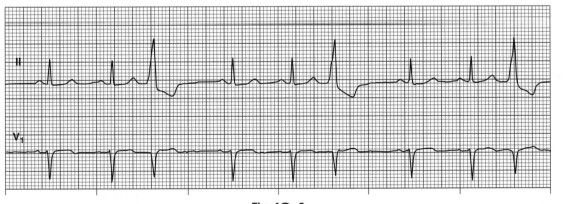

Fig. 10.4

Rhythm: _____ Rate: _____ P waves: _____
PR interval: _____ QRS duration: _____ QT interval: _____
Interpretation: _____

55. This rhythm strip is from a 59-year-old man complaining of poor circulation in his legs.

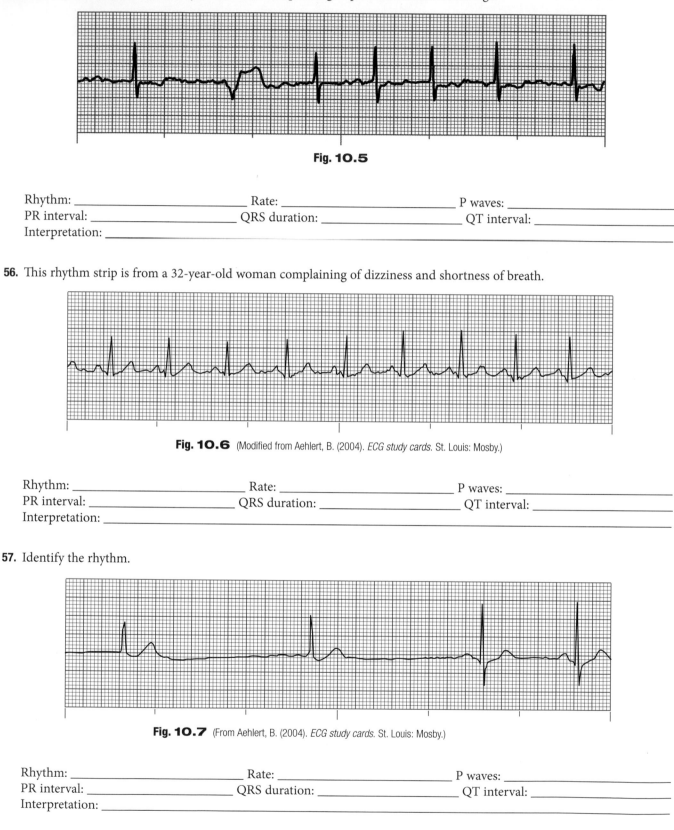

Fig. 10.5

Rhythm: _____ Rate: _____ P waves: _____
PR interval: _____ QRS duration: _____ QT interval: _____
Interpretation: _____

56. This rhythm strip is from a 32-year-old woman complaining of dizziness and shortness of breath.

Fig. 10.6 (Modified from Aehlert, B. (2004). *ECG study cards*. St. Louis: Mosby.)

Rhythm: _____ Rate: _____ P waves: _____
PR interval: _____ QRS duration: _____ QT interval: _____
Interpretation: _____

57. Identify the rhythm.

Fig. 10.7 (From Aehlert, B. (2004). *ECG study cards*. St. Louis: Mosby.)

Rhythm: _____ Rate: _____ P waves: _____
PR interval: _____ QRS duration: _____ QT interval: _____
Interpretation: _____

58. This rhythm strip is from a 76-year-old man who experienced a syncopal episode while playing golf.

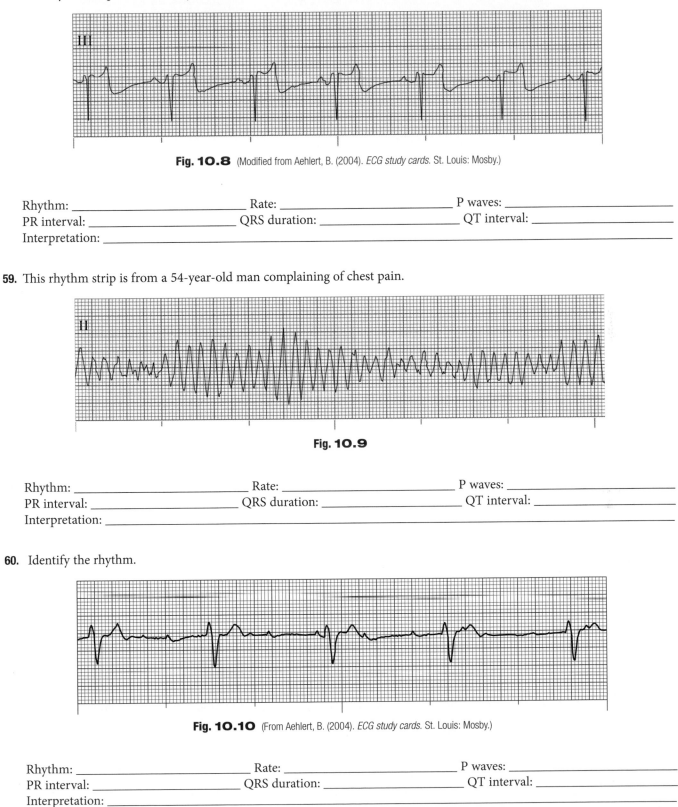

Fig. 10.8 (Modified from Aehlert, B. (2004). *ECG study cards*. St. Louis: Mosby.)

Rhythm: _____ Rate: _____ P waves: _____
PR interval: _____ QRS duration: _____ QT interval: _____
Interpretation: _____

59. This rhythm strip is from a 54-year-old man complaining of chest pain.

Fig. 10.9

Rhythm: _____ Rate: _____ P waves: _____
PR interval: _____ QRS duration: _____ QT interval: _____
Interpretation: _____

60. Identify the rhythm.

Fig. 10.10 (From Aehlert, B. (2004). *ECG study cards*. St. Louis: Mosby.)

Rhythm: _____ Rate: _____ P waves: _____
PR interval: _____ QRS duration: _____ QT interval: _____
Interpretation: _____

61. This rhythm strip is from a 70-year-old woman with chronic obstructive pulmonary disease.

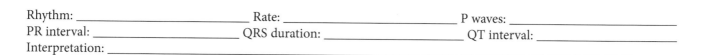

Fig. 10.11 (Modified from Aehlert, B. (2004). *ECG study cards.* St. Louis: Mosby.)

Rhythm: _____ Rate: _____ P waves: _____
PR interval: _____ QRS duration: _____ QT interval: _____
Interpretation: _____

62. This rhythm strip is from a 77-year-old man with chest pain. His chest hit the steering wheel during a motor vehicle crash.

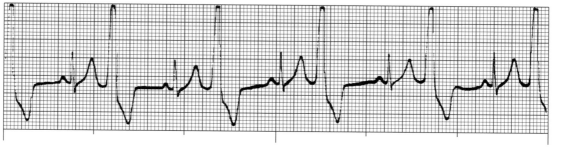

Fig. 10.12

Rhythm: _____ Rate: _____ P waves: _____
PR interval: _____ QRS duration: _____ QT interval: _____
Interpretation: _____

63. Identify the rhythm.

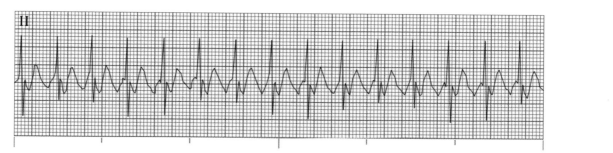

Fig. 10.13 (Modified from Aehlert, B. (2004). *ECG study cards.* St. Louis: Mosby.)

Rhythm: _____ Rate: _____ P waves: _____
PR interval: _____ QRS duration: _____ QT interval: _____
Interpretation: _____

64. This rhythm strip is from a 20-year-old woman who collapsed on the sidewalk of her residence. A family member states that she has a history of SVT and takes atenolol.

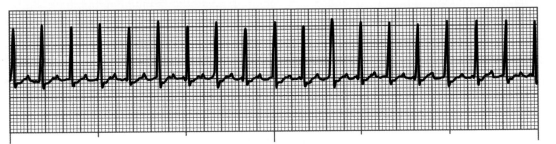

Fig. 10.14 (From Aehlert, B. (2004). *ECG study cards.* St. Louis: Mosby.)

Rhythm: _____ Rate: _____ P waves: _____
PR interval: _____ QRS duration: _____ QT interval: _____
Interpretation: _____

65. This rhythm strip is from a 42-year-old man with chest pain.

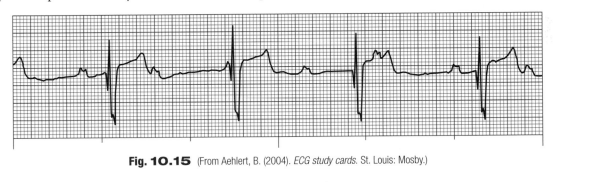

Fig. 10.15 (From Aehlert, B. (2004). *ECG study cards.* St. Louis: Mosby.)

Rhythm: _____ Rate: _____ P waves: _____
PR interval: _____ QRS duration: _____ QT interval: _____
Interpretation: _____

66. This rhythm strip is from a 76-year-old woman who is complaining of back pain. Her medical history includes an MI 2 years ago.

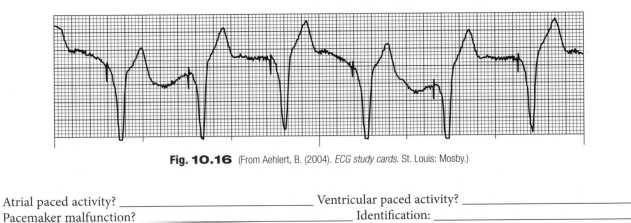

Fig. 10.16 (From Aehlert, B. (2004). *ECG study cards.* St. Louis: Mosby.)

Atrial paced activity? _____ Ventricular paced activity? _____
Pacemaker malfunction? _____ Identification: _____

67. Identify the rhythm.

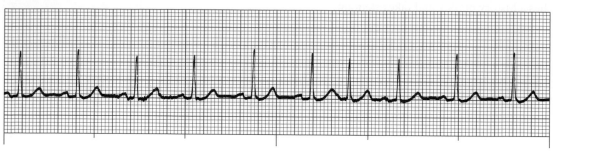

Fig. 10.17

Rhythm: _____ Rate: _____ P waves: _____
PR interval: _____ QRS duration: _____ QT interval: _____
Interpretation: _____

68. Identify the rhythm.

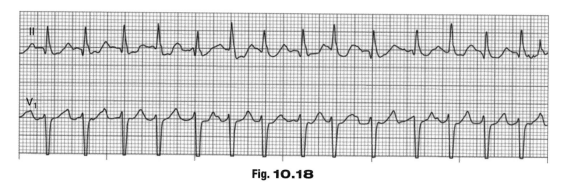

Fig. 10.18

Rhythm: _____ Rate: _____ P waves: _____
PR interval: _____ QRS duration: _____ QT interval: _____
Interpretation: _____

69. Identify the rhythm.

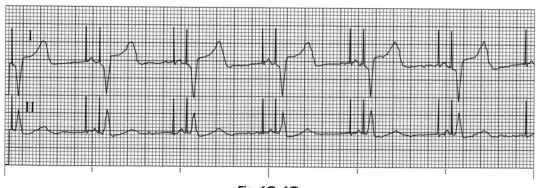
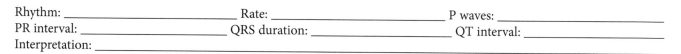

Fig. 10.19

Atrial paced activity? _____ Ventricular paced activity? _____
Pacemaker malfunction? _____ Identification: _____

70. Identify the rhythm.

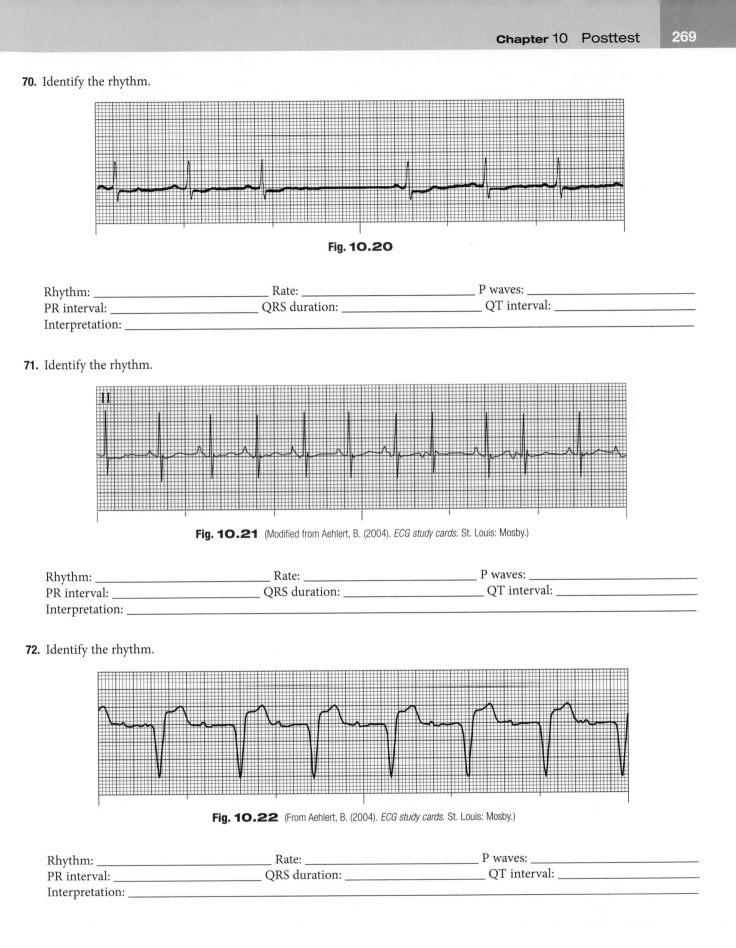

Fig. 10.20

Rhythm: _____ Rate: _____ P waves: _____

PR interval: _____ QRS duration: _____ QT interval: _____

Interpretation: _____

71. Identify the rhythm.

Fig. 10.21 (Modified from Aehlert, B. (2004). *ECG study cards.* St. Louis: Mosby.)

Rhythm: _____ Rate: _____ P waves: _____

PR interval: _____ QRS duration: _____ QT interval: _____

Interpretation: _____

72. Identify the rhythm.

Fig. 10.22 (From Aehlert, B. (2004). *ECG study cards.* St. Louis: Mosby.)

Rhythm: _____ Rate: _____ P waves: _____

PR interval: _____ QRS duration: _____ QT interval: _____

Interpretation: _____

73. Identify the rhythm.

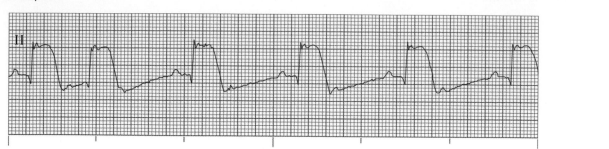

Fig. 10.23 (Modified from Aehlert, B. (2004). *ECG study cards*. St. Louis: Mosby.)

Rhythm: _____ Rate: _____ P waves: _____

PR interval: _____ QRS duration: _____ QT interval: _____

Interpretation: _____

74. This rhythm strip is from a 79-year-old man who experienced a syncopal episode. He has a history of seizures.

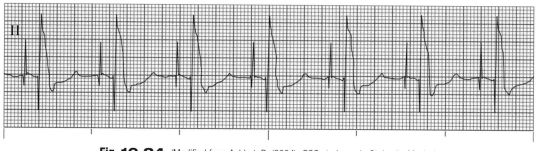

Fig. 10.24 (Modified from Aehlert, B. (2004). *ECG study cards*. St. Louis: Mosby.)

Atrial paced activity? _____ Ventricular paced activity? _____

Pacemaker malfunction? _____ Identification: _____

75. This rhythm strip is from an 81-year-old woman complaining of chest pain.

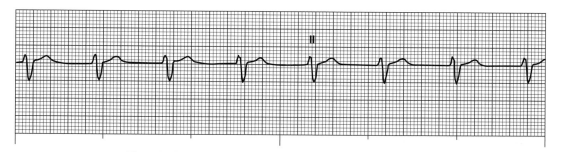

Fig. 10.25 (From Aehlert, B. (2004). *ECG study cards*. St. Louis: Mosby.)

Rhythm: _____ Rate: _____ P waves: _____

PR interval: _____ QRS duration: _____ QT interval: _____

Interpretation: _____

76. This rhythm strip is from a 74-year-old woman complaining of difficulty breathing.

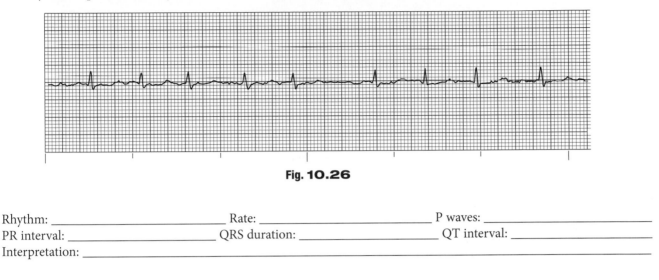

Fig. 10.26

Rhythm: _____ Rate: _____ P waves: _____
PR interval: _____ QRS duration: _____ QT interval: _____
Interpretation: _____

77. This rhythm strip is from a 63-year-old woman complaining of dizziness.

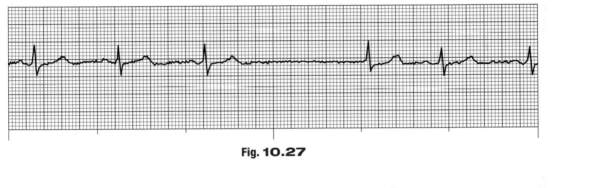

Fig. 10.27

Rhythm: _____ Rate: _____ P waves: _____
PR interval: _____ QRS duration: _____ QT interval: _____
Interpretation: _____

78. This rhythm strip is from a 53-year-old man complaining of chest pressure and shortness of breath. He has a history of a spinal cord injury and coronary artery disease.

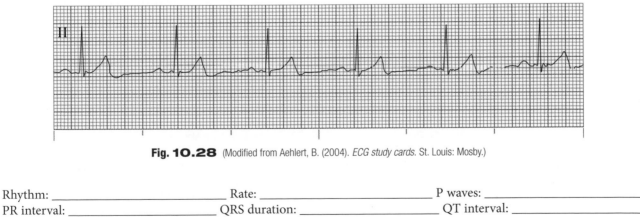

Fig. 10.28 (Modified from Aehlert, B. (2004). *ECG study cards*. St. Louis: Mosby.)

Rhythm: _____ Rate: _____ P waves: _____
PR interval: _____ QRS duration: _____ QT interval: _____
Interpretation: _____

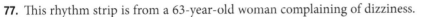

79. This rhythm strip is from an 82-year-old woman who had a ground-level fall.

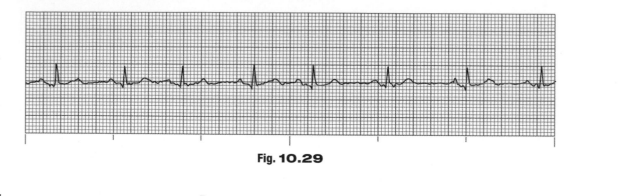

Fig. 10.29

Rhythm: _____ Rate: _____ P waves: _____
PR interval: _____ QRS duration: _____ QT interval: _____
Interpretation: _____

80. This rhythm strip is from a 70-year-old man who is complaining of a sharp pain across his shoulders.

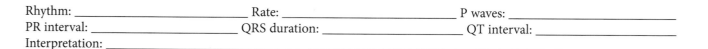

Fig. 10.30 (From Aehlert, B. (2004). *ECG study cards.* St. Louis: Mosby.)

Rhythm: _____ Rate: _____ P waves: _____
PR interval: _____ QRS duration: _____ QT interval: _____
Interpretation: _____

81. This rhythm strip is from a 17-year-old man who experienced a syncopal episode while playing baseball in 110° F heat for 4 hours. His core temperature is 101.8° F.

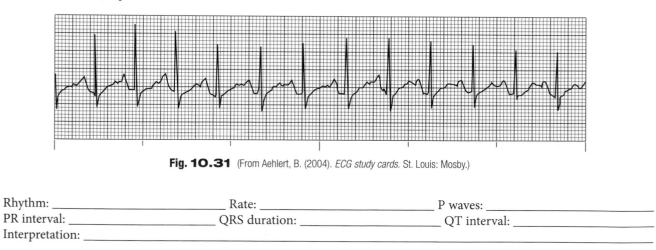

Fig. 10.31 (From Aehlert, B. (2004). *ECG study cards.* St. Louis: Mosby.)

Rhythm: _____ Rate: _____ P waves: _____
PR interval: _____ QRS duration: _____ QT interval: _____
Interpretation: _____

82. This rhythm strip is a 71-year-old man who is complaining of abdominal pain.

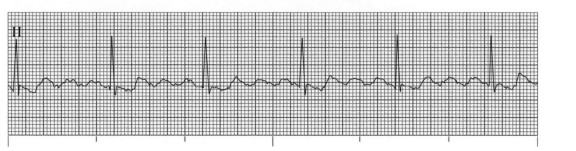

Fig. 10.32 (Modified from Aehlert, B. (2004). *ECG study cards.* St. Louis: Mosby.)

Rhythm: _____ Rate: _____ P waves: _____
PR interval: _____ QRS duration: _____ QT interval: _____
Interpretation: _____

83. Identify the rhythm.

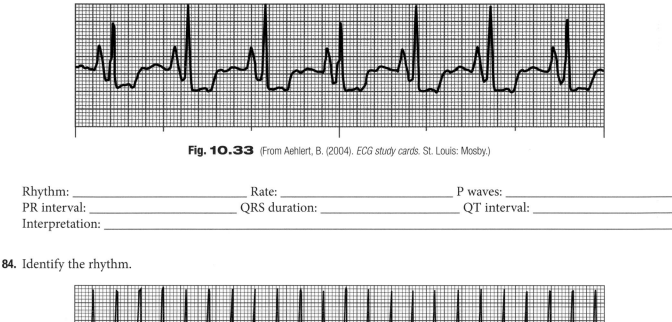

Fig. 10.33 (From Aehlert, B. (2004). *ECG study cards.* St. Louis: Mosby.)

Rhythm: _____ Rate: _____ P waves: _____
PR interval: _____ QRS duration: _____ QT interval: _____
Interpretation: _____

84. Identify the rhythm.

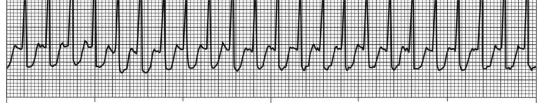

Fig. 10.34 (From Aehlert, B. (2004). *ECG study cards.* St. Louis: Mosby.)

Rhythm: _____ Rate: _____ P waves: _____
PR interval: _____ QRS duration: _____ QT interval: _____
Interpretation: _____

85. Identify the rhythm.

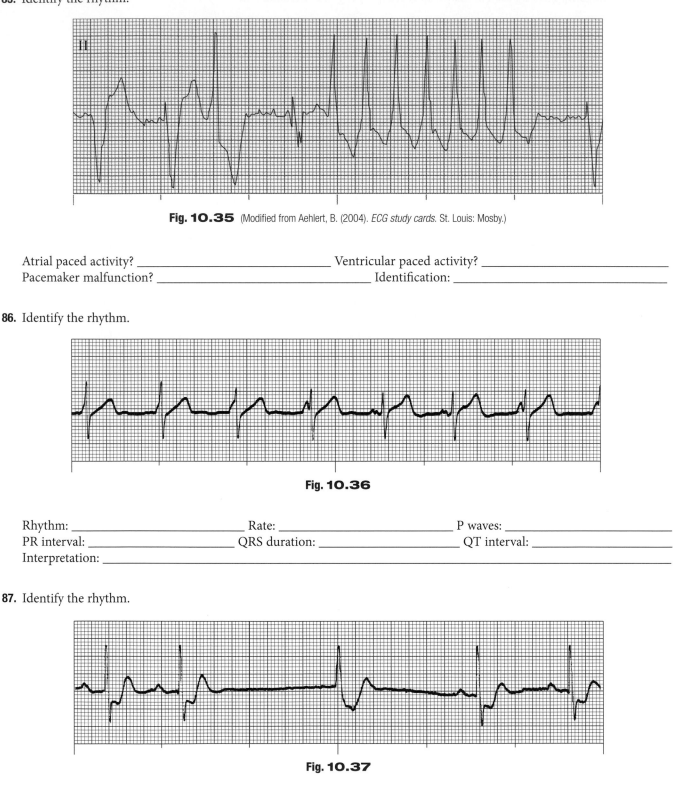

Fig. 10.35 (Modified from Aehlert, B. (2004). *ECG study cards.* St. Louis: Mosby.)

Atrial paced activity? _____ Ventricular paced activity? _____
Pacemaker malfunction? _____ Identification: _____

86. Identify the rhythm.

Fig. 10.36

Rhythm: _____ Rate: _____ P waves: _____
PR interval: _____ QRS duration: _____ QT interval: _____
Interpretation: _____

87. Identify the rhythm.

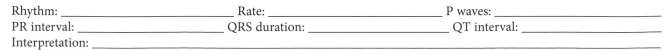

Fig. 10.37

Rhythm: _____ Rate: _____ P waves: _____
PR interval: _____ QRS duration: _____ QT interval: _____
Interpretation: _____

88. Identify the rhythm.

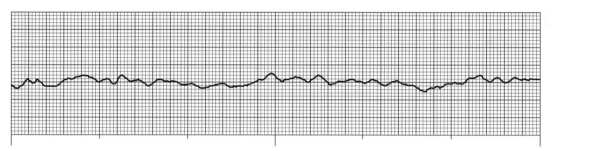

Fig. 10.38 (From Aehlert, B. (2004). *ECG study cards*. St. Louis: Mosby.)

Rhythm: _____ Rate: _____ P waves: _____
PR interval: _____ QRS duration: _____ QT interval: _____
Interpretation: _____

89. This rhythm strip is from an 18-year-old man with a gunshot wound to his chest.

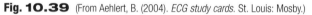

Fig. 10.39 (From Aehlert, B. (2004). *ECG study cards*. St. Louis: Mosby.)

Rhythm: _____ Rate: _____ P waves: _____
PR interval: _____ QRS duration: _____ QT interval: _____
Interpretation: _____

90. Identify the rhythm.

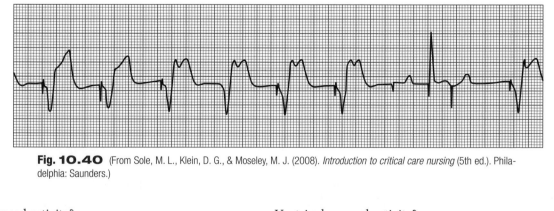

Fig. 10.40 (From Sole, M. L., Klein, D. G., & Moseley, M. J. (2008). *Introduction to critical care nursing* (5th ed.). Philadelphia: Saunders.)

Atrial paced activity? _____ Ventricular paced activity? _____
Pacemaker malfunction? _____ Identification: _____

91. Identify the rhythm.

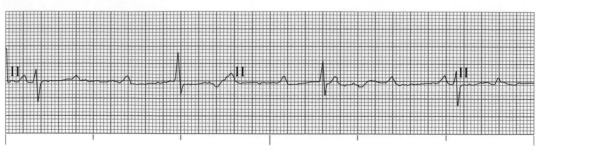

Fig. 10.41

Rhythm: _____ Rate: _____ P waves: _____
PR interval: _____ QRS duration: _____ QT interval: _____
Interpretation: _____

92. Identify the rhythm.

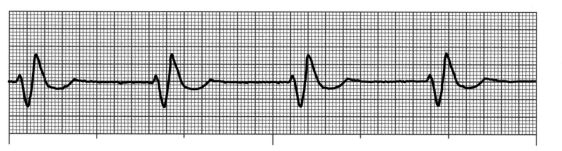

Fig. 10.42 (From Aehlert, B. (2004). *ECG study cards*. St. Louis: Mosby.)

Rhythm: _____ Rate: _____ P waves: _____
PR interval: _____ QRS duration: _____ QT interval: _____
Interpretation: _____

93. Identify the rhythm.

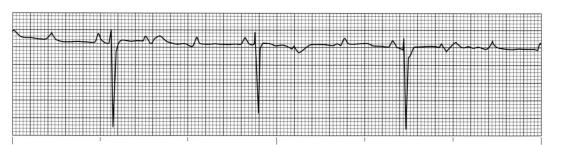
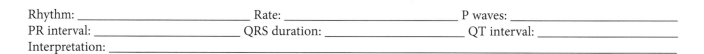

Fig. 10.43 (From Phillips, R. E., & Feeney, M. K. (1990). *The cardiac rhythms: A systematic approach to interpretation* (3rd ed.). Philadelphia: Saunders.)

Rhythm: _____ Rate: _____ P waves: _____
PR interval: _____ QRS duration: _____ QT interval: _____
Interpretation: _____

94. Identify the rhythm.

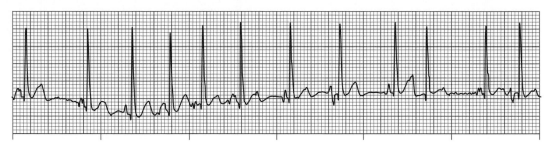

Fig. 10.44 (From Braunwald, E., Libby, P., Zipes, D. P., et al. (2001). *Heart disease: A textbook of cardiovascular medicine* (6th ed.). St. Louis: Mosby.)

Rhythm: _____ Rate: _____ P waves: _____
PR interval: _____ QRS duration: _____ QT interval: _____
Interpretation: _____

95. This rhythm strip is from an 88-year-old woman complaining of dizziness.

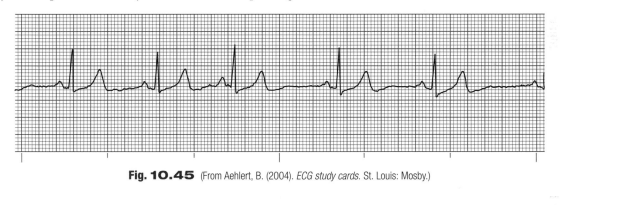

Fig. 10.45 (From Aehlert, B. (2004). *ECG study cards*. St. Louis: Mosby.)

Rhythm: _____ Rate: _____ P waves: _____
PR interval: _____ QRS duration: _____ QT interval: _____
Interpretation: _____

96. This rhythm strip is from a 70-year-old man who sustained second-degree burns over 20% of his body. He has a history of diabetes, coronary artery disease, and hypertension.

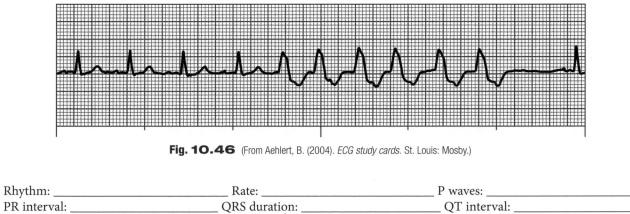

Fig. 10.46 (From Aehlert, B. (2004). *ECG study cards*. St. Louis: Mosby.)

Rhythm: _____ Rate: _____ P waves: _____
PR interval: _____ QRS duration: _____ QT interval: _____
Interpretation: _____

97. Identify the rhythm.

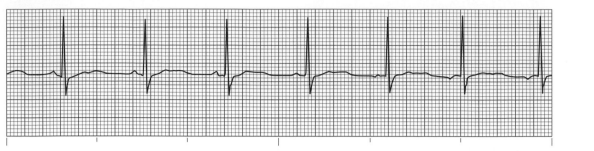

Fig. 10.47

Rhythm: _____ Rate: _____ P waves: _____
PR interval: _____ QRS duration: _____ QT interval: _____
Interpretation: _____

98. Identify the rhythm.

Lead II (continuous)

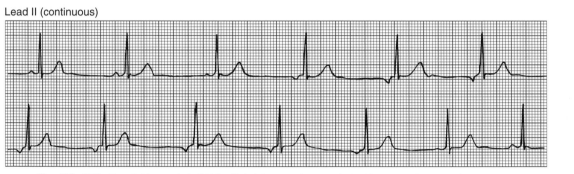

Fig. 10.48 (From Goldberger, A. L. (2006). *Clinical electrocardiography: A simplified approach* (7th ed.). St. Louis: Mosby.)

Rhythm: _____ Rate: _____ P waves: _____
PR interval: _____ QRS duration: _____ QT interval: _____
Interpretation: _____

99. Identify the rhythm.

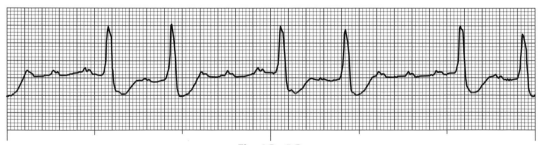

Fig. 10.49

Rhythm: _____ Rate: _____ P waves: _____
PR interval: _____ QRS duration: _____ QT interval: _____
Interpretation: _____

100. Identify the rhythm.

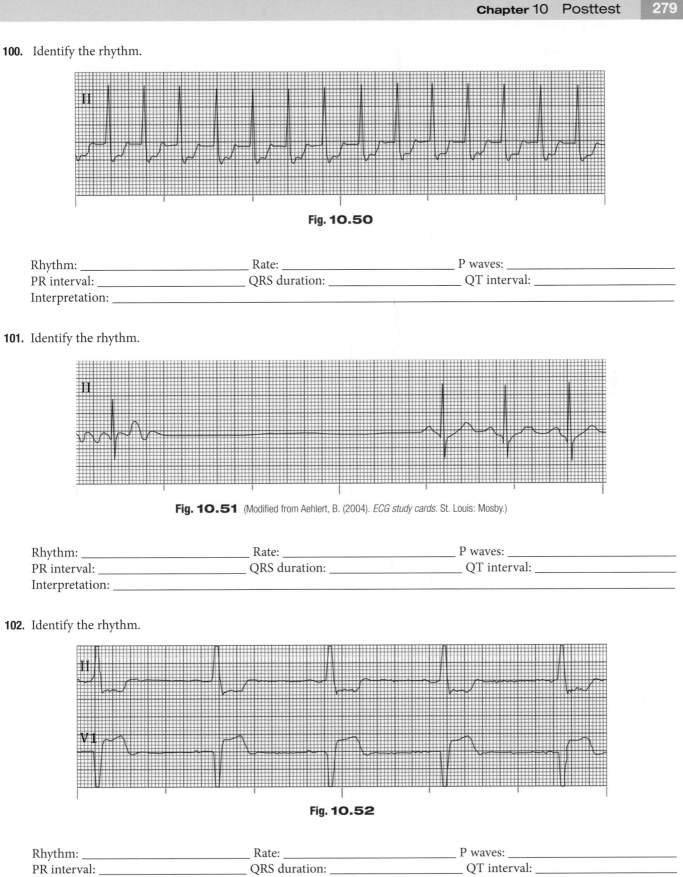

Fig. 10.50

Rhythm: _____ Rate: _____ P waves: _____
PR interval: _____ QRS duration: _____ QT interval: _____
Interpretation: _____

101. Identify the rhythm.

Fig. 10.51 (Modified from Aehlert, B. (2004). *ECG study cards*. St. Louis: Mosby.)

Rhythm: _____ Rate: _____ P waves: _____
PR interval: _____ QRS duration: _____ QT interval: _____
Interpretation: _____

102. Identify the rhythm.

Fig. 10.52

Rhythm: _____ Rate: _____ P waves: _____
PR interval: _____ QRS duration: _____ QT interval: _____
Interpretation: _____

103. Identify the rhythm.

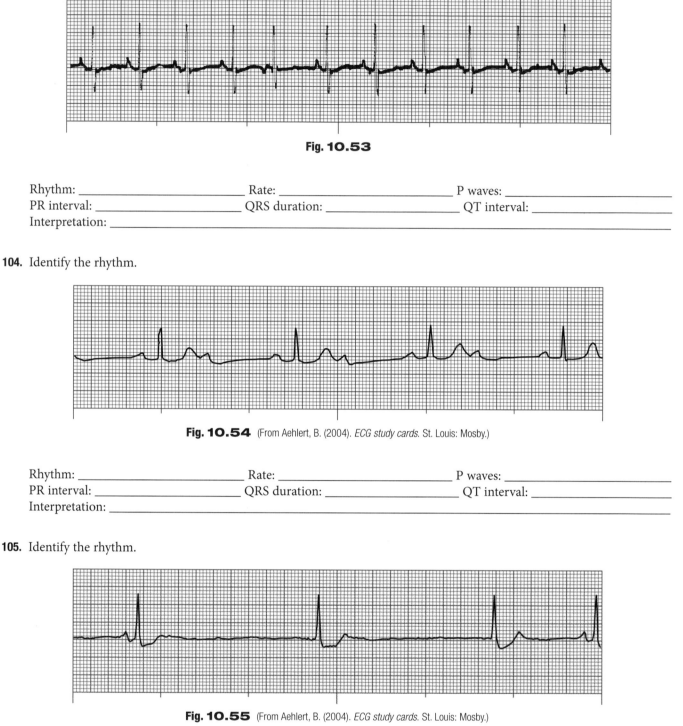

Fig. 10.53

Rhythm: _____ Rate: _____ P waves: _____
PR interval: _____ QRS duration: _____ QT interval: _____
Interpretation: _____

104. Identify the rhythm.

Fig. 10.54 (From Aehlert, B. (2004). *ECG study cards*. St. Louis: Mosby.)

Rhythm: _____ Rate: _____ P waves: _____
PR interval: _____ QRS duration: _____ QT interval: _____
Interpretation: _____

105. Identify the rhythm.

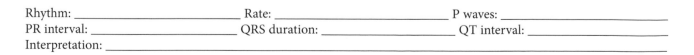

Fig. 10.55 (From Aehlert, B. (2004). *ECG study cards*. St. Louis: Mosby.)

Rhythm: _____ Rate: _____ P waves: _____
PR interval: _____ QRS duration: _____ QT interval: _____
Interpretation: _____

106. Identify the rhythm.

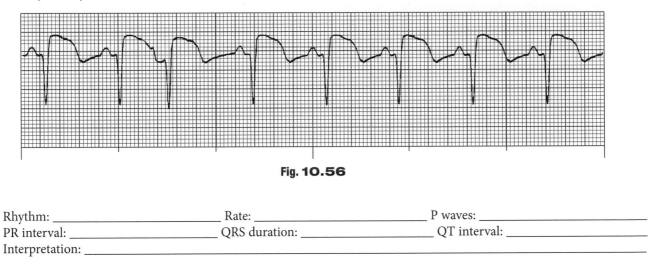

Fig. 10.56

Rhythm: _____ Rate: _____ P waves: _____
PR interval: _____ QRS duration: _____ QT interval: _____
Interpretation: _____

107. Identify the rhythm.

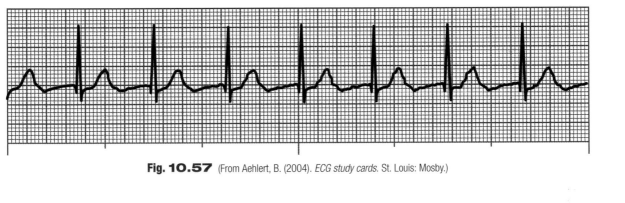

Fig. 10.57 (From Aehlert, B. (2004). *ECG study cards.* St. Louis: Mosby.)

Rhythm: _____ Rate: _____ P waves: _____
PR interval: _____ QRS duration: _____ QT interval: _____
Interpretation: _____

108. These rhythm strips are from a 67-year-old woman complaining of dizziness and chest pain. She has a history of a three-vessel coronary artery bypass graft and hypertension.

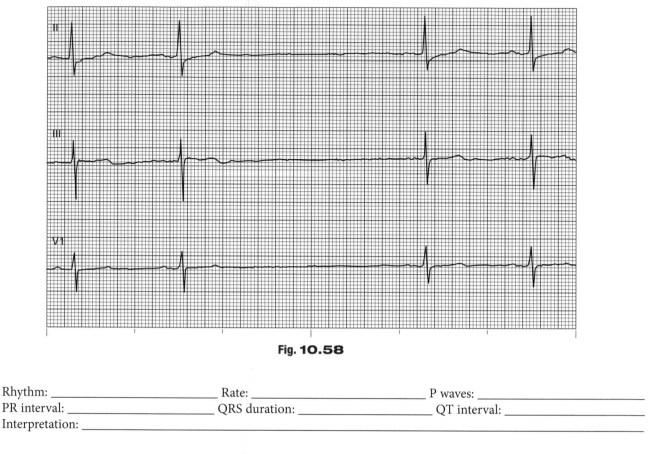

Fig. 10.58

Rhythm: _____ Rate: _____ P waves: _____

PR interval: _____ QRS duration: _____ QT interval: _____

Interpretation: _____

109. This rhythm strip is from a 59-year-old man who was driving to work on the freeway when his internal defibrillator discharged. He was asymptomatic at the time this ECG was obtained a few minutes after the event.

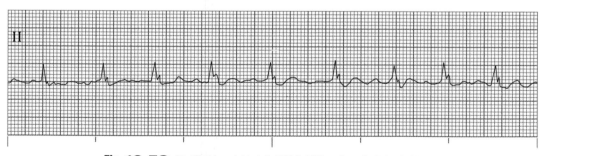

Fig. 10.59 (Modified from Aehlert, B. (2004). *ECG study cards*. St. Louis: Mosby.)

Rhythm: _____ Rate: _____ P waves: _____

PR interval: _____ QRS duration: _____ QT interval: _____

Interpretation: _____

110. This rhythm strip is from an 84-year-old man who is complaining of dizziness. He had a triple bypass 4 days ago.

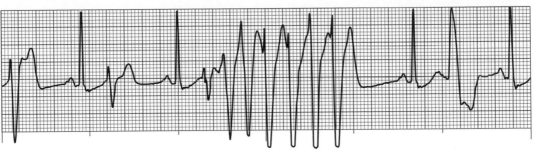

Fig. 10.60 (From Aehlert, B. (2004). *ECG study cards*. St. Louis: Mosby.)

Rhythm: _____ Rate: _____ P waves: _____
PR interval: _____ QRS duration: _____ QT interval: _____
Interpretation: _____

111. Identify the rhythm.

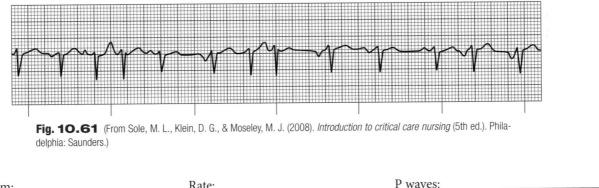

Fig. 10.61 (From Sole, M. L., Klein, D. G., & Moseley, M. J. (2008). *Introduction to critical care nursing* (5th ed.). Philadelphia: Saunders.)

Rhythm: _____ Rate: _____ P waves: _____
PR interval: _____ QRS duration: _____ QT interval: _____
Interpretation: _____

112. Identify the rhythm.

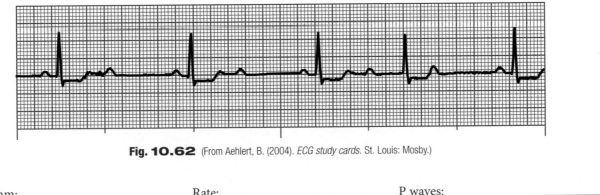

Fig. 10.62 (From Aehlert, B. (2004). *ECG study cards*. St. Louis: Mosby.)

Rhythm: _____ Rate: _____ P waves: _____
PR interval: _____ QRS duration: _____ QT interval: _____
Interpretation: _____

113. Identify the rhythm.

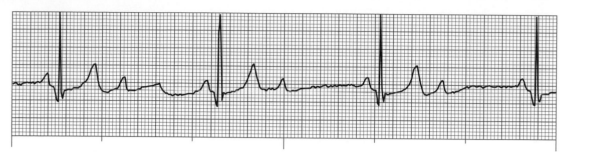

Fig. 10.63 (From Aehlert, B. (2004). *ECG study cards.* St. Louis: Mosby.)

Rhythm: _____ Rate: _____ P waves: _____
PR interval: _____ QRS duration: _____ QT interval: _____
Interpretation: _____

114. Identify the rhythm.

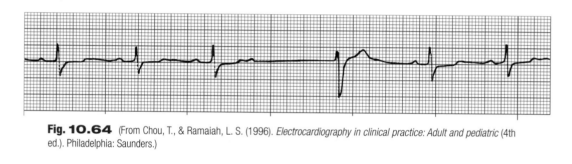

Fig. 10.64 (From Chou, T., & Ramaiah, L. S. (1996). *Electrocardiography in clinical practice: Adult and pediatric* (4th ed.). Philadelphia: Saunders.)

Rhythm: _____ Rate: _____ P waves: _____
PR interval: _____ QRS duration: _____ QT interval: _____
Interpretation: _____

115. Identify the rhythm.

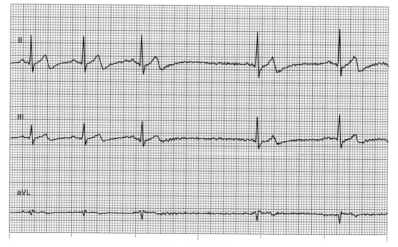

Fig. 10.65

Rhythm: _____ Rate: _____ P waves: _____
PR interval: _____ QRS duration: _____ QT interval: _____
Interpretation: _____

116. Identify the rhythm.

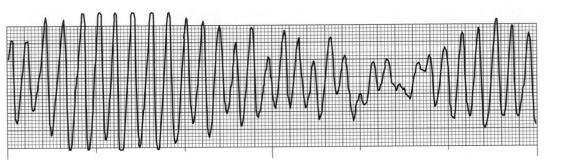

Fig. 10.66 (From Aehlert, B. (2004). *ECG study cards.* St. Louis: Mosby.)

Rhythm: _____ Rate: _____ P waves: _____
PR interval: _____ QRS duration: _____ QT interval: _____
Interpretation: _____

117. Identify the rhythm.

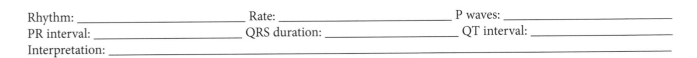

Fig. 10.67 (From Andreoli, T. E., Griggs, R., Wing, W., & Fitz, J. G. (2016). *Andreoli and Carpenter's Cecil essentials of medicine* (9th ed.). Philadelphia: Saunders.)

Rhythm: _____ Rate: _____ P waves: _____
PR interval: _____ QRS duration: _____ QT interval: _____
Interpretation: _____

118. This rhythm strip is from a 61-year-old woman complaining of chest pain. She has a history of asthma and chronic obstructive pulmonary disease.

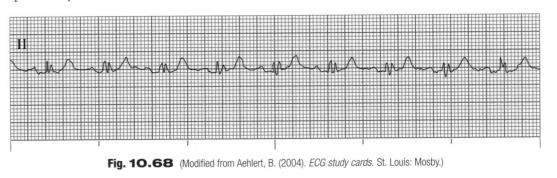

Fig. 10.68 (Modified from Aehlert, B. (2004). *ECG study cards.* St. Louis: Mosby.)

Rhythm: _____ Rate: _____ P waves: _____
PR interval: _____ QRS duration: _____ QT interval: _____
Interpretation: _____

119. This rhythm strip is from a 52-year-old man found unresponsive, apneic, and pulseless.

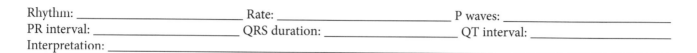

Fig. 10.69 (Modified from Aehlert, B. (2004). *ECG study cards.* St. Louis: Mosby.)

Rhythm: _____ Rate: _____ P waves: _____
PR interval: _____ QRS duration: _____ QT interval: _____
Interpretation: _____

120. Identify the rhythm.

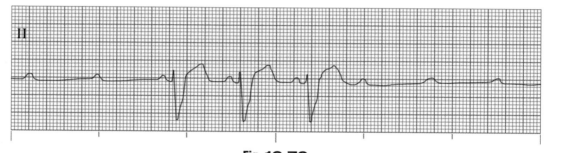

Fig. 10.70

Rhythm: _____ Rate: _____ P waves: _____
PR interval: _____ QRS duration: _____ QT interval: _____
Interpretation: _____

121. Identify the rhythm.

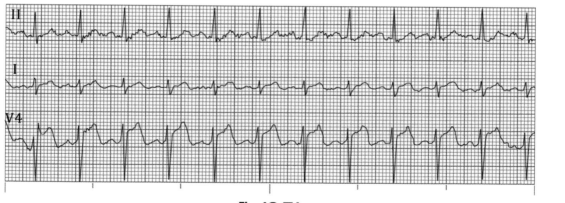

Fig. 10.71

Rhythm: _____ Rate: _____ P waves: _____
PR interval: _____ QRS duration: _____ QT interval: _____
Interpretation: _____

122. Identify the rhythm.

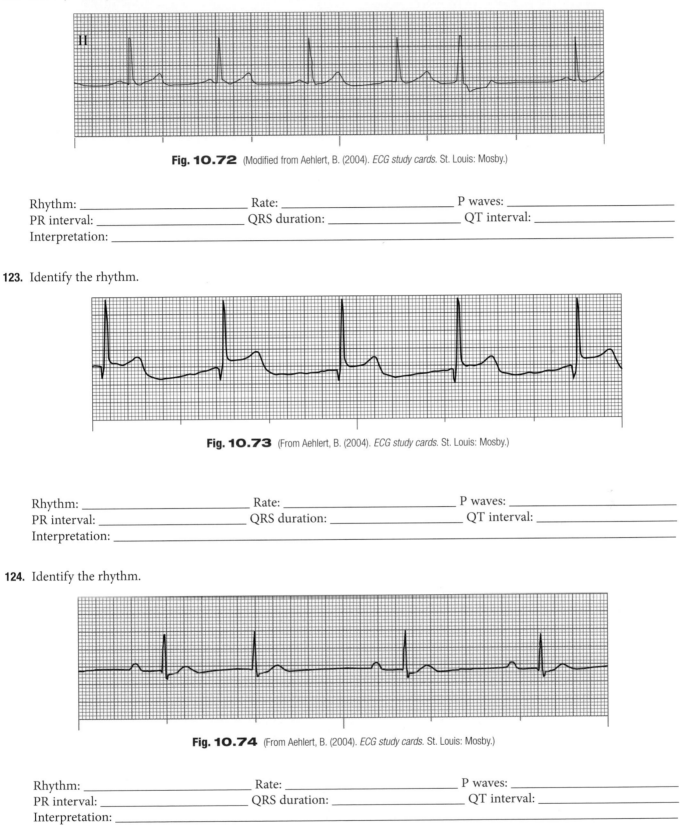

Fig. 10.72 (Modified from Aehlert, B. (2004). *ECG study cards.* St. Louis: Mosby.)

Rhythm: _____ Rate: _____ P waves: _____
PR interval: _____ QRS duration: _____ QT interval: _____
Interpretation: _____

123. Identify the rhythm.

Fig. 10.73 (From Aehlert, B. (2004). *ECG study cards.* St. Louis: Mosby.)

Rhythm: _____ Rate: _____ P waves: _____
PR interval: _____ QRS duration: _____ QT interval: _____
Interpretation: _____

124. Identify the rhythm.

Fig. 10.74 (From Aehlert, B. (2004). *ECG study cards.* St. Louis: Mosby.)

Rhythm: _____ Rate: _____ P waves: _____
PR interval: _____ QRS duration: _____ QT interval: _____
Interpretation: _____

125. These rhythm strips are from an 82-year-old man complaining of back pain.

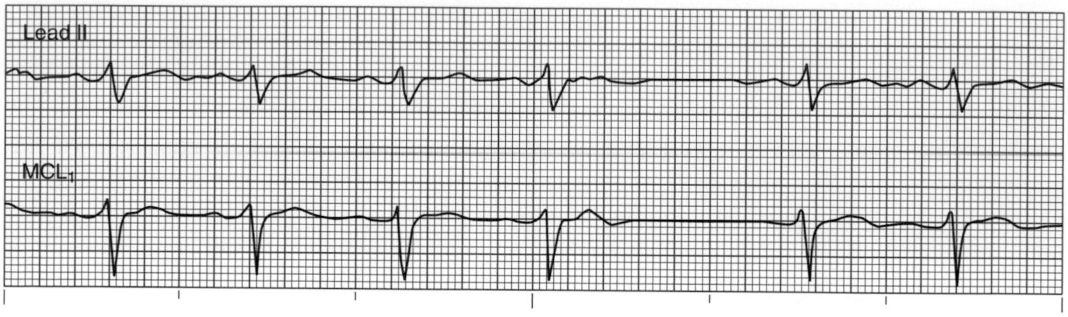

Fig. 10.75 (From Aehlert, B. (2004). *ECG study cards.* St. Louis: Mosby.)

Rhythm: _____ Rate: _____ P waves: _____

PR interval: _____ QRS duration: _____ QT interval: _____

Interpretation: _____

POSTTEST ANSWERS

1. **C.** The thick, muscular middle layer of the heart wall that contains the atrial and ventricular muscle fibers necessary for contraction is the myocardium.

2. **B.** A branch of the right coronary artery supplies the right atrium and right ventricle with blood.

3. **B.** The flow of blood from the superior and inferior venae cavae into the atria is normally continuous. About 70% of this blood flows directly through the atria and into the ventricles before the atria contract; this is called passive filling. When the atria contract, an additional 10% to 30% of the returning blood is added to filling of the ventricles. This additional contribution of blood resulting from atrial contraction is called atrial kick. Afterload is the pressure or resistance against which the ventricles must pump to eject blood. Cardiac output is the amount of blood pumped into the aorta each minute by the heart; it is defined as the stroke volume multiplied by the heart rate. Peripheral resistance is the resistance to the flow of blood determined by blood vessel diameter and the tone of the vascular musculature.

4. **B, C, D.** The right atrium receives deoxygenated blood from the superior vena cava (which carries blood from the head and upper extremities), the inferior vena cava (which carries blood from the lower body), and the coronary sinus (which receives blood from the intracardiac circulation).

5. **A, C.** The pulmonic and aortic valves are semilunar valves. The semilunar valves prevent backflow of blood from the aorta and pulmonary arteries into the ventricles. The tricuspid and mitral valves are AV valves, which separate the atria from the ventricles.

6. **D.** Parasympathetic (inhibitory) nerve fibers supply the SA node, atrial muscle, and the AV bundle of the heart by the vagus nerves. Parasympathetic stimulation has the following actions:
   - Slows the rate of discharge of the SA node
   - Slows conduction through the AV node
   - Decreases the strength of atrial contraction
   - Can cause a small decrease in the force of ventricular contraction

7. **A, B.** The left main coronary artery supplies oxygenated blood to its two primary branches: the LAD, which is also called the *anterior interventricular artery*, and the circumflex artery.

8. **C.** In general, cardiac cells have either a mechanical (i.e., contractile) or an electrical (i.e., pacemaker) function. Pacemaker cells are specialized cells of the electrical conduction system. Pacemaker cells also may be referred to as *conducting cells* or *automatic cells*. They are responsible for the spontaneous generation and conduction of electrical impulses.

9. **B.** During the absolute refractory period, the cell will not respond to further stimulation within itself. This means that the myocardial working cells cannot contract and that the cells of the electrical conduction system cannot conduct an electrical impulse, no matter how strong the internal electrical stimulus. On the ECG, the absolute refractory period begins with the onset of the QRS complex and terminates at approximately the apex of the T wave.

10. **C.** The portion of the ECG tracing between the QRS complex and the T wave is the ST segment. The term *ST segment* is used regardless of whether the final wave of the QRS complex is an R or an S wave. The ST segment represents the early part of repolarization of the right and left ventricles. The normal ST segment begins at the isoelectric line, extends from the end of the S wave, and curves gradually upward to the beginning of the T wave.

11. **D.** The QT interval, measured from the beginning of the QRS complex to the end of the T wave, represents the time from initial depolarization of the ventricles to the end of ventricular repolarization.

12. **C.** Lead III records the difference in electrical potential between the left leg (+) and left arm (−) electrodes. In lead III, the positive electrode is placed on the left leg, and the negative electrode is placed on the left arm.

13. **C.** Junctional escape beats and rhythms occur when the SA node fails to pace the heart or AV conduction fails.

14. **C.** To evaluate the rhythmicity of the atrial rhythm, the interval between two consecutive P waves is measured and compared to succeeding P to P intervals.

15. **A, B.** A bipolar lead is an ECG lead that has a positive and negative electrode. Each lead records the difference in electrical potential (i.e., voltage) between two selected electrodes. Although all ECG leads are technically bipolar, leads I, II, and III use two distinct electrodes, one of which is connected to the positive input of the ECG machine and the other to the negative input.

16. **C.** Leads II, III, and aVF view the heart's inferior surface.

17. **D.** The rate of a sinus bradycardia is less than 60 beats/min. R to R and P to P intervals are regular, P waves are positive in lead II, and one precedes each QRS complex. The PR interval is within normal limits and the QRS duration is 0.11 second or less unless it is abnormally conducted.

18. **A.** In sinus arrhythmia, the heart rate increases gradually during inspiration (R to R intervals shorten) and decreases with expiration (R to R intervals lengthen).

19. **B**. In SA block, which is also called sinus exit block, the pacemaker cells within the SA node initiate an impulse but it is blocked as it exits the SA node; thus, SA block is a disorder of impulse conduction. Sinus arrest, which is also called sinus pause or SA arrest, is a disorder of impulse formation. In sinus arrest, the pacemaker cells of the SA node fail to initiate an electrical impulse for one or more beats resulting in absent PQRST complexes on the ECG.

20. **D**. The heart's demand for oxygen increases as the heart rate increases. As the heart rate increases, there is less time for the ventricles to fill and less blood for the ventricles to pump out with each contraction, which can lead to decreased cardiac output. Because the coronary arteries fill when the ventricles are at rest, rapid heart rates decrease the time available for coronary artery filling. This decreases the heart's blood supply. Chest discomfort can result if the supplies of blood and oxygen to the heart are inadequate.

21. **B, C**. The terms *ectopic*, which means out of place, and *latent* are used to describe an impulse that originates from a source other than the SA node. Ectopic pacemaker sites include the cells of the AV junction and Purkinje fibers, although their intrinsic rates are slower than that of the SA node.

22. **C**. Multiformed atrial rhythm is an updated term for the rhythm formerly known as wandering atrial pacemaker. With this rhythm, the size, shape, and direction of the P waves vary, sometimes from beat to beat. The difference in the look of the P waves is a result of the gradual shifting of the dominant pacemaker between the SA node, the atria, and the AV junction. Wandering atrial pacemaker is associated with a normal or slow rate and irregular P to P, R to R, and PR intervals because of the different sites of impulse formation.

23. **D**. AVNRT is the most common type of SVT.

24. **A**. The two primary treatment strategies used to control symptoms associated with AFib are rate control and rhythm control. With rate control, the patient remains in AFib, but the ventricular rate is controlled to decrease acute symptoms, reduce signs of ischemia, and reduce or prevent signs of heart failure from developing. With rhythm control, sinus rhythm is reestablished.

25. **A**. The term *paroxysmal* is used to describe a rhythm that starts or ends suddenly. Atrial tachycardia that starts or ends suddenly is called paroxysmal supraventricular tachycardia (PSVT), once called paroxysmal atrial tachycardia (PAT). PSVT may last for minutes, hours, or days. If the onset or end of PSVT is not observed on the ECG, the dysrhythmia is simply called SVT.

26. **A**. AFib is the most common sustained dysrhythmia in adults and it occurs because of altered automaticity in one or several rapidly firing sites in the atria or reentry involving one or more circuits in the atria.

27. **B, C, E**. You can usually tell the difference between a PAC and a PJC by the P wave. A PAC typically has a positive P wave before the QRS complex in leads II, III, and aVF. A P wave may or may not be present with a PJC. If a P wave is present, it is inverted (retrograde) and may precede or follow the QRS. The QRS of the PAC or PJC is similar in shape to those of the underlying rhythm (i.e., usually narrow) unless the early beat is abnormally conducted.

28. **A, D, E**. Characteristic ECG findings with a Wolff-Parkinson-White pattern include a short PR interval, delta wave, and a wide QRS complex. A delta wave is an initial slurred deflection at the beginning of the QRS complex that results from the initial activation of the QRS by conduction over the accessory pathway.

29. **D**. In atrial flutter, atrial waveforms are produced that resemble the teeth of a saw, or a picket fence; these are called flutter waves, which are best observed in leads II, III, aVF, and V_1.

30. **B**. If the AV junction paces the heart, the electrical impulse must travel in a backward (retrograde) direction to activate the atria. If the atria depolarize before the ventricles, an inverted P wave will be seen *before* the QRS complex and the PR interval will usually measure 0.12 second or less. The PR interval is shorter than usual because an impulse that begins in the AV junction does not have to travel as far to stimulate the ventricles. If the atria and ventricles depolarize at the same time, a P wave will not be visible because it will be hidden in the QRS complex. When the atria are depolarized after the ventricles, the P wave typically distorts the end of the QRS complex and an inverted P wave will appear *after* the QRS.

31. **C**. Nonparoxysmal (i.e., gradual onset) junctional tachycardia usually starts as an accelerated junctional rhythm, but the heart rate gradually increases to more than 100 beats/min. The usual ventricular rate for nonparoxysmal junctional tachycardia is 101 to 140 beats/min. Paroxysmal junctional tachycardia, which is also known as focal or automatic junctional tachycardia, is an uncommon dysrhythmia that starts and ends suddenly and that is often precipitated by a PJC. The ventricular rate for paroxysmal junctional tachycardia is generally faster, at a rate of 140 beats/min or more.

32. **B**. Junctional (or ventricular) complexes may appear early (before the next expected sinus beat) or late (after the next expected sinus beat). If the complex is *early*, it is called a premature junctional (or ventricular) complex. If the complex is *late*, it is called a junctional (or ventricular) escape beat. To determine if a complex is early or late, you need to see at least two sinus beats in a row to establish the regularity of the underlying rhythm.

33. **C.** The term *symptomatic bradycardia* is used to describe a patient who experiences signs and symptoms of hemodynamic compromise related to a slow heart rate. Treatment of a symptomatic bradycardia should include assessment of the patient's oxygen saturation level and determining if signs of increased breathing effort are present. Give supplemental oxygen if oxygenation is inadequate and assist breathing if ventilation is inadequate. Establish intravenous access and obtain a 12-lead ECG. Atropine, administered intravenously, is the drug of choice for symptomatic bradycardia. Reassess the patient's response and continue monitoring the patient.

34. **A, C.** Junctional escape beats and rhythms occur when the SA node fails to pace the heart or AV conduction fails. Because a junctional rhythm starts from above the ventricles, the QRS complex is usually narrow, and its rhythm is very regular. A noncompensatory (incomplete) pause often follows a PJC. This pause represents the delay during which the SA node resets its rhythm for the next beat.

35. **A.** Three or more sequential PVCs are termed a *run* or *burst*, and three or more PVCs that occur in a row at a rate of more than 100 beats/min are considered a run of VT.

36. **A.** PVCs that look alike in the same lead and begin from the same anatomic site (i.e., focus) are called uniform PVCs.

37. **D.** PMVT is characterized by QRS complexes that vary in shape and amplitude from beat to beat and appear to twist from upright to negative or negative to upright and back, resembling a spindle. The ventricular rate is 150 to 300 beats/min and is typically 200 to 250 beats/min.

38. **B.** When a delay or interruption in impulse conduction from the atria to the ventricles occurs as a result of a transient or permanent anatomic or functional impairment, the resulting dysrhythmia is called an AV block. A BBB is a disruption in impulse conduction from the bundle of His through either the right or left bundle branch to the Purkinje fibers. With SA block, which is also called sinus exit block, the pacemaker cells within the SA node initiate an impulse but it is blocked as it exits the SA node. With sinus arrest, the pacemaker cells of the SA node fail to initiate an electrical impulse for one or more beats resulting in absent PQRST complexes on the ECG.

39. **B.** The rSR' pattern is characteristic of RBBB and is sometimes referred to as an "M" or "rabbit ear" pattern.

40. **B.** A first-degree AV block is present when there is a 1:1 relationship between P waves and QRS complexes and the PR interval is constant and more than 0.20 second in duration (prolonged).

41. **D.** Second-degree AV blocks are types of *incomplete* blocks because at least some of the impulses from the SA node are conducted to the ventricles. With third-degree AV block, there is a *complete* block in conduction of impulses between the atria and the ventricles.

42. **A, D.** Second-degree 2:1 AV block is characterized by P waves that are normal in size and shape, but every other P wave is not followed by a QRS. The atrial rate is twice the ventricular rate. Because there are no two PQRST cycles in a row from which to compare PR intervals, 2:1 AV block cannot be conclusively classified as type I or type II. To determine the type of block with certainty, it is necessary to continue close ECG monitoring of the patient until the conduction ratio of P waves to QRS complexes changes to 3:2, 4:3, and so on, which would enable PR interval comparison. With second-degree AV block in the form of 2:1 AV block, the level of the block can be located within the AV node or within the His-Purkinje system.

43. **B.** Once the presence of BBB is suspected, an examination of V_1 can reveal whether the block affects the right or the left bundle branch.

44. **D.** Capture refers to the successful conduction of an artificial pacemaker's impulse through the myocardium, resulting in depolarization. A pacemaker spike is a vertical line on the ECG that indicates the pacemaker has discharged. Sensitivity is the extent to which an artificial pacemaker recognizes intrinsic cardiac electrical activity. Inhibition is a pacemaker response in which the output pulse is suppressed when an intrinsic event is sensed.

45. **B.** The 12-lead ECG provides a 2.5-second view of each lead because it is assumed that 2.5 seconds is long enough to capture at least one representative complex. However, a 2.5-second view is not long enough to properly assess rate and rhythm, so at least one continuous rhythm strip is usually included at the bottom of the tracing.

46. **C.** Although an RVI may occur by itself, it is more commonly associated with an inferior MI and it should be suspected when ECG changes suggesting an inferior infarction are seen.

47. **B.** Poor R-wave progression is a phrase used to describe R waves that decrease in size from V_1 to V_4. This is often seen in an anteroseptal infarction but may be a normal variant in young persons, particularly in young women. Other causes of poor R-wave progression include LBBB, left ventricular hypertrophy, and severe chronic obstructive pulmonary disease (particularly emphysema).

48. **B.** A rapid, wide-QRS rhythm associated with pulselessness, shock, or heart failure should be presumed to be VT.

49. A, D. IVR, which is also called a ventricular escape rhythm, exists when three or more ventricular escape beats occur in a row at a rate of 20 to 40 beats/min (i.e., the intrinsic firing rate of the Purkinje fibers). The QRS complexes seen in IVR are wide because the impulses begin in the ventricles, bypassing the normal conduction pathway.

50. A. The first letter of a pacemaker identification code identifies the heart chamber (or chambers) paced (stimulated). A pacemaker used to pace only a single chamber is represented by either A (atrial) or V (ventricular). A pacemaker capable of pacing in both chambers is represented by D (dual).

Posttest Rhythm Strip Answers

Note: The rate and interval measurements provided here were obtained using electronic calipers.

51. Fig. 10.1
Rhythm: Regular
Rate: 88 beats/min
P waves: Inverted before each QRS; 1:1 relationship
PR interval: 0.14 second
QRS duration: 0.06 second
QT interval: 0.46 second
Interpretation: Accelerated junctional rhythm at 88 beats/min

52. Fig. 10.2
Rhythm: Irregular
Rate: 80 beats/min
P waves: Positive before each QRS; an early P wave distorts the T wave of beat 3
PR interval: 0.14 to 0.16 second
QRS duration: 0.07 second
QT interval: 0.36 second
Interpretation: Sinus rhythm at 80 beats/min with a nonconducted PAC and ST-segment depression

53. Fig. 10.3
Rhythm: Ventricular irregular; atrial regular
Rate: Ventricular about 70 beats/min; atrial 109 beats/min
P waves: Positive; more Ps than QRSs
PR interval: Lengthening
QRS duration: 0.10 second
QT interval: 0.33 second
Interpretation: Second-degree AV block type 1 at 70 beats/min

54. Fig. 10.4
Rhythm: Irregular
Rate: 90 beats/min
P waves: Positive before most QRS complexes; none visible for 3 early beats
PR interval: 0.14 second (sinus beats)
QRS duration: 0.05 second (sinus beats)

QT interval: 0.30 second (sinus beats)
Interpretation: Sinus rhythm at 90 beats/min with ventricular trigeminy

55. Fig. 10.5
Rhythm: Irregular
Rate: 70 beats/min
P waves: None visible; fibrillatory waves present
PR interval: None
QRS duration: 0.09 second (atrial beats)
QT interval: Unable to determine
Interpretation: AFib at 70 beats/min with a ventricular complex

56. Fig. 10.6
Rhythm: Regular
Rate: 92 beats/min
P waves: Positive before each QRS; 1:1 relationship
PR interval: 0.16 second
QRS duration: 0.08 second
QT interval: 0.33 second
Interpretation: Sinus rhythm at 92 beats/min; artifact is present

57. Fig. 10.7
Rhythm: Irregular
Rate: 30 beats/min (junctional beats) to 56 beats/min (sinus beats)
P waves: None with junctional beats; positive with sinus beats
PR interval: None with junctional beats; 0.18 second with sinus beats
QRS duration: 0.04 second (junctional beats); 0.07 second (sinus beats)
QT interval: 0.38 second
Interpretation: Junctional bradycardia at 30 beats/min to sinus bradycardia at 56 beats/min

58. Fig. 10.8
Rhythm: Regular
Rate: 65 beats/min
P waves: Positive before each QRS, some are notched; 1:1 relationship
PR interval: 0.19 second
QRS duration: 0.08 second
QT interval: 0.31 second
Interpretation: Sinus rhythm at 65 beats/min with ST-segment elevation (STE)

59. Fig. 10.9
Rhythm: Irregular
Rate: About 430 beats/min
P waves: None
PR interval: None
QRS duration: 0.12 to 0.14 second
QT interval: None
Interpretation: PMVT at about 430 beats/min

60. Fig. 10.10
Rhythm: Atrial and ventricular rhythms are essentially regular
Rate: Ventricular 45 beats/min; atrial 107 beats/min
P waves: Positive; more Ps than QRSs
PR interval: None
QRS duration: 0.15 second
QT interval: 0.40 second
Interpretation: Third-degree AV block at 45 beats/min with a wide QRS

61. Fig. 10.11
Rhythm: Regular
Rate: 83 beats/min
P waves: Inverted before each QRS
PR interval: 0.12 second
QRS duration: 0.08 second
QT interval: 0.38 second
Interpretation: Accelerated junctional rhythm at 83 beats/min with deeply inverted T waves; artifact is present

62. Fig. 10.12
Rhythm: Irregular
Rate: About 110 beats/min; 54 beats/min (sinus beats)
P waves: Sinus P waves; none with ventricular beats
PR interval: 0.12 second (sinus beats)
QRS duration: 0.07 second (sinus beats)
QT interval: 0.30 second (sinus beats)
Interpretation: Sinus bradycardia at 54 beats/min with ventricular bigeminy; rate about 110 beats/min if ventricular beats counted in the rate

63. Fig. 10.13
Rhythm: Regular
Rate: Ventricular 150 beats/min
P waves: Flutter waves visible
PR interval: None
QRS duration: 0.08 second
QT interval: Unable to determine
Interpretation: Atrial flutter with a ventricular response of 150 beats/min

64. Fig. 10.14
Rhythm: Regular
Rate: 180 beats/min
P waves: None visible
PR interval: Unable to determine
QRS duration: 0.06 second
QT interval: 0.23 second
Interpretation: AVNRT at 180 beats/min

65. Fig. 10.15
Rhythm: Regular
Rate: Ventricular 42 beats/min; atrial 71 beats/min
P waves: Positive; more Ps than QRSs
PR interval: None
QRS duration: 0.12 second
QT interval: 0.46 second
Interpretation: Third-degree AV block at 42 beats/min with a wide QRS, a prolonged QT interval, and STE

66. Fig. 10.16
Atrial paced activity? No
Ventricular paced activity? Yes
Pacemaker malfunction? No
Interpretation: Ventricular paced rhythm with 100% capture at 65 pulses/min

67. Fig. 10.17
Rhythm: Irregular
Rate: 100 beats/min
P waves: Positive before each QRS; the P wave of beat 7 is early and distorts the T wave of the preceding beat
PR interval: 0.15 second (sinus beats)
QRS duration: 0.05 second (sinus beats)
QT interval: 0.25 second (sinus beats)
Interpretation: Sinus rhythm at 100 beats/min with a PAC; beat 7 is the PAC; artifact is present

68. Fig. 10.18
Rhythm: Irregular
Rate: 140 beats/min
P waves: None consistently visible
PR interval: None
QRS duration: 0.09 second
QT interval: 0.29 second
Interpretation: AFib with a ventricular response of 140 beats/min; ST-segment depression in lead II

69. Fig. 10.19
Atrial paced activity? Yes
Ventricular paced activity? Yes
Pacemaker malfunction? No
Interpretation: Dual-chamber paced rhythm with 100% capture at 60 pulses/min

70. Fig. 10.20
Rhythm: Irregular
Rate: 60 beats/min
P waves: Positive before each QRS; a PQRST complex is missing
PR interval: 0.16 second
QRS duration: 0.08 second
QT interval: 0.33 second
Interpretation: Sinus rhythm at 60 beats/min with an episode of SA block

71. Fig. 10.21
Rhythm: Irregular
Rate: 110 beats/min
P waves: Positive before most QRSs; inverted with beats 8 and 10
PR interval: 0.13 second (sinus beats)
QRS duration: 0.06 second (sinus beats)
QT interval: 0.31 second (sinus beats)
Interpretation: Sinus tachycardia at 110 beats/min with two PJCs (beats 8 and 10)

72. Fig. 10.22
Rhythm: Irregular
Rate: 70 beats/min
P waves: Positive; 1:1 relationship
PR interval: 0.36 second
QRS duration: 0.12 second
QT interval: 0.38 second
Interpretation: Sinus arrhythmia at 70 beats/min with first-degree AV block and STE; artifact is present

73. Fig. 10.23
Rhythm: Ventricular irregular; atrial regular
Rate: Ventricular 60 beats/min; atrial 100 beats/min
P waves: Positive; more Ps than QRSs
PR interval: Lengthening
QRS duration: 0.04 second
QT interval: 0.28 second
Interpretation: Second-degree AV block type I at 60 beats/min with STE; although the complexes on the right side of the rhythm strip show 2:1 conduction, comparison of the PR intervals of beats 1 and 2 enable a diagnosis of second-degree type I AV block

74. Fig. 10.24
Atrial paced activity? Yes
Ventricular paced activity? Yes
Pacemaker malfunction? No
Interpretation: Dual-chamber paced rhythm with 100% capture at 70 pulses/min

75. Fig. 10.25
Rhythm: Regular
Rate: 73 beats/min
P waves: None visible
PR interval: None
QRS duration: 0.13 second
QT interval: 0.34 second
Interpretation: Accelerated IVR at 73 beats/min

76. Fig. 10.26
Rhythm: Irregular
Rate: 90 beats/min
P waves: No identifiable P waves; fibrillatory waves present
PR interval: None
QRS duration: 0.07 second
QT interval: Unable to determine; no consistently identifiable T waves
Interpretation: AFib at 90 beats/min

77. Fig. 10.27
Rhythm: Irregular
Rate: 60 beats/min
P waves: Positive before most QRSs; none visible with beat 4
PR interval: 0.17 second
QRS duration: 0.09 second
QT interval: 0.40 second

Interpretation: Sinus rhythm at 60 beats/min with an episode of sinus arrest and a junctional escape beat (beat 4); artifact is present

78. Fig. 10.28
Rhythm: Irregular
Rate: 60 beats/min
P waves: Positive before each QRS
PR interval: 0.20 to 0.22 second
QRS duration: 0.08 second
QT interval: 0.33 to 0.36 second
Interpretation: Sinus arrhythmia with first-degree AV block at 60 beats/min; artifact is present

79. Fig. 10.29
Rhythm: Irregular
Rate: 80 beats/min
P waves: Positive before each QRS; some are smooth and rounded, others are pointed
PR interval: 0.17 second
QRS duration: 0.07 second
QT interval: 0.33 second
Interpretation: Sinus rhythm at 80 beats/min with PACs (beats 3 and 5); artifact is present

80. Fig. 10.30
Rhythm: Irregular
Rate: 120 beats/min
P waves: Positive with sinus beats; none with ventricular beats
PR interval: 0.18 second (sinus beats)
QRS duration: 0.08 second (sinus beats)
QT interval: 0.30 second (sinus beats)
Interpretation: Sinus tachycardia at 120 beats/min with two uniform PVCs

81. Fig. 10.31
Rhythm: Regular
Rate: 130 beats/min
P waves: Positive; 1:1 relationship
PR interval: 0.16 second
QRS duration: 0.08 second
QT interval: 0.28 second
Interpretation: Sinus tachycardia at 130 beats/min with ST-segment depression; artifact is present

82. Fig. 10.32
Rhythm: Regular
Rate: Ventricular 55 beats/min
P waves: Flutter waves present
PR interval: None
QRS duration: 0.09 second
QT interval: Unable to determine
Interpretation: Atrial flutter at 55 beats/min

83. Fig. 10.33
Rhythm: Regular
Rate: 69 beats/min

P waves: Positive and peaked; 1:1 relationship
PR interval: 0.16 second
QRS duration: 0.08 second
QT interval: 0.32 second
Interpretation: Sinus rhythm at 69 beats/min with ST-segment depression and inverted T waves

84. Fig. 10.34
Rhythm: Regular
Rate: 230 beats/min
P waves: None visible
PR interval: None
QRS duration: 0.06 second
QT interval: Unable to determine
Interpretation: AVNRT at 230 beats/min with ST-segment depression

85. Fig. 10.35
Atrial paced activity? No
Ventricular paced activity? Yes
Pacemaker malfunction? No
Interpretation: Ventricular paced rhythm with a PVC, a paced beat, nonsustained monomorphic VT, and a paced beat; paced interval 71 pulses/min

86. Fig. 10.36
Rhythm: Irregular
Rate: 70 beats/min
P waves: Vary in size and shape
PR interval: Varies
QRS duration: 0.08 to 0.12 second
QT interval: 0.40 to 0.44 second
Interpretation: Underlying rhythm is sinus but pacemaker site varies; ventricular rate 70 beats/min; patient with known Wolff-Parkinson-White pattern; note the delta waves

87. Fig. 10.37
Rhythm: Irregular
Rate: 50 beats/min
P waves: Positive; none visible before the QRS with beat 3, but an inverted P wave appears after it
PR interval: 0.24 second
QRS duration: 0.08 second
QT interval: 0.33 second
Interpretation: Sinus rhythm at 50 beats/min with a first-degree AV block, an episode of sinus arrest, a junctional escape beat, and ST-segment depression

88. Fig. 10.38
Rhythm: Ventricular absent; atrial regular
Rate: Ventricular none; atrial 40 beats/min
P waves: Positive
PR interval: None
QRS duration: None
QT interval: None
Interpretation: P-wave asystole

89. Fig. 10.39
Rhythm: None
Rate: None
P waves: None
PR interval: None
QRS duration: None
QT interval: None
Interpretation: Ventricular fibrillation

90. Fig. 10.40
Atrial paced activity? Yes
Ventricular paced activity? Yes
Pacemaker malfunction? Yes—failure to capture and failure to sense
Interpretation: Dual-chamber pacemaker with failure to capture (seventh spike) and failure to sense (eighth spike) at 71 pulses/min

91. Fig. 10.41
Rhythm: Ventricular essentially regular; atrial essentially regular
Rate: Ventricular 37 beats/min; atrial 100 beats/min
P waves: Positive; more Ps than QRSs
PR interval: None
QRS duration: 0.09 second
QT interval: Unable to determine because T waves are not clearly visible
Interpretation: Third-degree AV block at 37 beats/min

92. Fig. 10.42
Rhythm: Regular
Rate: 39 beats/min
P waves: None visible
PR interval: None
QRS duration: 0.18 second
QT interval: 0.32 second
Interpretation: IVR at 39 beats/min

93. Fig. 10.43
Rhythm: Ventricular regular; atrial regular
Rate: Ventricular 36 beats/min; atrial 108 beats/min
P waves: Positive; more Ps than QRSs; 3:1 relationship
PR interval: 0.16 second
QRS duration: 0.09 second
QT interval: Unable to determine
Interpretation: Advanced second-degree AV block with 3:1 conduction at 36 beats/min

94. Fig. 10.44
Rhythm: Irregular
Rate: 120 beats/min
P waves: Vary in size, shape, and direction
PR interval: Varies
QRS duration: 0.08 second
QT interval: 0.25 second
Interpretation: Multifocal atrial tachycardia at 120 beats/min

95. Fig. 10.45
Rhythm: Irregular
Rate: 50 beats/min
P waves: Positive; the P wave of beat 3 is early
PR interval: 0.16 second
QRS duration: 0.08 second
QT interval: 0.40 second
Interpretation: Sinus rhythm at 50 beats/min with a PAC (beat 3)

96. Fig. 10.46
Rhythm: Irregular
Rate: 100 beats/min (sinus beats); 136 beats/min (ventricular beats)
P waves: Low amplitude but positive with sinus beats
PR interval: 0.16 second (sinus beats)
QRS duration: 0.08 second (sinus beats); 0.12 second (ventricular beats)
QT interval: 0.34 second (sinus beats)
Interpretation: Sinus rhythm at 100 beats/min with a run of monomorphic VT at 136 beats/min

97. Fig. 10.47
Rhythm: Irregular
Rate: 68 beats/min (sinus beats); 75 beats/min (junctional beats)
P waves: Positive with sinus beats; inverted with junctional beats
PR interval: 0.16 second (sinus beats)
QRS duration: 0.08 second
QT interval: 0.30 second
Interpretation: Sinus rhythm at 68 beats/min to an accelerated junctional rhythm at 75 beats/min

98. Fig. 10.48
Rhythm: Irregular
Rate: 50 beats/min (top strip)
P waves: Vary in size, shape, and direction
PR interval: Varies
QRS duration: 0.07 second
QT interval: 0.40 second
Interpretation: Wandering atrial pacemaker at 50 beats/min

99. Fig. 10.49
Rhythm: Ventricular irregular; atrial regular
Rate: Ventricular 50 beats/min; atrial 167 beats/min
P waves: Positive and notched; more Ps than QRSs
PR interval: 0.26 second; the PR intervals before and after the nonconducted P waves are constant
QRS duration: 0.12 second
QT interval: Unable to determine
Interpretation: Second-degree AV block type II at 60 beats/min with ST-segment depression

100. Fig. 10.50
Rhythm: Regular
Rate: 150 beats/min
P waves: One P wave appears after each QRS

PR interval: None
QRS duration: 0.06 second
QT interval: 0.20 second
Interpretation: Junctional tachycardia at 150 beats/min

101. Fig. 10.51
Rhythm: Irregular
Rate: 83 beats/min (sinus beats)
P waves: Flutter waves initially present; sinus P waves present for last 3 beats
PR interval: 0.20 second (sinus beats)
QRS duration: 0.10 second (sinus beats)
QT interval: 0.36 second (sinus beats)
Interpretation: Atrial flutter with a period of asystole to sinus rhythm at 83 beats/min

102. Fig. 10.52
Rhythm: Regular
Rate: 45 beats/min
P waves: Low amplitude but positive
PR interval: 0.22 second
QRS duration: 0.11 second
QT interval: 0.37 second
Interpretation: Sinus bradycardia at 45 beats/min with first-degree AV block and horizontal ST segments; artifact is present

103. Fig. 10.53
Rhythm: Irregular
Rate: 110 beats/min
P waves: Positive; the P wave of beat 5 is early and inverted
PR interval: 0.16 second (sinus beats)
QRS duration: 0.06 second (sinus beats)
QT interval: Unable to determine
Interpretation: Sinus tachycardia at 110 beats/min with a PJC (beat 5)

104. Fig. 10.54
Rhythm: Ventricular regular; atrial regular
Rate: Ventricular 40 beats/min; atrial 79 beats/min
P waves: Positive; more Ps than QRSs
PR interval: 0.26 second
QRS duration: 0.07 second
QT interval: 0.43 second
Interpretation: 2:1 AV block at 40 beats/min

105. Fig. 10.55
Rhythm: Irregular
Rate: 30 beats/min (junctional beats)
P waves: Positive (sinus beats); none with junctional beats
PR interval: 0.16 second (sinus beats); none (junctional beats)
QRS duration: 0.08 second
QT interval: 0.37 second
Interpretation: Sinus beat, two junctional beats, sinus beat; ST-segment depression; artifact is present

106. Fig. 10.56
Rhythm: Irregular
Rate: 80 beats/min
P waves: Positive; the P wave of beat 3 is early and distorts the previous T wave
PR interval: 0.16 second
QRS duration: 0.06 second
QT interval: Unable to determine
Interpretation: Sinus rhythm at 80 beats/min with a PAC (beat 3) and STE

107. Fig. 10.57
Rhythm: Regular
Rate: 79 beats/min
P waves: None visible
PR interval: None
QRS duration: 0.09 second
QT interval: 0.36 second
Interpretation: Accelerated junctional rhythm at 79 beats/min

108. Fig. 10.58
Rhythm: Irregular
Rate: 40 beats/min
P waves: Positive; some are notched
PR interval: 0.20 second
QRS duration: 0.08 second
QT interval: 0.44 second
Interpretation: Sinus bradycardia at 40 beats/min with an episode of sinus arrest

109. Fig. 10.59
Rhythm: Irregular
Rate: 90 beats/min
P waves: Fibrillatory waves are present
PR interval: None
QRS duration: 0.10 second and notched
QT interval: Unable to determine
Interpretation: AFib at 90 beats/min

110. Fig. 10.60
Rhythm: Irregular
Rate: 56 beats/min (sinus beats)
P waves: Positive with sinus beats; none with ventricular beats
PR interval: 0.16 second (sinus beats)
QRS duration: 0.06 second (sinus beats)
QT interval: Unable to determine
Interpretation: Sinus bradycardia at 56 beats/min with multiform ventricular bigeminy, a run of VT, and ST-segment depression

111. Fig. 10.61
Rhythm: Irregular
Rate: 130 beats/min
P waves: Vary in size, shape, and direction
PR interval: Varies
QRS duration: 0.08 second

QT interval: Varies
Interpretation: Multifocal atrial tachycardia at 130 beats/min

112. Fig. 10.62
Rhythm: Ventricular irregular; atrial regular
Rate: Ventricular 50 beats/min; atrial 83 beats/min
P waves: Positive; more Ps than QRSs
PR interval: Lengthens (visible in last three beats)
QRS duration: 0.07 second
QT interval: 0.40 second
Interpretation: Second-degree AV block type I at 50 beats/min with ST-segment depression; note the presence of 2:1 AV block at the start of the rhythm strip; artifact is present

113. Fig. 10.63
Rhythm: Ventricular regular; atrial regular
Rate: Ventricular 34 beats/min; atrial 68 beats/min
P waves: Positive; more Ps than QRSs; 2:1 relationship
PR interval: 0.16 second
QRS duration: 0.10 second
QT interval: 0.50 second (prolonged)
Interpretation: 2:1 AV block at 34 beats/min with ST-segment depression, a prolonged QT interval, and tall T waves; artifact is present

114. Fig. 10.64
Rhythm: Irregular
Rate: 60 beats/min
P waves: Positive; early P wave after beat 3; no P wave with beat 4
PR interval: 0.22 to 0.24 second
QRS duration: 0.08 second (sinus beats)
QT interval: 0.41 second
Interpretation: Sinus rhythm at 60 beats/min with a first-degree AV block, a nonconducted PAC, and a ventricular escape beat

115. Fig. 10.65
Rhythm: Irregular
Rate: 50 beats/min
P waves: Positive before each QRS; a PQRST complex is missing
PR interval: 0.16 second
QRS duration: 0.08 second
QT interval: 0.31 second
Interpretation: Sinus bradycardia at 50 beats/min with an episode of SA block; artifact is present

116. Fig. 10.66
Rhythm: Irregular
Rate: About 310 beats/min
P waves: None
PR interval: None
QRS duration: Varies
QT interval: Unable to determine
Interpretation: PMVT at about 310 beats/min

117. Fig. 10.67
Rhythm: Regular
Rate: Ventricular 90 beats/min; atrial 180 beats/min
P waves: Positive before each QRS; others are hidden in the T waves; 2:1 relationship
PR interval: 0.16 second
QRS duration: 0.06 second
QT interval: Unable to determine; P waves in T waves distort ST segment
Interpretation: Atrial tachycardia at 90 beats/min with 2:1 block and STE

118. Fig. 10.68
Rhythm: Regular
Rate: 88 beats/min
P waves: Positive
PR interval: 0.16 second
QRS duration: 0.10 to 0.12 second (notched)
QT interval: 0.32 second
Interpretation: Sinus rhythm at 88 beats/min with an incomplete BBB; artifact is present

119. Fig. 10.69
Rhythm: Regular
Rate: 57 beats/min
P waves: None visible
PR interval: None
QRS duration: 0.13 second
QT interval: 0.26 second
Interpretation: Accelerated IVR at 57 beats/min with tall T waves; artifact is present

120. Fig. 10.70
Rhythm: Ventricular irregular; atrial regular
Rate: Ventricular 30 beats/min; atrial 79 beats/min
P waves: Positive; more Ps than QRSs
PR interval: 0.15 second
QRS duration: 0.15 second
QT interval: 0.38 second
Interpretation: Advanced second-degree AV block at 30 beats/min with a wide QRS and STE

121. Fig. 10.71
Rhythm: Regular
Rate: 115 beats/min
P waves: Positive; 1:1 relationship
PR interval: 0.16 second
QRS duration: 0.08 second
QT interval: 0.28 second
Interpretation: Sinus tachycardia at 115 beats/min with STE in V_4; artifact is present

122. Fig. 10.72
Rhythm: Irregular
Rate: 60 beats/min
P waves: Positive (sinus beats); inverted after the QRS in beat 5
PR interval: 0.14 second (sinus beats)
QRS duration: 0.06 second
QT interval: 0.38 second
Interpretation: Sinus rhythm at 60 beats/min with a PJC (beat 5)

123. Fig. 10.73
Rhythm: Regular
Rate: 45 beats/min
P waves: None visible
PR interval: None
QRS duration: 0.10 second
QT interval: 0.48 second (prolonged)
Interpretation: Junctional rhythm at 45 beats/min with STE and a prolonged QT interval

124. Fig. 10.74
Rhythm: Irregular
Rate: 40 beats/min
P waves: Positive (sinus beats); none with beat 2
PR interval: 0.35 second (sinus beats)
QRS duration: 0.08 second (sinus beats)
QT interval: 0.35 second
Interpretation: Sinus bradycardia at 40 beats/min with first-degree AV block and a PJC (beat 2)

125. Fig. 10.75
Rhythm: Irregular
Rate 71: beats/min (sinus beats)
P waves: Positive before each QRS; one early P wave distorts the T wave of beat 4 (most clearly seen in lead MCL_1)
PR interval: 0.20 second (lead II)
QRS duration: 0.12 second (lead II)
QT interval: 0.40 second (lead II)
Interpretation: Sinus rhythm at 71 beats/min with a wide QRS and a nonconducted PAC

Index

Note: Pages followed by "*t*" or "*f*" refer to tables and figures, respectively.